SYLLABUS OF CLINICAL MEDICAL EDUCATION

FOR INTERNATIONAL MEDICAL STUDENTS (IN ENGLISH)

（The First Volume）

来华留学生
临床医学专业本科
（英语授课）教学大纲（上册）

中国教育国际交流协会国际医学教育分会 编

Edited by International Medical Education Committee,
China Education Association for International Exchange

清華大学出版社
北 京

图书在版编目(CIP)数据

来华留学生临床医学专业本科（英语授课）教学大纲. 上册：英文 / 中国教育国际交流协会国际医学教育分会编. — 北京:清华大学出版社，2019

ISBN 978-7-302-49760-8

Ⅰ.①来… Ⅱ.①中… Ⅲ.①临床医学–高等学校–教学大纲–英文 Ⅳ.①R4-41

中国版本图书馆CIP数据核字(2018)第037255号

责任编辑：李　君
封面设计：常雪影
责任校对：赵丽敏
责任印制：丛怀宇

出版发行：清华大学出版社
　　　　网　　　址：http://www.tup.com.cn, http://www.wqbook.com
　　　　地　　　址：北京清华大学学研大厦A座　　　邮　　编：100084
　　　　社 总 机：010-62770175　　　　　　　　邮　　购：010-62786544
　　　　投稿与读者服务：010-62776969, c-service@tup.tsinghua.edu.cn
　　　　质量反馈：010-62772015, zhiliang@tup.tsinghua.edu.cn
印 装 者：北京密云胶印厂
经　　销：全国新华书店
开　　本：185mm×260mm　　　印　张：18.25　　　字　数：437千字
版　　次：2019年6月第1版　　　印　次：2019年6月第1次印刷
定　　价：168.00元

产品编号：070678-01

《来华留学生临床医学专业本科（英语授课）教学大纲》参编院校名单

Anhui Medical University（安徽医科大学）

Army Medical University（陆军军医大学）

Capital Medical University（首都医科大学）

Central South University（中南大学）

China Medical University（中国医科大学）

Chongqing Medical University（重庆医科大学）

Dalian Medical University（大连医科大学）

Dongnan University（东南大学）

Fudan University（复旦大学）

Fujian Medical University（福建医科大学）

Guangxi Medical University（广西医科大学）

Guangzhou Medical University（广州医科大学）

Harbin Medical University（哈尔滨医科大学）

Hebei Medical University（河北医科大学）

Hebei University of Chinese Medicine（河北中医学院）

Huazhong University of Science and Technology（华中科技大学）

Jiangsu University（江苏大学）

Jiangxi University of Traditional Chinese Medicine（江西中医药大学）

Jilin University（吉林大学）

Jinan University（暨南大学）

Kunming Medical University（昆明医科大学）

Nanjing Medical University（南京医科大学）

Nanjing University（南京大学）

Nankai University（南开大学）

Nantong University（南通大学）

Ningbo University（宁波大学）

North China University of Science and Technology（华北理工大学）

North Sichuan Medical University（川北医学院）

Peking Union Medical College Hospital（北京协和医院）

Peking University（北京大学）

Qingdao University（青岛大学）

Shandong University（山东大学）

Shanghai Jiaotong University（上海交通大学）

Shanghai University of Traditional Chinese Medicine（上海中医药大学）

Shanxi Medical University（山西医科大学）

Sichuan University（四川大学）

Soochow University（苏州大学）

South China University of Technology（华南理工大学）

Southeast University（东南大学）

Southern Medical University（南方医科大学）

Sun Yat-sen University（中山大学）

The People's Hospital of Guangxi Zhuang Autonomous Region（广西壮族自
治区人民医院）

Tianjin Medical University（天津医科大学）

Tianjin University of Traditional Chinese Medicine（天津中医药大学）

Tongji University（同济大学）

University of Electronic Science and Technology of China（电子科技大学）

Weifang Medical University（潍坊医学院）

Wenzhou Medical University（温州医科大学）

Wuhan University（武汉大学）

Xi'an Jiaotong University（西安交通大学）

Xinjiang Medical University（新疆医科大学）

Xuzhou Medical University（徐州医科大学）

Yangzhou University（扬州大学）

Zhejiang University（浙江大学）

Zhengzhou University（郑州大学）

《来华留学生临床医学专业本科（英语授课）教学大纲》编审委员会名单

主　任　委　员　张岫美

常务副主任委员　李国霞

副 主 任 委 员　钟照华　刘　弋　付　蓉　高　静　万学红　王立伟　　樊立洁　姚继红

委　　　　　员　（按姓氏拼音排序）

边军辉　陈　君　陈　霞　陈挺玉　戴亚蕾　邓丹琪

高　见　高国全　龚朝辉　郭凤林　韩　菲　何　庆

贺桂琼　胡　臻　黄俊琪　黄黎玲　姜　宏　焦小民

金利泰　李　敏　梁忠宝　刘传勇　吕广明　吕嘉春

吕永震　孟　勇　朴立红　戚　峰　齐忠权　钱睿哲

任　蕾　单　彬　盛德乔　史宏灿　宋　扬　宋玉霞

孙　红　孙保亮　田启明　田庆宝　王　放　王　海

王　倩　魏　伟　吴　强　吴家红　吴希阳　肖凤玲

谢建新　徐　立　薛凤霞　燕　秋　杨　红　姚红红

姚小梅　于　丽　曾小云　张慧灵　张明宇　张雪梅

张义东　赵晓峰　赵永娜　郑　红　郑加麟　郑荣秀

周　雪

Foreword
序　　言

随着中国社会、经济、文化的快速发展，国际影响力的不断提升，"留学中国计划"的逐步实施，越来越多的外国人留学中国，来华留学生规模不断扩大。2018 年，有来自196 个国家和地区的 492 185 名各类外国留学生在我国的 1004 所高等院校学习，我国已经成为亚洲最大的留学目的地国家。来华学习医学的留学生人数增长迅速，目前来华学习医学的留学生人数已位居来华留学生人数的首位，2017 年来华学习医学本科的留学生 4.69万人，其中临床医学本科留学生 3.74 万人，来华医学留学生教育为生源国培养了大批的医学人才。

教育部历来高度重视来华医学留学生教育质量，不断加强对医学留学生教育的规范和管理，提出了"提质增效、质量优先"的发展战略。在 2007 年制定的《来华留学生医学本科教育（英语授课）质量控制标准暂行规定》基础上，教育部又委托中国教育国际交流协会国际医学教育分会制定了《来华留学生临床医学专业本科教育（英语授课）质量控制规定》，进一步规范和加强来华留学生临床医学本科教育。

2017 年 9 月，中国教育国际交流协会国际医学教育分会在浙江大学正式成立。2018年 3 月，教育部国际合作与交流司组织专家对 52 所招收临床医学留学生的高校实施调研。2018 年 10 月，中国教育国际交流协会又组织专家对部分高校的来华医学留学生教育的管理工作进行了专项调研，深入了解全国来华医学留学生教育的基本情况，为制定来华医学留学生教育政策提供依据。

由于来华留学生临床医学专业本科教育（MBBS）在我国较短的时间迅速发展，一些学校不能适应来华留学发展的需要，一些学校的办学资源和基础设施存在差异，课程设置差异也较大，有的学校开设课程不符合临床医学专业教育的基本要求，影响了来华留学生临床医学专业教育的健康发展，也影响了我们的国际声誉。新近公布的《中国本科医学教育标准——临床医学专业（2016 年版）》和即将公布实施的《来华留学生临床医学专业本科教育（英语授课）质量控制规定》对临床医学专业教育和来华留学生临床医学专业教育做出了具体规定和要求，教学大纲是教师和学生教学活动中重要的纲领性文件，制定MBBS 教学大纲就是落实两个标准的具体措施之一。

为规范来华留学生临床医学专业本科教育，提高来华医学留学生的教育质量，在教育部国际合作与交流司、中国教育国际交流协会领导和清华大学出版社的支持下，启动了MBBS 教学大纲的编写工作。2016 年 4 月，在天津医科大学召开了 MBBS 教学大纲编写会议，30 多所高校的领导和专家经过讨论、磋商，成立了"来华留学生临床医学专业本科（英语授课）教学大纲编审委员会"，制定了大纲编写的体例和编写原则，并收集了留学生主要生源国的教学大纲、执业医师资格考试要求等作为参考，会议确定了各科目教学大纲编写任务及牵头单位。在各科目主编的精心组织下，2017 年 5 月完成了来华留学生临床医学专业本科（英语授课）53 门课程教学大纲的初稿，2017 年 6 月在清华大学召开了大纲核心专家组的审稿会议，对大纲提出了修改意见，经各主编再次修改后，又进行了第三次修改，2018 年 9 月在清华大学举行大纲审定稿会，来自全国近 40 所高校的著名教授、大纲主编、课程负责人集聚一堂为来华留学生临床医学专业 53 门课程的英语教学大纲做了最后的审定。

现在，历时 3 年，各高校翘首期盼的《来华留学生临床医学专业本科（英语授课）教学大纲》由清华大学出版社正式出版，供全国使用。参加编写来华医学留学生 53 门课程英语授课教学大纲的专家由我国长期从事医学留学生教育的教授、学者和一线教师组成，他们在全国医学高等院校来华医学留学生教育领域里具有代表性和影响力，MBBS 教学大纲的编写出版凝聚了我国众多高校和专家的辛劳和努力。该套教学大纲主要供来华临床医学专业本科留学生，本土长学制医学生、医学本科生英语或双语教学使用。

来华留学生的教学质量是来华留学教育事业可持续发展的核心保障，教学大纲是来华医学留学生教育教材建设的重要组成部分。制定 MBBS 教学大纲是一件具有里程碑意义的工作，也是一件规范高校来华留学生临床医学专业教育的尝试性和探索性的工作，它不仅填补了我国来华医学留学生教学大纲的空白，而且对规范来华医学留学生教学，提高培养质量将发挥重要作用，同时也将对留学生系统性教材建设和教学改革发挥指导作用。

MBBS 教学大纲的出版是一个良好的开端，希望在今后的来华医学留学生教学中能够审视理解、多提意见、反馈信息、不断修改，使其日臻完善。

张岫美　李国霞

2019 年 5 月

Contents
目　　录

MEDICAL MATHEMATICS
医用高等数学

Chief Editors（主编）
  Liang Jin（梁进） Tongji University（同济大学）
  Hang Guoming（杭国明） Fudan University（复旦大学）

Deputy Chief Editors（副主编）
  Tu Xiaoming（屠小明） Nanjing Medical University（南京医科大学）
  Ke Zhenqing（柯振青） Jinan University（暨南大学）
  Tang Xiao（唐晓） Dalian Medical University（大连医科大学）

Editors（编委）（按姓氏拼音排序）
  Hang Guoming（杭国明） Fudan University（复旦大学）
  Ke Zhenqing（柯振青） Jinan University（暨南大学）
  Liang Jin（梁进） Tongji University（同济大学）
  Tang Xiao（唐晓） Dalian Medical University（大连医科大学）
  Tu Xiaoming（屠小明） Nanjing Medical University（南京医科大学）

Course Description

Medical Mathematics is a compulsory course for medicalstudents who are required to be fundamental scientifically trained. The course will provide the students with the essential advanced mathematical foundation for their future study and work. It serves their needs of mathematical concepts, logic thinking, analyzing ability and computation skill.

The course is designed to give the students basic knowledge in calculus, which includes: ①functions; ②limits; ③derivatives of single variable functions; ④integrations of single variable functions.

Objectives

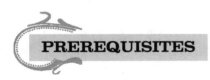

PREREQUISITES

The mathematical courses provided in the senior middle schools.

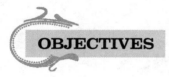

OBJECTIVES

In the process of imparting knowledge to students, it focus on the enhancement of the students'ability in abstract and logical reasoning, mental visualization of space figures and the ability of learning through self-study, and the students'computational competence. Special attention should also be given to developing the students'ability in applying the knowledge they have learnt in the course comprehensively to analyzing and solving the practical problems.

Teaching and Learning Methods

Teaching and learning methodology of this course are lectures, tutorials and exercises.

Recommended Textbooks

H. Anton, I. Blvens, S. Davis. 2008. Guo Jingming（郭镜明）ed. Calculus [M]. Beijing: Higher Education Press.

Schedule Table

Chapter	Contents	Presumptive Hours	Chapter	Contents	Presumptive Hours
0	Review of mathematical schools courses in the senior middle schoolsand and Introduction to Calculus	1	1	Properties and graphs of the basic elementary functions (polynomial, trigonometric, inversed trigonometric, exponential, logarithmic functions)	2
1	Concepts and denotations of sets, operations on sets and some important subsets of R	0.5	2	Concept of limits	1
1	Variables, definition of functions	0.5	2	One-sided limits	0.5
1	Domains and ranges of functions	1	2	Infinitesimals and infinities	0.5
1	Types of functions, Elementary functions	1	2	Rules for the limits of sums, products and quotients	1
1	Constructed a new function by arithmetic operations	1	2	Limits at infinity	1
1	Even and odd functions, piecewise defined functions, unbounded functions*	1	2	Cases that limit does not exist (unequal sides limits, unbounded and no single value approaching)*	1
1	Monotonicity, periodicity and boundedness of functions	1	2	Definitions of continuity of a function at a point and on an interval	2
1	Composite functions and inverse functions	1	3	Concept of derivatives	2

Continued

Chapter	Contents	Presumptive Hours	Chapter	Contents	Presumptive Hours
3	Geometric and physical interpretation of derivatives	2	4	Concept and properties of the primitive functions (antiderivatives) and indefinite integrals	2.5
3	Relationship between differentiability and continuity	1	4	Concept and properties of definite integrals	2.5
3	Basic rules for the derivatives of the sum, product and quotient of functions	3	4	Fundamental theorem of calculus	2
3	Derivative formulas of the basic elementary functions	1	4	Integration by substitution and by parts*	2
3	Chain rule	1	4	Calculations of simple indefinite and definite integrates	3
3	Computation of the derivatives of the elementary functions	3	5	Applications	2
3	High and implicit function derivatives*	2		Total	46

Course Contents

Chapter 1　Function

1. Concepts and denotations of sets, operations on sets and some important subsets of R.
2. Variables, definition of functions.
3. Domains and ranges of functions.
4. Types of functions, basic elementary functions.
5. Constructed a new function by arithmetic operations.
6. Even and odd functions, piecewise defined functions, unbounded functions*.
7. Monotonicity, periodicity and boundedness of functions.
8. Composite functions and inverse functions.
9. Properties and graphs of the basic elementary functions (polynomial, trigonometric, inversed trigonometric, exponential, logarithmic functions).

Chapter 2　Limits

1. Concept of limits.
2. One-sided limits.
3. Infinitesimals and infinities.
4. Rules for the limits of sums, products and quotients.
5. Limits at infinity.
6. Cases that limit does not exist (unequal sides limits, unbounded and no single value approaching)*.
7. Definitions of continuity of a function at a point and on an interval.

Chapter 3　Derivatives

1. Concept of derivatives.
2. Geometric and physical interpretation of derivatives.
3. Relationship between differentiability and continuity.
4. Basic rules for the derivatives of the sum, product and quotient of functions.
5. Derivative formulas of the basic elementary functions.
6. Chain rule.
7. Computation of the derivatives of the elementary functions.
8. High and implicit function derivatives*.

Chapter 4　Integrations

1. Concepts and properties of the primitive functions (antiderivatives) and indefinite integrals.
2. Concepts and properties of definite integrals.
3. Fundamental theorem of calculus.
4. Integrations by substitution and by parts*.
5. Calculations on simple indefinite and definite integrals.

Chapter 5　Applications

* The terms wish * are optional.

MEDICAL PHYSICS
医学物理学

Chief Editors（主编）
Hong Yang（洪洋） China Medical University（中国医科大学）
Song Ranran（宋然然） Qingdao University（青岛大学）
Zhang Meiling（张美玲） Tianjin Medical University（天津医科大学）

Deputy Chief Editors（副主编）
Min Kangli（闵康丽） Nanjing Medical University（南京医科大学）
Zeng Bing（曾兵） Qingdao University（青岛大学）
Zhang Yan （张燕） Guangxi Medical University（广西医科大学）

Editors（编委）（按姓氏拼音排序）
Hong Yang（洪洋） China Medical University（中国医科大学）
Min Kangli（闵康丽） Nanjing Medical University（南京医科大学）
Song Ranran（宋然然） Qingdao University（青岛大学）
Wu Yunping（吴运平） Qingdao University（青岛大学）
Zeng Bing（曾兵） Qingdao University（青岛大学）
Zhang Meiling（张美玲） Tianjin Medical University（天津医科大学）
Zhang Yan （张燕） Guangxi Medical University（广西医科大学）

Course Description

Medical Physics is an applied science combining the fields of physics, bioengineering, and electronics. The Medical Physics course is a one-semester introductory physics offered primarily for medical students. This course offers a core of fundamental physics together with an introduction to many medical applications. Topics covered will include: mechanics, vibrations and waves, ultrasound, fluids, electric fields and electric currents, geometric optics and wave optics, atomic and nuclear structure, and radioactivity.

Understanding of the basic principles involved and the ability to apply these principles in the solution of problems should be the major goals of the course. Consequently, the course should utilize guided inquiry and student-centered learning to foster the development of critical thinking skills.

Objectives

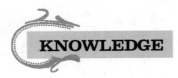

KNOWLEDGE

At the end of the course, the MBBS student shall be able to:

1. To describe the importance of physics in medicine.

2. Develop basic understanding of medical physics concepts.

3. To state and explain Newton's mechanics and its typical methods.

4. To master the basic concepts in vibrations and waves and state the application of ultrasound in medical imaging.

5. To master the basic concepts in fluid statics and fluid dynamics and state and apply the continuity and Bernoulli's Equation to the motion of blood.

6. To master the basic concepts in geometric optics and wave optics and understand the correction of the common defects in human eyes.

7. To understand the basic concepts in atomic and nuclear structure and describe the medical applications of laser.

8. To understand the basic concepts in radioactivity and describe the medical applications of radioactivity.

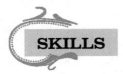

SKILLS

At the end of the course, the student shall be able to:

1. Practice the following experiments and master the common used methods of physics experiments.

2. Develop problem-solving and critical-thinking skills.

3. Develop scientific communication skills.

4. Learn to integrate and apply various physics concepts to a single problem, especially medical application problems.

Teaching and Learning Methods

Theory: Teaching medical physics to MBBS students is provided with the help of lectures and tutorials that deal with the principles of fundamental physics. The lecturer use PowerPoint for the lectures; show the titles, topics, sentences and pictures in the slides.

Practical: Practical training asks for medical students are to know the basic principles, methods and techniques, strategies, and skills by the typical physics experiments and experimental design. The student is advised to pay attention to the regulation and safety rules in the physics laboratory.

Recommended Textbooks

Zhang Meiling（张美玲）, Li Zengzhi（李增智）, Ji Qiang（吉强）. 2016. Medical Physics（医学物理学）[M]. Beijing: Qinghua University Press.

Zhang Meiling（张美玲）, Yang Jiumin（杨久敏）, Li Zengzhi（李增智）. 2016. Laboratory Experiments and Study Guide to Accompany Medical Physics（医用物理学实验与学习指导）[M]. Beijing: Qinghua University Press.

Schedule Table

Chapter	Contents	Hours	Chapter	Contents	Hours
1	Describing motion	2	13	Magnetism	2
2	Dynamics: Newton's laws of motion	2	14	Electromagnetic induction	2
3	Work and energy	2	15	The laws of reflection and refraction	2
4	Linear momentum	2	16	Image formation by a mirror	2
5	Vibrations	2	17	Image formation with lenses	4
6	Waves	6	18	Interference	2
7	Fluids in static	2	19	Diffraction	2
8	Fluids in motion	2	20	Polarization	2
9	Viscosity	2	21	Early quantum theory and models of the atom	2
10	Surface tension	2	22	Nuclear physics and radioactivity	2
11	Electric charge and electric field	2	23	Nuclear effects and uses of radiation	2
12	Electric currents	2		Total	52

Course Contents

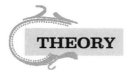

THEORY

Chapter 1　Describing Motion

Particle, frame of reference, coordinates system, position vector, displacement, velocity, speed, acceleration, equation of motion, graphical presentation, position vector, velocity vector, acceleration vector, 3D kinematics, projectile motion.

Chapter 2　Dynamics: Newton's Laws of Motion

Newton's laws of motion, inertia, Newton's universal law of gravitation, free body diagram, resistive forces, air drag, terminal velocity.

Chapter 3　Work and Energy

Work done by variable force, power, energy, kinetic energy, potential energy, mechanical energy, conservative and non-conservative forces, conservation of energy, static equilibrium, stability.

Chapter 4　Linear Momentum

Momentum, impulse, impulse-momentum theorem, conservation of momentum, elastic and inelastic collision, center of mass.

Chapter 5　Vibrations

Hooke's law, simple harmonic motion, equation of S.H.M, spring-mass system, amplitude, period, angular frequency, simple harmonic motion and the uniform circular motion, phase, simple pendulum, physical pendulum, small angle approximation, damped oscillation, forced oscillation. resonance and natural frequencies.

Chapter 6　Waves

Transverse wave, longitudinal wave, progressive wave, energy transport via mechanical waves, wavelength, wave speed, reflection of waves, superposition of waves, interference, sound waves, intensity level, decibels, loudness, beats, beat frequency, infrasonic wave, ultrasonic wave, ultrasonic medical imaging, Doppler effect.

Chapter 7　Fluids in Static

Phases of matter, pressure in fluids, measurement of pressure, buoyancy and Archimedes'principle.

Chapter 8　Fluids in Motion

Ideal fluid, streamline, tube of flow, unsteady flow, steady flow, flow rate, equation of continuity, Bernoulli's principle, applications of Bernoulli's principle, measurement of blood pressure.

Chapter 9　Viscosity

Laminar flow and turbulent flow, Reynolds number, viscosity, flow in tubes, Poiseuille's equation, Stokes's law, terminal velocity, blood flow.

Chapter 10　Surface Tension

Surface tension, surface tension coefficient, surface energy, capillarity, contact angle, cohesive force, adhesive force, air embolism, surfactant, surface absorption.

Chapter 11　Electric Charge and Electric Field

Electric charge, Coulomb's law, electric field, electric field line, electric potential and electric potential energy, electric potential difference, equipotential surfaces.

Chapter 12   Electric Currents

Current, current density, drift velocity, resistivity, Ohm's law, resistance, superconductivity, transition temperature, batteries, EMF, Kirchhoff's rules, electric hazards.

Chapter 13   Magnetism

Magnet, magnetic field, magnetic field lines, magnetic force on moving charges, magnetic force on current carrying wires, Hall effect, mass spectrometer.

Chapter 14   Electromagnetic Induction

Faraday's law of electromagnetic induction, Lentz's law, electromotive force, induced electromotive force , motional emf, induced electric field, induced emf, eddy current.

Chapter 15   The Laws of Reflection and Refraction

The laws of reflection and refraction, index of refraciton, total internal reflection, optical fiber, endoscope.

Chapter 16   Image Formation by a Mirror

Graphical ray-trace method, paraxial rays, the mirror formula, sign convention, diopter, coaxial spherical system, magnification of a mirror image.

Chapter 17   Image Formation with Lenses

Types of lenses, thin lens, focal points of thin lenses, lens makers'equation, image location by ray tracing, lens formulas for thin lenses, sign convention, magnification, visual acuity, simple magnifier, compound microscope, angular magnification. Structure and function of human eye, accommodation, visual angle, visual acuity, near point and far point, hyperopia, myopia, astigmatism.

Chapter 18   Interference

Huygen's principle, interference, Young's double-slit experiment, intensity distribution, optical path difference, thin film interference, anti-reflective coating, Newton's ring, wedge-shaped film.

Chapter 19   Diffraction

Single-slit Fraunhofer diffraction, circular apertures, limits of resolution.

Chapter 20   Polarization

Polarized light, Malus's law, Brewster's law.

Chapter 21   Early Quantum Theory and Models of the Atom

Early models of the atom, atomic spectra, the Bohr model of hygrogen atom, atomic energy levels, electron absorption and emission, the production of laser, lasic and PRK.

Chapter 22   Nuclear Physics and Radioactivity

Structure and properties of the nucleus,binding energy and nuclear forces, radioactivity, alpha decay, beta decay, gamma decay, conservation of nucleon number and other conservation laws,half-life and rate of decay. X-ray, computed tomography, radiology.

Chapter 23   Nuclear Effects and Uses of Radiation

Nuclear reaction,passage of radiation through matter, radiation damage, radiation therapy,tracers and imaging in medicine,emission tomography,nuclear magnetic resonance (NMR) and magnetic resonance imaging (MRI).

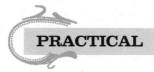

PRACTICAL

1. The adjustment and use of ultrasonic diagnositic instruments.
2. Application and study in characteristic of wheatstone bridge.
3. Measurement of resistance by voltmeter-ammeter method.
4. Determination of the focal length of the lenses.
5. Oscilloscope and measuring the speed of ultrasonic wave.
6. Measurement of human audible threshold curve.
7. Research on polarization of light.
8. Use Abbe refractometer to measure index of refraction of liquids.

MEDICAL BASIC CHEMISTRY
医学基础化学

Chief Editors（主编）

Ou Zhongping（欧忠平） Jiangsu University（江苏大学）

Chen Zhenghua（陈正华） Tianjin Medical University（天津医科大学）

Deputy Chief Editors（副主编）

Liu Yu（刘誉） Jinan University（暨南大学）

Xue Zhaoli（薛兆历） Jiangsu University（江苏大学）

Fang Yuanyuan（房媛媛） Jiangsu University（江苏大学）

Editors（编委）（按姓氏拼音排序）

Chen Zhenghua（陈正华） Tianjin Medical University（天津医科大学）

Fang Yuanyuan（房媛媛） Jiangsu University（江苏大学）

Liu Yu（刘誉） Jinan University（暨南大学）

Ou Zhongping（欧忠平） Jiangsu University（江苏大学）

Xue Zhaoli（薛兆历） Jiangsu University（江苏大学）

Course Description

Medical Basic Chemistry is a subject which studies the law of matter and its change, and it is one of the indispensable and basic courses for medical students. The basic concepts, methods and principles about the composition and properties of matter, together with the chemical change rules of matter transformation will be introduced. The most important task of the course is to explain the structure and properties of elements, the formation and changes of matter, basic concepts of chemical reaction and the related calculations. This course includes three parts: the first part mainly introduces the atomic structure, chemical bond (valence bond theory, hybrid orbital theory and valence shell electron pair repulsion theory) and the characteristics of crystal type and its influence on properties of materials; the second part mainly introduces the basic knowledge of chemical thermodynamics and the basic principle; the third part mainly introduces some important elements, physical and chemical properties of the compounds and the periodic regularity. In laboratory practice, basic quantitative chemical experimental techniques, principles of chemical reactions and physical measurements are illustrated.

The purpose for the Medical Basic Chemistry learning is to master the basic theory of chemistry and to build a solid foundation for medical students. Therefore, Basic

Chemistry is an essential course in the curriculum of medical students.

Objective

The main objectives are of making students complete basic foundations in chemical reactions and the rules that govern chemical reactions, and become familiar with the scope, methodology and applications of modern chemistry. After study of this course, students will understand that all matters consist of atoms which form molecules via different chemical bonds; will become adept at problem solving by learning to interpret experimental data, to utilize suitable and efficient analytic methods, and to assess whether or not the results of calculations are reasonable; will understand the principles in atomic and molecular theories, as well as the formation of equilibrium in chemical reactions and the factors that affect equilibrium; will generalize the analytical and quantitative skills gained in this course and apply them in the advanced courses and throughout their careers.

Teaching and Learning Methods

Theory: Teaching Basic Chemistry to medical students is provided with the help of lectures and tutorials that deal with the basic principles of chemistry.

Practical: Practical training asks for medical students to know the basic principles, methods, techniques and skills by the typical chemical experiments. The student is especially advised to pay attention to the regulations and safety of the chemical laboratory.

Recommended Textbooks

Fu Xiancai (傅献彩).1999. College Chemistry [M]. Beijing: Higher Education Press.

John W. Hill, Ralph H. Petrucci, Terry W. Mcceary et al. 2005. General Chemistry [M]. 4th ed. New York: Pearson.

John W Moore, Conrad L Stanitski, Peter C Jurs. 2008. Principles of Chemistry: The Molecular Science [M]. Boston: Cengage.

Theodore L Brown, H Eugene Lemay, Bruce E Bursten Jr et al. 2013. Chemistry: The Central Science [M]. 10th ed. New York: Pearson.

William L. Masterton, Cecile N. Hurley, Edward Neth. 2013. Chemistry: Principles and Reactions [M]. 7th ed. Boston: Cengage.

Schedule Table of Lecture

Chapter	Contents	Class Hours	Chapter	Contents	Class Hours
1	Introduction	2	4	Molecules and Ions	2
2	Matter and Measurement	3	5	Stoichiometry: Calculations with Chemical Formulas	2
3	Atoms	2	6	Calculations with Equations	2

Continued

Course Contents

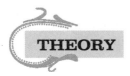

THEORY

Chapter 1　Introduction: Matter and Measurement

1. Concept of matter and properties.
2. Composition of matter, element, compound, mixture and classification of matter.
3. Physical states of matter, gas, liquid and solid.
4. Physical properties, chemical properties.
5. Separation of mixture.
6. Units of measurements, seven SI base units, derived SI units.
7. Precision and accuracy.
8. Significant figures and significant figures in calculations.
9. Dimensional analysis.

Chapter 2　Atoms, Molecules and Ions

1. The atomic theory of matter: Dalton's four postulates, the law of conservation of mass.

2. Discovery of atomic structure, cathode rays, electrons, radioactivity and discovery of the nucleus.

3. Size of atoms, subatomic particles, atomic mass unit, charges in an atom.

4. Symbols of elements, atomic number, isotopes and average atomic mass.

5. Periodic Table, groups, nonmetals, metalloids, metals.

6. Molecules and molecular compounds, chemical formulas, allotrope, diatomic molecules and types of formulas.

7. Cations, anions, predicting ionic charges, empirical formulas for ionic compounds.

8. Inorganic nomenclature, names and formulas of ionic compounds, patterns in oxyanion nomenclature.

Chapter 3　Stoichiometry–Calculations with Chemical Formulas and Equations

1. Concept of law of conservation of mass.

2. Balancing chemical equations, the information of subscripts and coefficients in chemical equations.

3. Reaction types: combination reactions; decomposition reactions and combustion reactions.

4. Mole, Avogadro's number, mole relationships.

5. Molar mass and using of moles.

6. Finding empirical formulas.

7. Stoichiometric calculations.

8. Limiting reactants and percent yield.

Chapter 4　Aqueous Reactions and Solution Stoichiometry

1. The formation of solution.

2. Electrolytes, nonelectrolytes, strong electrolyte and weak electrolyte.

3. Precipitation reactions and solubility guidelines of ionic compounds.

4. Molecular equation, ionic equation and net ionic equation.

5. Concept of acid and base.

6. Strong acids and bases; indicator; acid-base reactions; neutralization reactions.

7. Oxidation-reduction reactions.

8. Oxidation numbers, activity series, displacement reactions.

9. Concentrations of solutions, molarity.

10. Preparing a solution, expressing the concentration, diluting a solution.

11. Titration.

Chapter 5　Electronic Structure of Atoms

1. Electromagnetic radiation, wavelength, frequency, nature of energy.

2. Line spectrum, the energy states of hydrogen atom, pharmacokinetics, the wave behavior of matter, pharmacological actions, action mechanism, uses adverse reactions and the uncertainty principle.

3. Four quantum numbers: n, l, m_l, m_s; electron shell and subshell.

4. Representations of orbitals: s, p, d.

5. Energies of orbitals.

6. Pauli Exclusion Principle, Hund's rule.

7. Electron configuration.

Chapter 6　Periodic Properties of Elements

1. Development of periodic table, periodic trends, effective nuclear charge.

2. Covalent radii, sizes of ions.

3. Ionization energy, periodic trends in ionization energies and electron affinities.

4. Metals, nonmetals, metalloids, summary of oxides.

5. Alkali metals, reacting with O_2, flame test.

6. Alkaline earth metals, reacting with water and Cl_2, O_2.

7. Group 6A: oxygen, sulfur.

8. Group 7A: halogens.

9. Group 8A: noble gases.

Chapter 7　Basic Concepts of Chemical Bonding

1. Concept of basic types of chemical bonds: ionic bonds, covalent bond and metallic bond.

2. Ionic bonding, lattice energy, electron configuration of ions and transition metal ions.

3. Covalent bonding: multiple bonds, electronegativity, bond polarity, polar covalent bonds.

4. Lewis structures and writing the structures.

5. Resonance.

6. Exceptions to the octet rule: odd number of electrons, fewer than eight electrons and more than eight electrons.

7. Average bond enthalpies, bond length and enthalpies of reaction.

Chapter 8　Molecular Geometry and Bonding Theories

1. Concept of VSEPR theory and molecular geometry and VSEPR model.

2. The effect of nonbonding electrons and multiple bonds on bond angles.

3. Molecular shape and molecular polarity.

4. Covalent bonding and orbital overlap.

5. Hybrid orbitals: sp, sp^2 and sp^3, dsp^3 and d^2sp^3.

6. Multiple bonds: σ and π bonds, delocalized π bonding.

7. Molecular orbitals, bond order.

8. Electron configurations and molecular properties.

Chapter 9　Gases

1. Characteristics of gases, pressure and units of pressure.

2. Gas law: Boyle's Law, Charles's Law, Avogadro's Law.

3. Ideal-gas equation and relating the Ideal-Gas Equation and the gas laws, Charles's Law, Avogadro's Law, and further applications of the Ideal-Gas Equation.

4. Densities of gases and the properties of codeine.

5. Pharmacological actions and molecular mass.

6. Dalton's law of partial pressures.

Chapter 10　Properties of Solutions

1. Solutions process, solute, solvent and energy changes in solution.

2. Types of solutions: saturated, unsaturated and supersaturated.

3. Factors affecting solubility.

4. Gases in solution, Henry's law.

5. Solid solubility with temperature.

Chapter 11　Chemical Equilibrium

1. Concept of equilibrium and depicting equilibrium.

2. The equilibrium constants, K_c and K_p, relationship between the K_c and K_p.

3. Manipulating equilibrium constants.

4. Heterogeneous equilibrium.

5. Equilibrium calculations, the reaction quotient (q), predicting the direction of approach to equilibrium.

6. Calculating equilibrium concentrations from the equilibrium constant.

7. Le Châtelier's principle, effects of volume, pressure and temperature changes.

8. The Haber process.

Chapter 12　Acid - base Equilibria

1. Concept of acid, base (Arrhenius, Brønsted–Lowry theory) and conjugate acid and base.

2. Acid and base strength.

3. Autoionization of water (K_w), pH values, solution type and other "p" scales (pOH, pK_w).

4. Weak acid (K_a): dissociation constants, equilibrium expression, calculating K_a from the pH, calculating percent ionization, calculating pH from K_a.

5. Weak base (K_b): dissociation constants, calculating pH from K_b, types of weak bases.

6. Relationship between the K_a and K_b.

7. Reactions of anions and cations with water.

8. Factors affecting acid strength.

Chapter 13　Additional Aspects of Aqueous Equilibria

1. The common-ion effects and buffers.

2. Buffer calculations, Henderson-Hasselbalch Equation, pH range of a buffer, calculating pH changes in buffers.

3. Titration of a strong acid with a strong base.

4. Titration of a weak acid with a strong base.

5. Titration of a weak base with a strong acid.

6. Titrations of polyprotic acids.

7. Factors affecting solubility: pH value, temperature, etc.

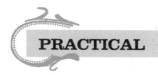

PRACTICAL

Chemistry is an experimental science, which means that, in general, chemical theories followed observations made in the lab. That is why the laboratory work is important for students. The laboratory course is intended to help students to see the connections between the theory and practice.

Students are required to have team work, and each group may have two or more students, depending on the size of class. Students in a group are encouraged to work on their lab reports together but they must write their lab reports independently. Each lab report must include the following sections: Introduction (a statement of the problem or investigation, including necessary background information and hypotheses), Materials, Procedure, Qualitative and/or Quantitative Data, Results and Conclusions.

Schedule Table of Experiment

Experiment	Contents	Class Hours	Experiment	Contents	Class Hours
1	Introduction to Measuring Techniques	4	4	Properties Associated with Changes in Physical State	4
2	Properties of Matter	4	5	Acid-Base Titration Curves Using a pH Meter	4
3	An Introduction to Chemical Reaction	4		Total	20

Experiment 1　Introduction to Measuring Techniques

1. Purpose.

(1) To learn the methods of measuring amounts of solids and liquid.

(2) To learn how to use balance, pipet and buret.

(3) To understand how and why need to choose proper equipment for a measurement.

2. Procedure.

(1) Identification of Apparatus.

● Show students some equipment which they may not know.

(2) Balance.

● Show students how to use a balance.

● Explain the methods for obtaining the mass of a substance.

● Stress that a beaker should be dry when put it into the balance.

(3) Dispensing Liquid.
- Show students how to use the pipet and buret.
- How to transfer solutions and how to get a reading.

Experiment 2　Properties of Matter

1. Purpose.
(1) To observe how different substances have different properties.
(2) To understand the different types of properties.
(3) To familiarize yourself further with the lab environment.
2. Procedure.
(1) Physical Properties.
- Appearance and odor.
- Density.
- Boiling point.
- Solubility.
(2) Chemical Properties.
- Combustion in air.
- Reaction with sodium (to be done in the hood).
- Sample calculations.

Experiment 3　An Introduction to Chemical Reaction

1. Purpose.
(1) To examine different types of chemical reactions.
(2) To examine the principle of conservation of mass.
2. Procedure.
Total 6 reactions.
Reaction 1-Formation of Lead Iodide.
$$Pb(NO_3)_2(s) + 2KI(s) \rightarrow PbI_2(s) + 2KNO_3(s)$$
$$\text{white}\quad\text{white}\quad\text{yellow}\quad\text{white.}$$
- Mix two solids and compare mass before and after.
- Note: put one glove on your hand that stirs the mixture.
Dispose product from this reaction in a "Lead Waste" bottle only.
Reaction 2-Combustion of Magnesium.
$$2Mg(s) + O_2 \rightarrow 2MgO(s)$$
- Burn the magnesium in air and see the mass increased.
Reaction 3-Dehydration Reaction.
$$CuSO_4 \cdot 5H_2O \rightarrow CuSO_4(s) + 5H_2O$$
$$\text{blue}\qquad\text{white}$$
- Heat the blue solid and see the mass lost.
Reaction 4 and 5-Complexation Reactions.
$$[Cu(H_2O)_4]^{2+}(aq) + 4NH_3(aq) \rightarrow [Cu(NH_3)_4]^{2+} + 4H_2O(l)$$
$$[Co(H_2O)6]^{2+}(aq) + 6NH_3(aq) \rightarrow [Co(NH_3)_6]^{2+}(aq) + 6H_2O(l)$$
Colored complexes formed.

Don't inhale ammonia fumes.

Reaction 6-Acid-base Reaction.

$$NaOH(aq) + HCl(aq) \rightarrow NaCl(aq) + H_2O(l)$$

● Neutralization reaction: salt and water formed.

Make sure NaOH solution does not splatter since it is caustic.

Experiment 4　Properties Associated with Changes in Physical State

1. Purpose.

To learn how to determine the normal melting and boiling points.

2. Procedure.

(1) Determine the Melting Point of Naphthalene.

Set up a water bath.

Get a small amount sample of naphthalene on a watch glass-use scoopula.

Get several capillary melting point tubes.

Note: naphthalene is toxic by ingestion and skin contact, be careful!

● Show students how to introduce the sample into the capillary.

● Show students how to attach the capillary to the thermometer.

(2) Determine the Boiling Point of Methanol.

Obtain 1 mL methanol in a small dry beaker.

Note: methanol is flammable and should be considered toxic by inhalation, ingestion or skin contact.

(3) Determine the Boiling Point of an Unknown Liquid.

Obtain 1 mL unknown liquid and record its number in line 3

Note: you should assume the unknown liquid is flammable and toxic.

● Dispose any residual liquid unknown in "Liquid Solvent" bottle.

● Return the washed culture tube to the place from which you obtained it.

Experiment 5　Acid–Base Titration Curves Using a pH Meter

1. Purpose.

(1) To learn the titration technique.

(2) To learn how to use the pH meter.

(3) To learn how to determine the equivalence point and pK_a.

(4) To understand the differences between the titration curves of strong, weak and polyprotic acids with base.

2. Procedure-you will carry out titrations of three different acids: a strong acid, a weak acid and a polyprotic acid. For each titration, you should plot two graphs, one of pH vs V_{NaOH} and the other of DpH/DV vs average volume of NaOH.

(1) Titration Curve of a Strong Acid.

● Care with electrode and don't hit it when you stir the solution.

● Add titrant (here the NaOH solution) in increments of 2 mL at the beginning points, and then you should add the NaOH in increments of 1 mL or 0.5 mL, which is based on the changes of pH value.

● Only small additions of titrant are needed when the titration closes to the equivalence point. You must add the titrant drop by drop and stir well at that time.

● Record your readings (the volume of NaOH from buret and the corresponding pH value from the pH meter) immediately.

(2) Titration Curve of a Weak Acid.

● Titration of an unknown weak acid.

● Some procedure as the titration of a strong acid.

(3) Titration Curve of a Polyprotic Acid.

● You should have two equivalence points in the titration curve.

● Pay attention to the calculation of K_{a1} and K_{a2}.

MEDICAL ORGANIC CHEMISTRY
医学有机化学

Chief Editors（主编）
    Ye Xiaoxia（叶晓霞）　Wenzhou Medical University（温州医科大学）
    Lü Wei（吕伟）　Tianjin Medical University（天津医科大学）

Deputy Chief Editors（副主编）
    Guo Jinxin（郭今心）　Shandong University（山东大学）
    GuoYunping（郭蕴萍）　Kunming Medical University（昆明医科大学）
    Li Wei（李伟）　Chongqing Medical University（重庆医科大学）

Editors（编委）（按姓氏拼音排序）
    Guo Jinxin（郭今心）　Shandong University（山东大学）
    GuoYunping（郭蕴萍）　Kunming Medical University（昆明医科大学）
    Li Wei（李伟）　Chongqing Medical University（重庆医科大学）
    Liu Lei（刘磊）　JiLin University（吉林大学）
    Lü Wei（吕伟）　Tianjin Medical University（天津医科大学）
    Ye Xiaoxia（叶晓霞）　Wenzhou Medical University（温州医科大学）

Course Description

This course is a one-semester introduction to organic chemistry that is designed for students preparing to become a physician, dentist, nurse, pharmacist, veterinarian, and so on. This subject deals primarily with the basic principles to understand the structure and reactivity of organic molecules. This course focuses on allowing students to gain an understanding and appreciation for simple organic compounds. It introduces them to the various classes of aliphatic and aromatic carbon compounds, their nomenclature, structures and properties. This course also conveys information that provides students with an understanding and appreciation of the following functional groups of the simple organic molecules found in living systems: Alcohols, Diols, Thiols, Phenols, Ethers, Epoxides, Sulfides, Aldehydes, Ketones, Amides, Esters, Amines, Carboxylic Acids and Carboxylic Acid Derivatives. The importance of these molecules in living systems is described and stressed. The major constituents of human bodies—carbohydrates, lipids, amino acids, proteins, nucleotides, and nucleic acids are also covered. The class presents the diversity of functional groups with regard to reactivity and reaction mechanisms, in particular free radical, nucleophilic and electrophilic mechanisms. Students learn stereochemistry as it relates to chemical structure and function. Additionally, they develop an understanding of hydrophobicity and hydrophilicity, and the utility of these properties in medicine.

Almost all of reactions in living things involve organic compounds, and it is impossible to understand life without some knowledge of organic chemistry. Therefore this subject is an essential course in the clinical medical curriculum.

Objectives

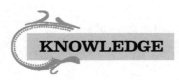

KNOWLEDGE

1. Grasp the structural formulas and nomenclature of organic compounds.
2. Grasp the properties of the different functional groups in organic chemistry.
3. Grasp the products by name and/or structure for major organic reactions.
4. Be familiar with the relationship between the structures and the properties of organic compounds.
5. Be familiar with the uses of some important organic compounds.
6. Be familiar with hazards of some important organic compounds.
7. Be familiar with some important biological pathways that the student will encounter in his/her professional studies.
8. Understand the relationship between organic chemistry and medicine.

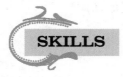

SKILLS

Grasp the basic techniques and concepts in organic chemistry through laboratory experiments.
1. Be able to do the experiment of the separation and purification of chemical mixtures.
2. Be able to do the experiment synthesis of some organic compounds, and master the techniques of the organic chemistry laboratory, such as reflux, distillation and so on.

Teaching and Learning Methods

Theory: Teaching organic chenistry to medical students is provided with the help of lectures and tutorials that deal with the structure and reactions of common organic functional groups with significant emphasis on the biochemical context of the chemical properties of organic molecules.

Practical: Practical training asks for medical students are to know the basic principles, methods and techniques, strategies, and skills by the typical experiments and experimental design of organic chemistry. The student is advised to pay attention to the regulation and safety of the laboratory of organic chemistry.

"*The more you practice, the more proficient you will become.*"

Recommended Textbooks

Janice Gorzynski Smith. 2011. Organic chemistry [M]. 3rd ed. New York: The McGraw-Hill Companies, Inc.

Jonathan Clayden , Nick Greeves, Stuart Warren. 2012. Organic Chemistry [M]. 2nd ed. London: Oxford University Press.

Peng Shiqi (彭师奇). 2012. Organic Chemistry [M]. Beijing: Higher Education Press.

William H. Brown, Brent L. Iverson, Eric V. Anslyn, et al. Foote. 2013. Organic Chemistry[M]. 7th ed. Boston: Cengage Learning.

Xia Shunzhen (夏淑珍), Luo Yiming (罗一鸣), Feng Wenfang (冯文芳). 2012. Organic Chemistry for Students of Medicine and Biology [M]. 2nd ed. Wuhan: Huazhong University of Science and Technology Press.

Schedule Table

Chapter	Contents	Hours	Chapter	Contents	Hours
1	Introduction	2	10	Derivatives of Carboxylic Acids	4
2	The Alkanes and Cycloalkanes	4	11	Amines	4
3	Alkenes and Alkynes	4	12	Spectroscopy of Organic Compounds	2
4	Aromatic Compounds	4	13	Heterocycles	4
5	Enantiomerism	4	14	Carbohydrates	4
6	Halohydrocarbons	4	15	Lipids	2
7	Alcohols, Phenols and Ethers	4	16	Amino Acids, Peptides and Proteins	2
8	Aldehydes and Ketones	4	17	Nucleic Acids	2
9	Carboxylic Acids and Substituted Acids	4		Total	58

Course Contents

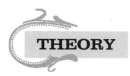

THEORY

Chapter 1　Introduction

1. Organic compounds and organic chemistry.

The basic concepts of organic compounds and organic chemistry, the characteristic, classification and structure of organic compounds.

2. Bonding in organic compound.

The valence theory and hybridization, three kinds of hybridization, hydrogen bonding.

3. Classification and reaction types of organic compounds.

The features of the organic compounds and the organic reaction types, two kinds of cleavage, the relationship between organic chemistry and medicine.

4. Acid-base theory.

Lewis acid and base, electrophilic reagents and nucleophilic reagents.

Chapter 2　The Alkanes and Cycloalkanes

1. Alkanes.

(1) Structure of alkanes.

(2) Skeletal isomerism in alkanes.

(3) Nomenclature of alkanes.

(4) Conformational isomerism, conformation of ethane and butane.

(5) Physical properties of alkanes.

(6) Reactions of alkanes, the mechanisms of radical reaction, stability of free radical, the reactivity and selectivity of alkanes in the halogenations.

2. Cycloalkanes.

(1) Nomenclature of cycloalkanes.

(2) Relative stability of cycloalkanes.

(3) *Cis-Trans* isomerism of cycloalkanes.

(4) Conformational isomerism of cyclohexane.

(5) Physical properties of cycloalkanes.

(6) Reactions of cycloalkanes.

Chapter 3　Alkenes and Alkynes

1. Structure of alkenes and alkynes.

2. Nomenclature of alkenes and alkynes.

3. *Cis-Trans* isomerism in alkenes, sequence rules, Markovnikov's rule.

4. Electronic effect.

5. Physical Properties of Alkenes and Alkynes.

6. Reactions of alkenes and alkynes, the mechanisms of electrophilic addition reaction(X_2, HX, H_2O, HOX, H_2SO_4, etc), oxidation reaction ($KMnO_4$, O_3), acidity of terminal alkynes.

7. Conjugated dienes, electrophilic additions to conjugated dienes.

Chapter 4　Aromatic Compounds

1. Benzene: structure and bonding.

2. Nomenclature of aromatic compounds.

3. Physical properties of aromatic compounds.

4. Reactions of aromatic compounds: the electrophilic substitution reactions (halogenation, nitration, sulfonation and Friedel-Crafts alkylation and acylation),the

reactions of side chain of alkylbenzene (halogenation and oxidation), orientation rules of electrophilic substituent reaction in substituted aromatic rings (orientation effect, orientation in disubstituted benzenes, synthetic application of orienting effects and the explanation of orienting effects), oxidation and reduction of aromatic compounds.

5. Fused-ring aromatic hydrocarbons: the nomenclature of fused-ring arenes and the structure of naphthalene, the chemical properties of the polycyclic aromatic compounds.

6. Aromaticity-Hückel's rule.

Chapter 5 Enantiomerism

1. Chirality and enantiomers: the classification of the isomerism, the conceptions in stereochemistry: chirality, chiral carbon atom, chiral molecule, achiral molecule and enantiomers , recognition of chirality.

2. Measurement of optical activity.

3. Representation of enantiomers—Fischer projection formula.

4. Nomenclature of enantiomers: nomenclature of enantiomers (D/L representation and R/S representation).

5. Stereoisomers with two chiral carbon atoms: stereoisomers with two different chiral carbon atoms, stereoisomers with two simliar chiral carbon atoms, the concepts of racement, diastereomer, *meso* compound.

6. Enantiomers without chiral carbon atoms.

7. Properties of enantiomers , resolution of enantiomers, reform of chiral molecules and biological function of chiral molecules.

Chapter 6 Halohydrocarbons

1. Classification and nomenclature of halohydrocarbons, the structure of alkyl halides.

2. Physical properties of halohydrocarbons.

3. Reactions of halohydrocarbons: the mechanisms of nucleophilic substitution reaction: S_N1 and S_N2, the comparison between S_N1 and S_N2 and factors influencing S_N1 and S_N2, the elimination reactions (E) and Zaitsev's rule, the mechanisms of and impact factors of E1 and E2 reaction; the nucleophilic substitution versus elimination; nucleophilic substitution of halogenated alkenes and benzenes, reaction with metals (preparing Grignard reagents).

Chapter 7 Alcohols, Phenols, and Ethers

1. Alcohols.

(1) Structure and classification of alcohols.

(2) Nomenclature of alcohols.

(3) Physical properties of alcohols, hydrogen bonding.

(4) Reactions of alcohols: acidity and basicity of alcohols, esterification of alcohols with inorganic acids, dehydration of alcohols, halogenation of alcohols, oxidation of alcohols.

2. Phenols.

(1) Structure and nomenclature of phenols.

(2) Physical properties of phenols.

(3) Chemical properties of phenols: acidity of phenols, electrophilic substitution in aromatic ring of phenols (bromination, nitration, and sulfonation), esterification of phenols with organic acids, reaction of phenols with $FeCl_3$, oxidation of phenols.

3. Ethers.

(1) Structure and nomenclature of ethers.

(2) Physical properties of ethers.

(3) Chemical properties of ethers: oxonium salts, cleavage of ether bond.

4. Epoxides, thiols and sulfides.

Chapter 8　Aldehydes and Ketones

1. Classification and nomenclature of aldehydes and ketones.

2. Structure of aldehydes and ketones: structure of carbonyl groups.

3. Physical properties of aldehydes and ketones.

4. Reactions of aldehydes and ketones: nucleophilic addition reaction of aldehydes and ketones (mechanism of addition reaction, various nucleophilic addition reaction of aldehydes and ketones—cyanide addition/ addition of water /reaction with sodium bisulfite/ reaction with alcohols/addition of Grignard reagent/ reaction with nitrogen nucleophilic reagents).

5. Reaction involving α-hydrogens: keto-enol tautomerism, aldol condensation, halogenations.

6. Oxidation and hydride addition: oxidation, reduction.

Chapter 9　Carboxylic Acids and Substituted Acids

1. Carboxylic acids.

(1) Structure and nomenclature of carboxylic acids.

(2) Physical properties of carboxylic acids.

(3) Chemical properties of carboxylic acids: acidity of carboxylic acids, formation of derivatives of carboxylic acids, replacement of α-Hydrogen, reduction of carboxylic acids, decarboxylation of carboxylic acids.

2. Hydroxy acids.

(1) Structure and nomenclature of hydroxy acids.

(2) Physical properties of hydroxy acids.

(3) Chemical properties of hydroxy acids: acidity, alcohol acids (oxidation reaction, dehydration—α-hydroxy acids/β-hydroxy acids/γ-hydroxy acids and δ-hydroxy acids), phenol acids.

3. Keto-acids.

(1) Nomenclature of keto-acids.

(2) Chemical properties of keto-acids, acidity, α-keto-acids, β-keto-acids.

Chapter 10　Carboxylic Acids Derivatives

1. Classification and structure of carboxylic acid derivatives (acyl halides/ carboxylic acid anhydrides/esters/amides).

2. Nomenclature of carboxylic acid derivatives.

3. Physical properties of carboxylic acid derivatives.

4. Reactions of carboxylic acid derivatives: nucleophilic acyl substitution reactions (hydrolysis/alcoholysis/aminolysis), the mechanism for nucleophilic acyl substitution reactions, Claisen condensation of esters.

5. Imide.

6. Urea and barbiturates (weak basicity/ hydrolysis/reaction of urea with HNO_2 / biuret reaction, formation of barbiturates acid and its derivatives).

Chapter 11　Amines

1. Classification and nomenclature of amines.

2. Structure of amines.

3. Physical properties of amines.

4. Chemical properties of amines: basicity of amines (the electronic effect/ the solvation effect /the steric hindrance effect), amines as nucleophiles (alkylation of amines/acylation of amines/sulfonylation of amines), reaction with nitrous acid, electrophilic aromatic substitution.

5. Aromatic diazonium salts: replacement of nitrogen/coupling of diazonium salts—synthesis of azo compounds.

6. Alkaloids.

Chapter 12　Spectroscopy of Organic Compounds

1. General principle of absorption spectra.

2. Ultraviolet-visible spectra: ultraviolet-visible absorption spectra, interpreting ultraviolet absorption spectra.

3. Infrared spectra: molecular vibration and IR absorption—the modes of stretching and bending, vibrational equation, the characteristic infrared absorption of groups of some functional groups (infrared spectra of hydrocarbons/other functional groups —carbonyl functional groups, alcohols and phenols, carboxylic acids, amines), interpretation of IR spectra.

4. Nuclear magnetic resonance spectra: basic concept for nuclear magnetic resonance—nuclear spin states, nuclear magnetic resonance, ^1H nuclear magnetic resonance (^1H NMR) spectroscopy and chemical shifts (shielding and deshielding of protons, chemical shift, the factors affecting the chemical shifts, integration of peak areas; signal splitting—the spin-spin splitting phenomenon, the origin of spin-spin splitting; carbon-13 spectroscopy).

5. Mass spectrometry.

6. How to identify the structure of organic compound by these spectroscopies.

Chapter 13　Heterocycles

1. Classification and nomenclature of heterocycles.

2. Structure and properties of five-membered aromatic heterocycles: structure of five-membered aromatic heterocycles, properties of five-membered aromatic

heterocycles (acidity and basicity of pyrrole, electrophilic substitution), derivatives of pyrrole, structure and function of imidazole.

3. Structure and properties of pyridine and pyrimidine: structure and properties of pyridine and pyrimidine (solubility of pyridine, basicity of pyridine, electrophilic reaction and nucleophilic reaction, oxidation on the side chain of pyridine, pyrimidine and its derivatives.

4. Fused-heterocyclic compounds.

5. The sulfa drugs.

Chapter 14　Carbohydrates

1. Classification and nomenclature of carbohydrates, the structure of monosaccharides—open chain structure, mutarotation and cyclic structure of monosaccharides.

2. Monosaccharides: the physical properties of monosaccharides, the chemical.

properties of monosaccharides—glycoside formation, oxidation of monosaccharides, dehydration.

3. Disaccharides and polysaccharides: lactose , sucrose, maltose, cellobiose, starch , glycogen and cellose.

Chapter 15　Lipids

1. Fats and oils—triacylglycerols : the structure and composition of triacylglycerols, classification and nomenclature of fatty acids, physical properties of triacylglycerols, chemical properties of triacylglycerols (addition reactions, oxidation reactions, and saponification).

2. Waxes.

3. Phospholipids: the structure and nomenclature of phosphoglycerides, lecithins, cephalins, sphingolipids, phospholipids, cell membrane.

4. Steroids: the structure of steroids(base structure of steroids, stereochemistry of steroids), sterols, cholic acid, bile acids, steroid hormones(sex hormones, adrenal cortical hormones).

5. Steroid hormones.

Chapter 16　Amino Acids, Peptides and Proteins

1. Amino acids.

(1) Classification and nomenclature of amino acids.

(2) Structure and configuration of amino acids.

(3) Properties of amino acids: physical properties of amino acids, chemical properties of amino acids (acid/base nature and the isoelectric point, dehydration, decarboxylation, reaction with nitrous acid, the ninhydrin reaction, reactions with linking R groups).

2. Peptides.

(1) Structure and nomenclature of peptides.

(2) Plane of peptide bond.

(3) Biological active peptide.

3. Proteins.

(1) Element composition and classification of proteins.

(2) Hierarchy of protein structure.

(3) Properties of proteins.

Chapter 17　Nucleic Acids

1. Chemical structure and classification of nucleic acids.

2. Nucleosides and nucleotides.

3. The hierarchy of nucleic acid structure.

4. Physical and chemical properties of nucleic acids.

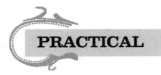

PRACTICAL

1. Column Chromatography.

To understand the basic principle of column chromatography and learn how to operate the column chromatography.

2. Extraction.

To understand the principle of liquid-liquid extraction and learn about handling the of separatory funnel.

3. Recrystallization.

To learn about the theory and technique of the purification of solid organic compounds by recrystallization and master the operation of hot filtration and vacuum filtration.

4. Refractive Index Determination of Liquids.

To learn the significance of refractive index in research of organic liquids and master the determination method of refractive index by using an Abbe refractometer.

5. Distillation.

To be familiar with the principle of simple distillation and the determination method of boiling point, to learn about assembling the apparatus for simple distillation.

6. Dehydration of Rectified Spirit.

To know the basic principles of the drying of organic compounds, and varieties and usage of the drying agents. To learn about the preparation method of absolute ethanol.

7. Synthesis of n-Butyl Acetate.

To understand the principle of esterification reactions of organic acid with alcohol and to learn the isolation and purification methods of synthetic liquid products by extraction, washing, drying and distillation procedures.

8. Synthesis of Acetyl Salicylic Acid(Aspirin).

To learn the method of preparing aspirin by acetylation reaction, to master the techniques of purification for solid products, to learn the identification of purity of the solid product by determination of melting point or some specific reaction and to be familiar with the operation of vacuum filtration and recrystallization.

ELEMENTARY CHINESE

基 础 汉 语

Chief Editors（主编）

Zhou Jian（周健） Jinan University（暨南大学）

Zhang Xi（张曦） Nanjing Medical University（南京医科大学）

Li Xinchao（李新朝） Jiangsu University（江苏大学）

Deputy Chief Editors（副主编）

Xu Fuping（徐富平） Jinan University（暨南大学）

Deng Shulan（邓淑兰） Sun Yat-sen University（中山大学）

Wang Meiling（王美玲） Xi'an Jiaotong University（西安交通大学）

Editors（编委）（按姓氏拼音排序）

Deng Shulan（邓淑兰） Sun Yat-sen University（中山大学）

Li Xinchao（李新朝） Jiangsu University（江苏大学）

Liang Shuang（梁爽） Guangxi Medical University（广西医科大学）

Wang Meiling（王美玲） Xi'an Jiaotong University（西安交通大学）

Wang Shuhui（王树蕙） Jinan University（暨南大学）

Xu Fuping（徐富平） Jinan University（暨南大学）

Zhang Xi（张曦） Nanjing Medical University（南京医科大学）

Zhou Jian（周健） Jinan University（暨南大学）

Course Description

As an integrated language course, Elementary Chinese provides the beginners with phonetics, vocabulary, grammar and characters knowledge and helps them develop the language skills as well as adapt to the new campus environment. As a compulsory course for medical students, Elementary Chinese focuses on daily conversations closely related to campus life and daily settings, which can be put into practice immediately after the class. This course firstly devotes to the pronunciation drill which is a key to language learners' learning and communication success outside the classroom. Chinese characters stroke order is also emphasized and character writing is involved in class. Vocabulary learning is the most important task in classroom teaching, and the course will offer many opportunities to highlight the collocation and variation of the target words. The most frequently used grammatical rules are explained to the learners, mostly taught in the context of practical communication. Along with the above Elementary Chinese attaches importance to developing learners'cross-cultural awareness.

The course is aimed at supporting the learners to reach high levels of Chinese language competence when they use it to talk, read and write about their own needs, experiences, opinions, and interests, which lays a solid foundation for their further Medical Chinese learning.

Objectives

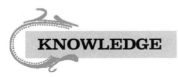

At the end of the course, the MBBS students shall be able to:

1. Know the rules of Chinese Pinyin that basically comprise of initial, final, intonation, light tone, modified tone and retroflex final.

2. Know the rules about Chinese character writing.

3. Know some rules about Chinese syntax, in particular basic sentence patterns.

4. Master the common grammar items such as modal verbs, prepositions and particles.

5. Master over 1,800 words and know how to use them appropriately in the verbal and written communications.

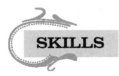

At the end of the course, the student shall be able to:

1. Identify and produce pronunciation appropriately in daily conversations.

2. Be aware of rhythms, the word stress and sentence stress.

3. Introduce personal information (name, age, dwelling, hobby, family, ability, appearance, character, and so on).

4. Understand simple dialogues, requests and statements related to general topics.

5. Process daily routines, give instructions and make arrangements.

6. Read and understand brief textual materials related to daily life.

7. Write short message to complete the introduction and description on familiar topics.

Teaching and Learning Methods

Classroom teaching: A communicative approach will be used throughout the course with an emphasis on daily situations. The language teaching in classroom will be activity based and learner centered. Some audio/video-based listening exercise will take place in the class. Students will be required to obtain a textbook to support their studies.

Practical: Students will be suggested to catch every chance to do language practical. Taking part in the classroom interaction with teacher and completing the classroom language tasks can promote the internalization of knowledge. As far as students'task is concerned, they are expected to do review and preparation for new lessons. Students will be encouraged to establish connection with native speakers.

Recommended Textbooks

戴桂芙，刘立新，李海燕．2014.（博雅）初级汉语口语（第一、第二册）［M］. 3 版. 北京：北京大学出版社.

Dai Guifu, Liu Lixin, Li Haiyan. 2014. (Boya) Elementary Spoken Chinese (Vol.1 & Vol. 2) [M]. 3rd ed. Beijing: Peking University Press.

黄立，钱旭菁．2012. 博雅汉语（准中级加速篇1）［M］. 2 版. 北京：北京大学出版社.

Huang Li, Qian Xujing. 2012. Boya Chinese (Quasi-intermediate, Vol.1) [M], 2nd ed. Beijing: Peking University Press.

刘德联，刘晓雨．2014.（博雅）中级汉语口语（第一、第二册）［M］. 3 版. 北京：北京大学出版社.

Liu Delian, Liu Xiaoyu. 2014. (Boya) Intermediate Spoken Chinese (Vol.1 & Vol.2) [M]. 3rd ed. Beijing: Peking University Press.

马箭飞，李德均，成文．2006. 汉语口语速成（基础篇）［M］. 2 版. 北京：北京语言大学出版社.

Ma Jianfei, Li Dejun, Chengwen. 2006. Short-Term Spoken Chinese (Elementary) [M]. 2nd ed. Beijing: Beijing Language and Culture University Press.

马箭飞，苏英霞，翟艳．2015. 汉语口语速成（入门篇，上、下册）［M］. 3 版. 北京：北京大学出版社.

Ma Jianfei, Su Yingxia, Zhaiyan. 2015. Short-Term Spoken Chinese (Threshold, Vol.1 & Vol. 2) [M]. 3rd ed. Beijing: Peking University Press.

任雪梅，徐晶凝．2013. 博雅汉语（初级，上、下册）［M］. 2 版. 北京：北京大学出版社.

Ren Xuemei, Xu Jingning. 2013. Boya Chinese (Elementary, Vol.1 & Vol. 2) [M]. 2nd ed. Beijing: Peking University Press.

杨寄洲，邱军，朱庆明．2006. 汉语教程（第1册，上、下）［M］. 北京：北京语言大学出版社.

Yang Jizhou, Qiu Jun, Zhu Qingming. 2006. Hanyu Jiaocheng(Volume one, I & II) [M]. Beijing: Beijing Language and Culture University Press.

杨寄洲，邱军，朱庆明．2006. 汉语教程（第2册，上、下）［M］. 北京：北京语言大学出版社.

Yang Jizhou, Qiu Jun, Zhu Qingming. 2006. Hanyu Jiaocheng(Volume two, I & II) [M]. Beijing: Beijing Language and Culture University Press.

Schedule Table

Chapter	Contents	Hours	Chapter	Contents	Hours
Part one	Knowledge and skills	268	26	Calling for repair	6
1	Rules of Chinese Pinyin	6	27	Making an appointment	6
2	Chinese character stroke	2	28	Purchase in market	6
3	Classroom Chinese	2		Review	2
4	Greetings	4	29	Reporting a case in police station	6
5	Chinese numerals	4	30	Reservation	6
6	Eating in canteen	4	31	Seeing a doctor	6
7	Asking for phone number	4	32	I have a date with China	6
8	Self-introduction	4	33	Taking a taxi for the first time	6
	Review	2		Review	2
9	Buildings on campus	4	34	Summer holidays	6
10	Telling the time	4	35	Farewell party	6
11	Family photo	4	36	Three days to see	6
12	Friend's birthday	4	37	Being happy is actually quite easy	6
13	Money exchange in bank	4	38	Three e-mails	6
	Review	2		Review	2
14	Accommodation	4	39	Color and character	6
15	Hobby	4	40	What should I do	6
16	Calling for foods	4	41	Education of love	6
17	Daily talk: Favorites	4	42	Do as the Romans do	6
18	What do you study	4	43	Yu Gong removed the mountains	6
	Review	2		Review	2
19	Making time schedule	6	44	Low-carbon life	6
20	Asking for class leave	6	45	The ideal career	6
21	Shopping online	6	46	When the day comes	6
22	A wonderful competition	6	47	Set the watch forward by three minutes	6
23	How was your quiz	6	48	Going to Berlin by hitchhiking	6
	Review	2		Review	2
24	School life	6	Part two	Language practical	20
25	A lucky day	6		Total	288

Course Contents

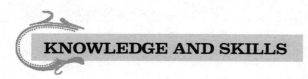

KNOWLEDGE AND SKILLS

Chapter 1   Rules of Chinese Pinyin

1. Target words: Pīnyīn, shēngmǔ, yùnmǔ, shēngdiào, qīngshēng, biàndiào, érhuàyīn.
2. Formation of Chinese syllables.
3. Rules of combination of the initials, finals and tones.
4. The four tones and a neutral tone in Mandarin.
5. Rules of tone change.
6. Rules of retroflex final.
7. Identify and produce the basic sounds of Chinese Phonetic Alphabet.
8. Language tasks: Differentiate similar initials, finals and syllables.

Chapter 2   Chinese Character Stroke

1. Target words: Hànzì, bǐhuà, bùjiàn, bǐshùn.
2. Basic strokes of Chinese character.
3. Combinations of Chinese character stroke.
4. The orders of stroke for writing Chinese character.
5. The relationships between the radicals and Chinese character.
6. The semantic functions of character radical.
7. Chinese character exercise (write down the characters in correct stroke order).

Chapter 3   Classroom Chinese

1. To begin a class: Kāishǐ shàngkè ba.
2. In class: Diǎnmíng; Zhǔnbèi hǎo le ma; Qǐng ānjìng; Qǐng gēn wǒ dú; Qǐng yìqǐ dú; Dǎkāi shū; Fāndào dì jiǔ yè; Shuí kěyǐ shì yí xià; Zuò wán le ma? Jìxù; Zhùyì.
3. Comments: Hěn hǎo; Hěn bàng; Fēicháng hǎo; Duì le; Cuò le.
4. Exercise and homework: Liànxí, chāoxiě, sān biàn, tīngxiě.
5. To dismiss the class: Shíjiān dào le; Xiàkè.
6. Examinations: Kǎoshì,fùxí, kǒushì, bǐshì, fēnshù, chéngjì.
7. Others: Qǐng zài shuō yí biàn; Shénme yìsi? Wǒ bù míngbái.

Chapter 4   Greetings

1. Target temporal words: Zǎoshang, shàngwǔ, zhōngwǔ, xiàwǔ, wǎnshang.
2. Expressions of greeting: Nǐ(men) hǎo; Zǎoshang hǎo; Wǎnshang hǎo; Wǎn ān.
3. Target politeness formulae: Xièxie; Bú kèqi; Duìbuqǐ; Méi guānxi; Zàijiàn; Qǐng jìn; Rènshi nǐ hěn gāoxìng.

4. Personal Pronouns: Nǐ, wǒ, tā, dàjiā.

5. Usage of the interrogative question words: Ma, Ne.

6. Usage of the adverb words: Yě, dōu, hěn.

7. Usage of the pluralities: Men, nǐmen, wǒmen, tāmen.

8. Chinese character exercise.

Chapter 5　Chinese Numerals

1. Target units of quantity: Gè, shí, bǎi, qiān, wàn.

2. Numeral expressions: From 1 to 101.

3. Monetary units of RMB: Kuài/yuán, máo/jiǎo, fēn.

4. Expressions for giving price and enquiring price.

5. Demonstrative pronouns: Zhè, nà.

6. Question words for number: Duōshao, jǐ.

7. Oral language task: Play games of counting number.

8. Chinese character exercise.

Chapter 6　Eating in Canteen

1. Target words: Shítáng, mǐfàn, miàntiáo, jīròu, chǎo, jīdàn, yú, niúròu, zhūròu, qīngcài, tāng, làjiāo, dòufu, xīhóngshì, húluóbo, mógū, dǎbāo, wèidào, xiāng, kěkǒu, zǎofàn, wǔfàn, wǎnfàn.

2. Target measure words: Gè, píng, bēi, pán, hé, bāo, zhāng, shuāng, kuài, bǎ.

3. Expression of tablewares: Kuàizi, wǎn, sháozi, pánzi, bēizi, cāndāo, cānchā.

4. The particular interrogative word "shénme".

5. Negative words: "Bù" and "méi".

6. Intension verbs: "Yào", "xiǎng" and "xǐhuan".

7. Oral language task: Introduce your favorite foods and beverages.

8. Chinese character exercise.

Chapter 7　Asking for Phone Number

1. Target words: Qǐngwèn, qǐng, gàosù, shǒujī, diànhuà, hàomǎ, shì, fángjiān, dòng, lóu, zhīdào, búyòng.

2. Tell the phone number/ room number/ building number.

3. Tell the floor of building.

4. The sentences with "shì".

5. Particular interrogatives: "Nǎr", "nǎli".

6. The difference between "èr" and "liǎng".

7. Word order of the narrative sentences and the general questions.

8. Oral language tasks: Design a dialogue to ask for phone/room number.

9. Chinese character exercise.

Chapter 8　Self-introduction

1. Target words: Jièshào, yíxià, míngzì, guójiā, zhuānyè, àihào, dàxué, xuéxí, zài, xìng, dōu, de.

2. Usage of the preposition "zài".

3. Usage of the modal particle "le".

4. Construction "Shì……de".

5. The word order in Chinese sentence: "Dōu bù" and "bù dōu".

6. Location as adverbial modifier.

7. Oral language task: Make self-introduction.

8. Chinese character exercise.

Chapter 9　Buildings on Campus

1. Main buildings on campus: jiàoxuélóu, túshūguǎn, sùshèlóu, bàngōnglóu, xíngzhènglóu, shítáng, tǐyùguǎn, lǐtáng, nánmén.

2. Usage of the prepositional construction "cóng……dào……".

3. Usage of the particle "de" (wǒ de shū).

4. Geographic locations: Dōngbian, nánbian, xībian, běibian.

5. Relative locations: Zuǒbian, yòubian, qiánbian, hòubian, zhōngjiān, duìmiàn, pángbiān, fùjìn.

6. Location expressions: "A zài B de zuǒbian"; "B de zuǒbian shì A".

7. Oral language task: Introduce your campus to a new comer.

8. Chinese character exercise.

Chapter 10　Telling the Time

1. Target words: Diǎn, fēn, bàn, yíkè, chà……, rì, yuè, nián, xīngqī, jīntiān, zuótiān, míngtiān, xiànzài.

2. Expressions of the clock time and the date.

(1) The sequence of clock time expression: "……diǎn……fēn".

(2) The sequence of date expression: "……nián……yuè……rì".

3. The time of Chinese traditional festivals.

4. Chinese zodiac culture.

5. Description of the class schedule.

6. Oral language task: Tell some big days such as your parents'birthday, or time of the traditional festivals in your country.

7. Chinese character exercise.

Chapter 11　Family Photo

1. Target words: Zhàopiān, jiā, kǒu, yǒu, bàba, māma, gēge, jiějie, dìdi, mèimei, háizi, yéye, nǎinai, hái, gǒu, tiáo, yīshēng, jiàoshī, gōngchéngshī, zhíyuán, jīnglǐ, huàjiā, shāngren, gēn.

2. Usage of the verb "yǒu (have)".

3. Expressions about age.

4. Usage of the adverb "hái".

5. Pepositions: "Gēn" and "hé".

6. Oral language task: Describe a family photo.

7. Chinese character exercise.

Chapter 12   Friend's Birthday

1. Target words: Péngyǒu, shēngrì, máng, zhèngzài, zhǔnbèi, lǐwù, dàngāo, qiǎokèlì, tián, huā, xīnyì, nán(male), wǎnfàn, yǐhòu, shuí, sòng, tóngxué, tóngwū, yǐjīng.

2. Particular interrogative: Shuí/shéi.

3. Degree adverbs: Hěn, fēicháng, bǐjiào, jíle.

4. Alternative question construction "shì……háishì……".

5. Usage of the present tense adverbs: Zhèngzài, yǐjīng.

6. Usage of locations as adverbial modifier.

7. Oral language task: Introduce one of your friends.

8. Chinese character exercise.

Chapter 13   Money Exchange in Bank

1. Target words: Tiánbiǎo, duìhuàn, huìlǜ, xiànjīn, yínhángkǎ, zhànghào, cúnkuǎn, qǔqián, qiānmíng, hùzhào, qiānzhèngyè, fùyìn.

2. Expression of the major currencies: Rénmínbì, Měiyuán, Yīngbàng, ōuyuán, Rìyuán.

3. Construction "Měi……dōu……".

4. Affirmative-negative question construction: Adjective + bù + Adjective.

5. Affirmative-negative question construction: Verb + bù + verb.

6. Usage of modal particle "Ba".

7. Usage of particular interrogatives: "Wèishénme", "zěnme".

8. Oral language task: Design a dialogue about exchanging money in bank.

9. Chinese character exercise.

Chapter 14   Accommodation

1. Target words: Zhùsù, sùshè, gōngyù, huánjìng, tiáojiàn, guǎnlǐ, dǎsǎo, gānjìng, shūfu, ānquán, chuáng, xǐshǒujiān, chúfáng, yángtái, sùguǎn, shuākǎ, dēngjì, fúwù.

2. Expressions of campus community service: Chāoshì, gānxǐdiàn, lǐfàdiàn, kuàidì zhōngxīn, cānguǎn, xiūlǐdiàn, yīyuàn.

3. The measure words for organization: "Jiā", "suǒ".

4. The classifier "xiē" and "yìxiē".

5. Usage of adverb "zhǐ(only)".

6. Numeral-classifier compounds as attributives of the nouns.

7. Oral language task: Describe the environment of your dormitory.

8. Chinese character exercise.

Chapter 15   Hobby

1. Target words: Yuèdú, dǎlánqiú, dǎpáiqiú, dǎwǎngqiú, tīzúqiú, yóuyǒng, lǚxíng, túbù, kàndiànyǐng, chànggē, tiàowǔ, shàngwǎng, wǎngyóu, yújiā.

2. Usage of auxiliary verbs: "Néng", "huì", "kěyǐ".

3. Usage of verbal reduplication: An informal or casual tone of voice.

4. Word stress and sentence stress.

5. Construction "Tài……le".

6. Oral language task: Introduce your hobby.

7. Short composition: My hobbies.

Chapter 16   Calling for Foods

1. Target words: Wàimài, diǎndān, sòng, shāodǐng, yóu, qīngdàn, wēilà, mǎshàng, shú, fèn (measure word), yíngyǎng, yuánliào.

2. The usual patterns of Enumeration.

3. Usage of particular interrogative "Zěnmeyàng".

4. Comparison: "yǒudiǎnr + Adjective" and "Sth. + Adjective + yìdiǎnr".

5. "De" structure (Wǒ yào bú là de).

6. Oral language task: Design a dialogue about ordering lunch by mobile phone.

7. Chinese character exercise.

Chapter 17   Daily Talk: Favorites

1. Target words: Yánsè, lánsè, hóngsè, huángsè, zǐsè, báisè, hēisè, lǜsè, shēn, hǎokàn, piàoliang, gèng, tǐyù, yùndòng, yǔmáoqiú, bǎnqiú, táiqiú, huáxuě, bèngjí, cìjī, hǎowán, xīngfèn, nánwàng, chàyidiǎn.

2. Alternative questions with verbs: "VP1 + háishì + VP2".

3. Degree adverbs: "Zuì", "tài", "tǐng".

4. Usage of adverb "gèng".

5. Construction "Yìbānláishuō".

6. Oral language task: Which sport games do you like?

7. Short composition: My roommate's favorites.

Chapter 18   What Do You Study

1. Target words: Yīxué, réntǐ jiěpōuxué, shēnglǐxué, xīnlǐxué, shēngwùhuàxué, wàikēxué, nèikēxué, fùchǎnkē, érkē, yàolǐxué, yīxuéyíchuánxué, zhēnjiǔxué, shèqū yīxué, yǎnkēxué, shénjīngbìngxué, jīchǔ hànyǔ, yīxué hànyǔ, xuéqī.

2. Classifiers: "Mén" (for course) and "jié" (for class).

3. Usage of adverb "quán" and "quánbù".

4. Construction "Yǒude……, yǒude……".

5. Construction "Yìbiān……, yìbiān……".

6. Oral language task: Introduce your daily course arrangement.

7. Chinese character exercise.

Chapter 19   Making Time Schedule

1. Target words: Shàngkè, zìxiū, hànyǔjiǎo, kāihuì, xuǎnjǔ, bǐsài, jiànshēn, cānjiā, huódòng.

2. Temporal words as adverbial modifier: "Gāngcái", "gānggāng", "mǎshàng".

3. Construction "Xiān……, ránhòu……".

4. Adverbs: "Zài" (once more) and "yòu" (again).

5. Sentences with "subject-predicate" predicate.

6. Oral language task: Introduce your class schedule of this week.

7. Short composition: A busy day.

Chapter 20　Asking for Class Leave

1. Target words: Qǐng bìngjià, bànlǐ, shǒuxù, bùshūfu, fārè, késou, sǎngzi téng, gǎnmào, kāiyào, jiànyì, xiūxi, zuìhǎo, bānzhǔrèn, tóngyì, xīwàng, pīzhǔn, qǐngjiàtiáo.

2. Temporal construction: "Yìkāishǐ……, hòulái……".

3. Usage of the aspect particle "le".

4. Construction "Yīnwèi……, suǒyǐ……".

5. Construction "……le……jiù……".

6. Sentences with adjectival predicates.

7. Oral language task: Design a dialogue about asking for class leave.

8. Composition: Class leave note writing.

Chapter 21　Shopping Online

1. Target words: Mǎi, dōngxī, shāngchǎng, wǎnggòu, fāngbiàn, xuǎnzé, zhìliang, kuǎnshì, táobǎo, jīngdōng, kuàidì, dìzhǐ, zhīfù, zhīfùbǎo, wēixìn.

2. Classifiers: Jiàn, tái, bǎ, dài, tiáo, bù.

3. Expressions for approximate number: "Dàgài", "zuǒyòu".

4. Usage of adverbs: "Děi", "yīnggāi".

5. Construction "Suīrán……, dànshì……".

6. Construction "Yào……le".

7. Oral language task: Retell the text.

8. Chinese character exercise.

Chapter 22　A Wonderful Competition

1. Target words: Qiúduì, jìngōng, duìshǒu, lìhài, shàng bànchǎng, xià bànchǎng, jīliè, jīngcǎi, lālāduì, guānzhòng, jiāyóu, pīnqiǎng, shèmén, défēn, bǐfēn, cáipàn, yíng, shū, yǒuyì, kāixīn, fàngsōng.

2. Compound degree complement: Verb + "de" + comment word.

3. Compound directional complement: Verb + "shàngqù/xiàlái"; Verb + "qǐlái"; Verb + "jìnqù/chūlái".

4. Compound durational complement: Verb + "le" + durational phrase.

5. Asking questions with "duō": duōdà, duōyuǎn, duōcháng, duōgāo, duōjiǔ, duōnán.

6. Constructions: "Hǎo róngyì"/ "Hǎo bù róngyì".

7. Oral language task: Describe a cricket competition.

8. Composition: Extensive writing about a cricket final.

Chapter 23　How Was Your Quiz

1. Target words: Cèyàn, wán, yǒuxiē, jǐnzhāng, jiéguǒ, fàngsōng, xiàoguǒ, dào(measure word), tí, shíjiān, gòu, nán, màn, quèshí, yuèdú, fùxí, bāngzhù, dānxīn, jiějué, dǎsuan, gèngjiā, nǔlì.

2. Construction "Kuàiyào……le".

3. Complements clarifying state or degree using "de".

4. Construction "Duì······láishuō".

5. Construction "bù A bù B"(bù duō bù shǎo).

6. Oral language task: Retell the text.

7. Composition: The final exam is coming.

Chapter 24　School Life

1. Target words: Xíguàn, shēnghuó, gāng, bùhǎoyìsi, qǐchuáng, shuì, zǎo, shuì, zǎoqǐ, máobìng, gǎi, yǐnshí, zhōngguó, cài, yóunì, yíngyǎng, fēngfù, tiānqì, xiàyǔ, jìjié, cháoshī, qiūtiān, gānshuǎng, dōngtiān, wēnnuǎn.

2. Usage of adverb "zǎojiù" (Zǎojiù xíguàn le zhèli de yǐnshí).

3. Usage of rhetorical question: "Búshì······ma".

4. Construction "shì······de"(emphasize the time/place/manner/purpose).

5. Usage of adverbs: "Cái" and "jiù".

6. The exclamation construction "duō······ā".

7. Oral language task: Introduce your campus life.

8. Chinese character exercise.

Chapter 25　A Lucky Day

1. Target words: Xìngyùn, guǎnggào, chángshì, yóujiàn, qǐngqiú, liánmáng, huífù, jīhuì, liúxué, zhēnxī, chúle······yǐwài, lèishuǐ, xīwàng, gūfù, bìngqiě, yídìng.

2. Location words "shàng" and "lǐ".

3. Adverb "huì": A usage of speculation of events that will occur.

4. Construction "Chúle······yǐwài, hái······".

5. Construction "Búshì······jiùshì······".

6. Imperative sentences: Issuing an order, giving a suggestion, making a request.

7. Oral language task: Retell the text.

8. Composition (Diary writing).

Chapter 26　Calling for Repair

1. Target words: Kōngtiáo, huài, nánshòu, sùguǎn, dēngjì, bàoxiū, wéixiūgōng, tōngzhī, zhǐhǎo , děng, jímáng, kànyàngzi, yàoshì, huīfù, bìxū, gǎnxiè, xīnkǔ, bǎoxiū.

2. Construction "yàoshì······dehuà".

3. Usage of the particle "le" (duration complement).

4. Usage of the adverb "zhǐhǎo" (having no choice but to).

5. Consequential complements.

6. The negative expressions of consequential complement.

7. Oral language task: Design a dialogue about calling for repair.

8. Chinese character exercise: Fill in a repairs application form.

Chapter 27　Making an Appointment

1. Target words: Qiānzhèng, yùyuē, dàoqī, zhōngxīn, xùqiān, yáncháng, guīdìng,

jiǎofèi, xiédài, zhèngjiàn, lí, dìtiězhàn, tóngyì, ānpái, xiǎngbudào, diào.

    2. Usage of the adverb "jiù": Action 2 takes place immediately after action 1.

    3. Usage of the aspect particle "guo": Verb + guo.

    4. Measure words: "Biàn", "cì".

    5. Preposition "lí": A usage of distance.

    6. Oral language task: Make an appointment with your friend to discuss the coming cricket competition.

    7. Chinese character exercise.

Chapter 28   Purchase in Market

    1. Target words: Ròucài shìchǎng, guīmó, pǐnzhǒng, qíquán, fēngfù, guàng, zhōumò, jùhuì, fènliàng, shūcài, tǔdòu, yángcōng, huánjià, gālífěn, zīránfěn, yángròu, gǎnlǎnyóu, sāimǎn, pēngtiáo, dàxiǎn shēnshǒu, fēngwèi, jiāxiāng, tèsè.

    2. "Bǐ" sentence.

    3. Reduplications of numeral ("yí gè gè", "yí gè yí gè").

    4. Expressions of approximate number ("qī bā gè", "liǎng sān jīn").

    5. Construction "Yòu……yòu……".

    6. Mark of result complement "zhù": "Jìzhù", "tíngzhù", "zhànzhù".

    7. Oral language task: Design a dialogue between a seller and a customer in market.

    8. Chinese character exercise.

Chapter 29   Reporting a Case in Police Station

    1. Target words: Diàndòngchē, diū, jǐngchájú, bàoàn, jiēdài, jiānkòng, shèxiàngtóu, tíngfàng, lùbiān, suǒ, xiǎotōu, liúxià, liánxì fāngshì, cházhǎo, tōngzhī, cūxīn.

    2. "Bǎ" sentence.

    3. Construction: "Yī……jiù……".

    4. Temporal words: "Yǐqián", "yǐhòu".

    5. Construction "Yìdiǎnr yě bù……".

    6. Usage of durative aspect "zhe".

    7. Oral language task: Design a dialogue between a police and a victim.

    8. Chinese character exercise.

Chapter 30   Reservation

    1. Target words: Fùmǔ, lǚxíng, kànwàng, jiǔdiàn, fāngbiàn, yùdìng, qiántái, kōngfáng, biāozhǔnjiān, zhùsù, fángfèi, dǎzhé, bǎoliú, tuìdìng, dàodá, zhèngjiàn, fángkǎ, xìnyòngkǎ.

    2. Adjective reduplication: AA + de (dàdàde), AABB (gāngānjìngjìng).

    3. Construction "yuèláiyuè".

    4. Construction "Gāi……le".

    5. Mark of complement of result "dào": "Dìngdào", "huídào", "zhǎodào".

    6. Oral language task: Reserve a playground from university for the sake of the cricket competetion and training.

7. Chinese character exercise.

Chapter 31　Seeing a Doctor

1. Target words: Guòmǎlù, zhuàng, bèi, qíxíng, hónglǜdēng, liúxuè, pò, gǎnjǐn, shàngyào, bāozā, shāngkǒu, dǎzhēn, xiāoyán, búyàojǐn, yùfáng, gǎnrǎn, kǒufúyào.

2. "Bèi" sentence.

3. Usage of compound directional complement.

4. Construction "Verb + qǐlái".

5. Prepositions: "Wǎng", "duì".

6. Oral language task: Retell the text.

7. Composition: Seeing a doctor.

Chapter 32　I Have a Date with China

1. Target words: Yuēhuì, yuánfèn, búdàn, érqiě, xīyǐn, kǎolù, zhīchí, dàolǐ, xuǎnzé, rùxué, hàoqí, wénhuà, fēnwéi, jīdòng, rènzhēn, jìnbù, qíshí, gēn······yǒuguān.

2. Construction "Búdàn······, érqiě······".

3. Existential sentences: Place + verb + zhe + measure word + noun.

4. Construction "Verb + lái + verb + qù".

5. Usage of the adverb: "Qíshí" (actually).

6. Constructions: "Yì tiān bǐ yì tiān······", "Yì nián bǐ yì nián······".

7. Oral language task: Impression on the city where you study now.

8. Chinese character exercise.

Chapter 33　Taking a Taxi for the First Time

1. Target words: Dǎdi, fēijīchǎng, jiē, dǔchē, wǎndiǎn, cōngmáng, bēibāo, wàngjì, chēpáihào, jiāojí, lǐngqǔ, xìnghǎo, jiāohuí, wánhǎo, guǒrán, jīnglì, yìnxiàng, shànliáng, yǒuhǎo.

2. "Ràng"/"jiào" sentence.

3. Usage of adverb: "Xìnghǎo".

4. Usage of the structural particle: "De" (jiāojí de děngdài).

5. Decimal number, fractional number and percentage.

6. Construction "Xiàng······yíyàng".

7. Oral language task: Design a dialogue between a passenger and a taxi driver.

8. Composition: One-day city tour.

Chapter 34　Summer Holidays

1. Target words: Kǒuyǔ, jìnbù, qǐng, fǔdǎo, lǎoshī, shǔjià, lǚxíngtuán, tígāo, liǎojiě, lìshǐ, wénhuà, liànxí, dǎoyóu, chúle······yǐwài, nánguài, yìjǔliǎngdé, chéngyǔ;

2. Construction "Nǎr ā".

3. constructions: "Chúle······yǐwài, hái······"; "Chúle······yǐwài, dōu······".

4. Sentences with an adjectival predicate;

5. Modal adverb "de" (Hànyǔ shuō de hěn liúlì).

6. Oral language task: Introduce the ways to improve Chinese speaking.

7. Chinese character exercise.

Chapter 35　Farewell Party

1. Target words: Gàobié, bìyè, xíngli, shōushi, dǎbāo, chéngzuò, hángbān, wàng, hǎoxiàng, yǒukōng, fēijīchǎng, guānzhào, bāngzhù, gǎnjī, sòngxíng, huānyíng, yílùpíng'ān.

2. Adverb: "Hǎoxiàng" (a usage of tentative judgment).

3. Usage of adverb "cái": Small amount on the speaker's opinion.

4. Construction "Yì fāngmiàn······, lìng yì fāngmiàn······".

5. Construction "Zhǐyào······jiù······".

6. Construction "Bǎ······verb chéng······".

7. Oral language task: Retell the text.

8. Composition: We are friends.

Chapter 36　Three Days to See

1. Target words: Jiànkāng, zhòngyào, shùlín, yǒuyìsi, yǎnjīng, shīmíng, ěrduo, shīcōng, yīkào, chùjué, chùmō, dàzìrán, xiānhuā, fāngxiāng, huāwén, lànghuā, zhēnxī, tǐhuì, qīnqiè, xìngfú, rèqíng.

2. Construction "A + hé/gēn + B + yíyàng······".

3. The negative expression of comparative construction: "A + méiyǒu + B ······".

4. Potential complement: Verb + de + dào (tīng de dào, kàn de dào).

5. Oral language task: Retell the text.

6. Chinese character exercise.

Chapter 37　Being Happy Is Actually Quite Easy

1. Target words: Cóngqián, gèzhǒnggèyàng, jiǎnféi, pàng, kāixīn, zhěngtǐ, shòubuliǎo, xīnkǔ, píng'ān, wēnróu, yízhènzi, zuìhǎo, mǎnzú, zhùfú, tóngnián.

2. Usage of adverb: "Zuìhǎo" (giving suggestion).

3. Construction: Yī + measure (noun) + Yī + measure (noun) + de + verb (a movement or an action is repeated in a one-by-one manner).

4. Usage of verbal reduplication.

5. Sentences with two connected actions: VP1 + VP2.

6. Oral language task: Retell the text.

7. Composition: A big day.

Chapter 38　Three E-mails

1. Target words: Diànzǐ yóujiàn, yóuxiāng, chīsù, sùcài, zuòfǎ, qiézi, huīfù, xuèyā, jiéhūn, lǎobǎn, chǎojià, shēngqì, dānxīn, diànnǎo, huífù, fāsòng, shōudào, kěndìng, shèjì.

2. Construction: "Bùjǐn······, érqiě······".

3. Usage of separable words ("Jié le hūn", "chǎo guo jià").

4. Usage of conjunction: "Búguò".

5. Potential complement: Verb + de + liǎo; verb + bù + liǎo.

6. Preposition "Wèile······" (purpose).

7. Oral language task: Retell the text.

8. Composition: Write a letter to say thanks to your classmate, and reply to them if you received a letter of acknowledgement.

Chapter 39　Color and Character

1. Target words: Dàibiǎo, rèqíng, lèguān, chéngshí, xiǎngshòu, chángshì, qīngsōng, jījí, shuōmíng, nèixiàng, wàixiàng, mèngxiǎng, jiānqiáng, chénggōng, yìnxiàng, chéngrèn, chéngshú, niánlíng, dúlì, lěngjìng.

2. Constructions: "Cónglái dōu……"; "Cónglái dōu bù……".

3. Construction: Adjective + de + hěn ("kuài de hěn").

4. Construction "Zài yě méi/bù……".

5. Construction "Lián……yě/dōu……".

6. Construction discrimination: "Zài + location + VP" and "VP + zài + location".

7. Oral language task: Retell the text.

8. Composition: The ideal character.

Chapter 40　What Should I Do

1. Target words: shìyìng, kǔnǎo, shúxī, guānxì, lǐjiě, lǎoshi, rěnràng, jiāoliú, gōutōng, lìchǎng, huànwèi, sīkǎo, máodùn, lìrú, bìyào, fàngqì.

2. Verb used as a mark in existential sentence: "Yǒu".

3. Simple directional complement "lái" and "qù".

4. Construction "Zhǐyào……jiù……".

5. Construction "Máfán nín……".

6. Usage of adverb: "Yóuqí".

7. Chinese character exercise.

Chapter 41　Education of Love

1. Target words: Wǎnhuì, qìfēn, gāozhǎng, jǐmǎn, yíkè, jiāzhǎng, xīnqíng, yǎnjiǎng, qīnwěn, tèshū, xīnqíng, wēixiào, bùrú, rèliè, zhǎngshēng, jīdòng, yǎnlèi.

2. Construction discrimination: "Cónglái méi", Cónglái bù".

3. The compound directional complement with "Lái" and "qù": "shànglái/qù", "xiàlái/qù", "jìnlái/qù", "chūlái/qù", "huílái/qù", "guòlái/qù", "qǐlái".

4. Construction "Jì……yě/yòu……"(states exist simultaneously).

5. Construction "Bǎ + object + verb + directional complement".

6. Oral language task: Retell the text.

7. Chinese character exercise.

Chapter 42　Do As the Romans Do

1. Target words: Rùxiāngsuísú, jiànjiàn, chídào, nàozhōng, dǎzhāohu, wènhǎo, qíguài, línjū, duìhuà, kěndìng, sǎn, qīnqiè, shúrén, huídá, shìyìng, fēngsú.

2. Construction: Interrogative + yě/dōu……(anybody or anything is included).

3. Negative forms of "bǐ" sentence: A + méiyǒu + B + adjective; A + bù + bǐ/rú + B + adjective.

4. Construction "Wúlùn……yě/dōu……".

5. Rhetorical questions ("Zhème duō, nǐmen chī de wán ma? ").

6. Oral language task: Retell the text.

7. Chinese character exercise.

Chapter 43　Yu Gong Removed the Mountains

1. Target words: Yúgōng yíshān, dǎng, bùguǎn, fānshān, fāngbiàn, dàilǐng, sūnzi, zànchéng, tóngyì, niánjì, shítou, shāngliáng, bàntiān, wā, bāngmáng, shénxiān, jīngshén, gǎndòng, pài, yìlì.

2. Construction: "Jíshǐ……yě/dōu……"(emphasize the result or conclusion will not change under such a supposition).

3. Approximate number mark "lái"("shí lái gè rén").

4. Metaphor construction "Hǎoxiàng……sìde".

5. Construction "Zhǐyǒu……cái……".

6. Disscusion: What can we learn from Yugong's story?

7. Chinese character exercise.

Chapter 44　Low-carbon Life

1. Target words: Dītàn, shěng, jiéyuē, gōngjiāochē, jiénéngdēng, yòngdiànliàng, shǐyòng, shòumìng, diànqì, bá diànyuán, zìláishuǐ, píngzhuāngshuǐ, jiāohuā, shuǐgāng, diàntī, yícìxìng, tōngfēng, xiánshì, guǎn.

2. Usage of reduplication of the measure word: "Gègè dōu "(all without exception).

3. Construction: "A shì A, jiùshì……"(raise an opposing viewpoint).

4. The adverb of modal particle: "Dàodǐ"(emphasize the final outcome after a long process).

5. Construction: "Jǐn guǎn……, dànshì/kěshì……".

6. Oral language task: Retell the task.

7. Composition: Environment protection.

Chapter 45　The Ideal Career

1. Target words: Lǐxiǎng, zhíyè, guānjiàn, fāngmiàn, shōurù, huánjìng, guānxì, kànfǎ, niánqīng, jiànshi, jīnglì, jiātíng, wúsuǒwèi.

2. Usage of adverb "hǎozài", "xìngkuī".

3. Imperative adverb: "Qiānwàn".

4. Construciton: "Bùguǎn……dōu……. " (emphasize the result or conclusion will not change).

5. Conjunction "……zàishuō……. "(add an additional reason).

6. Oral language task: Talking about the ideal career.

7. Chinese character exercise.

Chapter 46　When the Day Comes

1. Target words: Chúfáng, nánchī, yǎo, cuì, fǎnyìng, zhēnde, zhàogù, guānxīn, péibàn, qìwèi, yáchǐ, xián, hòuhuǐ, jīhu.

2. Constructions: "Zhǐyào……, jiù…… "; "Jìrán……, jiù……".

3. Construction: Zěnme yě/dōu + verb + bù + result (emphasize there is no way to achieve the desired result).

4. Expressions of fractions and multiples.

5. Construction "Lián…… yě/dōu…… ".

6. Construction "Nǎpà…… yě/dōu…… ".

7. Language task: Retell the text.

8. Chinese character exercise.

Chapter 47　Set the Watch Forward by Three Minutes

1. Target words: Bō, mìshū, yōudiǎn, shǒushí, àixī, làngfèi, qǔdé, chénggōng, jiǔdiàn, zhǔnshí, jìsuàn, xūyào, tíqián, dāngshí, xiàbān, dǔchē, fàngqì, jiěshì, nándù, hǎochu.

2. Construction: Bǎ + object + verb phrase + numerals (a change happens to the objects as a result of an action or behavior).

3. Usage of the modal particle of rhetorical question: "Nándào".

4. Oral languge task: Ways to save time in daily life.

5. Chinese character exercise.

Chapter 48　Going to Berlin by Hitchhiking

1. Target words: Dāchē, zhāoshǒu, chuānyuè, xíngchéng, gōnglǐ, mùdì, jìngrán, niándǐ, shěbude, biànchē, lǚtú, shuōfú, qiānzhèngguān, jùjué, xiǎngxiàng, yōngbào, màncháng, yóu, xiàng.

2. Usage of the modal particle: "Jìngrán" (something happened beyond imagination or expectation).

3. Construction: Yī + verb/adjective, ……. (a result merges right after a very short action or feeling.).

4. Oral language task: Arrangement in gap year.

5. Chinese character exercise.

LANGUAGE PRACTICAL

1. To learn Chinese songs.

2. To watch Chinese movies.

3. To learn how to make Chinese foods.

4. City tour.

5. Chinese language and culture show.

6. Chinese text reading competition.

7. Chinese calligraphy learning.

8. Campus culture activities.

9. To celebrate the traditional Chinese festivals with Chinese friends.

10. To visit companies or farms.

ELEMENTARY CHINESE
医 学 汉 语

Chief Editors（主编）
Zong Shihai（宗世海） Jinan University（暨南大学）
Wang Xingyue（王星月） Sichuan University（四川大学）
Deng Shulan（邓淑兰） Sun Yat-sen University（中山大学）

Deputy Chief Editors（副主编）
Xu Fuping（徐富平） Jinan University（暨南大学）
Tong Xun（佟迅） Southeast University（东南大学）
Li Jing（李静） Dalian Medical University（大连医科大学）

Editors（编委）（按姓氏拼音排序）
Deng Shulan（邓淑兰） Sun Yat-sen University（中山大学）
Li Jing（李静） Dalian Medical University（大连医科大学）
Tong Xun（佟迅） Southeast University（东南大学）
Wang Xingyue（王星月） Sichuan University（四川大学）
Xu Fuping（徐富平） Jinan University（暨南大学）
Zhao Changying（赵长鹰） Jinan University（暨南大学）
Zong Shihai（宗世海） Jinan University（暨南大学）

Course Description

As a cross-disciplinary language course, Medical Chinese provides intermediate level learners with Chinese terms of medical diagnosis and treatment, and helps them to develop the language knowledge and skills applied in a hospital environment. The learners are taught terms with respect to case inquiry, symptom description, physical examinations, test results, diagnosis and analysis, treatments and precautions in the context of practical communication. This course will offer many opportunities to improve the learners'listening and speaking skills. Listening skills include understanding common dialogues and conversations with a variety of accents related to common activities in the hospital; Speaking skills include being able to take part in discussions or present a position on patients'case with clarity and continuity. Reading and writing skills on familiar medical topics are also required. Along with the above the course will attach importance to developing learners'cross-cultural awareness.

The course is aimed at helping the learners to establish the comprehensive language competence with a goal to pursue internship. By studying this course, the learners will be able to undertake medical internship training smoothly, and work efficiently with their Chinese workmates in the hospital.

Objectives

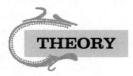

THEORY

At the end of the course, the MBBS students shall be able to:

1. Know the name of the major departments in hospital.
2. Know the terms about human body and organs.
3. Know the disease name encountered in the different departments of hospital.
4. Know the professional terms about disease symptoms, examinations, test results, diagnosis and treatments.
5. Know the drugs'name used for the treatment of different diseases.
6. Know the basic structure and content about writing a case record.
7. Master over 1,800 general words and medical terms high frequently used in medical affairs.

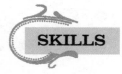

SKILLS

At the end of the course, the student should be able to:

1. Understand common conversations related to daily medical works.
2. Produce clear and natural pronunciation to deal with patients'affairs in a hospital.
3. Take part in discussions or present a position on patients'case.
4. Understand the texts of descriptive material such as prescriptions, drug labels.
5. Write out patient's case record independently.
6. Learn the new expressions used in hospital as needed.

Teaching and Learning Methods

Classroom teaching: A communicative approach will be used throughout the course with an emphasis on daily communieation. Some audio/video-based listening exercise will take place in the class. Students will be required to obtain a textbook to support their studies.

Practical: Students will be encouraged to catch every chance to do language practical. Some activities will be held such as hospital visit, role-play performance and case record writing competition.

Recommended Textbooks

陈丽萍，张哲，孙景辉. 2009. 实用医学汉语（临床篇，妇儿科）［M］. 北京：外语教学与研究出版社.

Chen Liping, Zhang Zhe, Sun Jinghui. 2009. Practical Medical Chinese (Clinical, Gynecology, Obstetrics & Neonatal Dept.)[M]. Beijing: Foreign Language Teaching and Research Press.

陈孝平，汪建平. 2014. 外科学［M］. 北京：人民卫生出版社.

Chen Xiaoping, Wang Jianping. 2014. Surgery [M]. Beijing: People's Medical Publishing House.

葛均波，徐永健. 2013. 内科学［M］. 北京：人民卫生出版社.

Ge Junbo, Xu Yongjian. 2013. Internal Medicine [M]. Beijing: People's Medical Publishing House.

莫秀英. 2007. 医学汉语（实习篇Ⅰ、Ⅱ、Ⅲ）［M］. 北京：北京大学出版社.

Mo Xiuying. 2007. Medical Chinese (Vol.1, Vol. 2 & Vol. 3)[M]. Beijing: Beijing University Press.

万学红，卢雪峰. 2013. 诊断学［M］. 北京：人民卫生出版社.

Wan Xuehong, Lu Xuefeng. 2013. Diagnostics [M]. Beijing: People's Medical Publishing House.

王卫平. 2013. 儿科学［M］. 北京：人民卫生出版社.

Wang Weiping. 2013. Pediatrics [M]. Beijing: People's Medical Publishing House.

王星月，易江，张哲. 2009. 实用医学汉语（临床篇，外科）［M］. 北京：外语教学与研究出版社.

Wang Xingyue, Yi Jiang, Zhang Zhe. 2009. Practical Medical Chinese (Clinical,Surgery) [M]. Beijing: Foreign Language Teaching and Research Press.

谢幸，苟文丽. 2013. 妇产科学［M］. 北京：人民卫生出版社.

Xie Xing, Gou Wenli. 2013. Obstetrics and Gynecology [M]. Beijing: People's Medical Publishing House.

张忠双，李聪，张哲. 2010. 实用医学汉语（临床篇，内科）［M］. 北京：外语教学与研究出版社.

Zhang Zhongshuang, Li Cong, Zhang Zhe. 2010. Practical Medical Chinese (Clinical, Internal Medicine) [M]. Beijing: Foreign Language Teaching and Research Press.

Schedule Table

Chapter	Contents	Hours	Chapter	Contents	Hours
Part one	Knowledge and skills	4	4	Respiratory medicine 2: Pneumonia	6
1	Main departments and sections in hospital	2	5	Respiratory medicine 3: Asthma	6
2	Body parts and organs	2	6	Respiratory medicine 4: Bronchiectasis	6
Part two	Case study	264		Review	2
3	Respiratory medicine 1: Influenza	6	7	Department of gastroenterology 1: Gastroenteritis	6

Continued

Chapter	Contents	Hours	Chapter	Contents	Hours
8	Department of gastroenterology 2: Acute pancreatitis	6	27	Orthopedics 2: Lumbar disc herniation	6
9	Department of gastroenterology 3: Gall stone	6	28	Urologic surgery: Acute cystitis	6
10	Department of gastroenterology 4: Gastric ulcer	6	29	Thoracic surgery: Esophageal cancer	6
	Review	2	30	Burns surgery: Burn injury	6
11	Cardiology department: Coronary artery disease	6		Review	2
12	Neurology department: Apoplexy	6	31	Obstetrics and Gynecology 1: Pelvic inflammatory disease	6
13	Hematology department: Leukemia	6	32	Obstetrics and Gynecology 2: Menstrual disorder	6
14	Nephrology department: Chronic nephritis	6	33	Obstetrics and Gynecology 3: Pregnancy and labor	6
15	Hematology and Rheumatology: Rheumatoid arthritis	6	34	Obstetrics and Gynecology 4: Ectopic pregnancy	6
	Review	2	35	Obstetrics and Gynecology 5: Postpartum complications	6
16	Endocrinology and Metabolism 1: Hyper-thyroidism	6	36	Obstetrics and Gynecology 6: Uterine tumor	6
17	Endocrinology and Metabolism 2: Diabetes mellitus	6		Review	2
18	Department of infectious disease: Chronic hepatitis	6	37	Pediatrics 1: Jaundice	6
19	Neurology 1: Epilepsy	6	38	Pediatrics 2: Viral myocarditis	6
20	Cardiothoracic surgery: Malignant tumor	6	39	Pediatrics 3: Nutritional diseases	6
	Review	2	40	Pediatrics 4: Pertussis	6
21	General surgery 1: Acute appendicitis	6		Review	2
22	General surgery 2: Hernia	6	41	E.N.T department: Tympanitis	6
23	Cardiac surgery: Congenital heart disease	6	42	Department of dermatology: Exanthematous diseases	6
24	Hepatobiliary surgery 2: Rupture of spleen	6	43	Department of ophthalmology: Senile cataract	6
25	Hepatobiliary surgery 3: Hepatic carcinoma	6		Review	2
	Review	2	Part three	Language practical	20
26	Orthopedics 1: Humerus fracture	6		Total	288

Course Contents

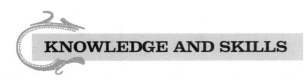

KNOWLEDGE AND SKILLS

Chapter 1　Main Departments and Sections in Hospital

The core target words include the followings:

1. Zhùyuànbù, Ménzhěnbù.

2. Nèikē: Hūxī nèikē, Xiāohuà nèikē, Xīnxuèguǎn nèikē, Xuèyèkē, Shènnèikē, Zhǒngliú nèikē, Nèifēnmìkē.

3. Wàikē: Pǔwàikē, Gāndǎn wàikē, Xīnxiōng wàikē, Mìniào wàikē, Jiǎoxíng wàikē, Shénjīng wàikē, Shāoshāng zhěngxíng wàikē.

4. Fùkē, Chǎnkē.

5. Érkē.

6. Jízhěnkē.

7. Chuánrǎnkē, ěrbíhóukē, Yǎnkē, Pífūkē, Jīngshén xīnlǐkē.

8. Guāncháshì, Shǒushùshì, Zhòngzhèng jiānhùshì, Huàyànshì, Fàngshèkē, Bìng'ànshì.

9. Dǎozhěntái, Guàhàochù, Shōufèichù, Yàofáng, Hùshizhàn.

10. Qítā: Zhǐdǎo lǎoshī, zhǔzhì yīshēng, shíxíshēng, hùshi, hùshizhǎng.

Chapter 2　Body Parts and Organs

The core target words include the followings:

1. Tóubù: Nǎo, ébù, tóufa, méimao, yǎnjīng, bí, ěr, liǎn, chún, yáchǐ, shé, xiàhé.

2. Jǐngbù: Yān, hóu, jiǎzhuàngxiàn.

3. Jiānbèibù.

4. Xiōngbù: Xīnzàng, fèi, qìguǎn, zhīqìguǎn, lèigǔ.

5. Fùbù: Gān, pí, wèi, shèn, dǎn, yíxiàn, xiǎocháng (shí'èrzhǐcháng , kōngcháng, huícháng), dàcháng (mángcháng, lánwěi, jiécháng, zhícháng).

6. Túnbù.

7. Shàngzhī: Shàngbì, zhǒu, qiánbì, shǒuwàn, shǒuzhǎng, shǒuzhǐ, zhǐjia.

8. Xiàzhī: Dàtuǐ, xīgài, xiǎotuǐ, jiǎohuái, jiǎo, jiǎozhǐ.

9. Qítā: Gǔ, jīròu, guānjié, shénjīng, xuèguǎn, jìngmài, dòngmài, xuèyè, gǔsuǐ.

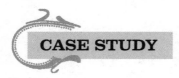

CASE STUDY

Chapter 3　Influenza

1. Core target words: Liúgǎn, zhòngzhèng, bìngdú, gǎnrǎn, bìngfāzhèng, yǐnqǐ, gāorè, fálì, hūxīdào, liúbítì, bísè, jiāzhòng, sǔnhài, chōuxuè, tuìrèyào, niào, jiǎnxiào, guānchá, hùlǐ, chūyuàn.

2. Case in the text: A patient diagnosed as severe influenza is transferred to the Respiratory Medicine.

(1) Zhèngzhuàng hé tǐzhēng: Gāorè, quánshēn téngtòng, fálì.

(2) Tǐgé jiǎnchá: Shìzhěn, chùzhěn.

(3) Fǔzhù jiǎnchá: Xuèchángguī, xuèyè shēnghuà jiǎnchá, xiōngpiàn.

(4) Zhěnduàn jiéguǒ: Zhòngdù liúgǎn.

(5) Zhìliáo fāng'àn: Yàowù zhìliáo (kàngbìngdú).

(6) Qítā: Bìngren xūyào gélí, yào wòchuáng xiūxi, fángjiān yào tōngfēng.

3. Oral language task: Retell the text.

4. Case record writing.

Chapter 4　Pneumonia

1. Core target words: Fèiyán, bìnglì(case record), zhǔsù, zhèngzhuàng, tǐzhēng, tán, gānké, tīngzhěn, hūqì, xīqì, shīluóyīn, X guāngpiàn, jiǎnchá jiéguǒ, yīnyǐng, zhěnduàn, yánzhòng, fùzé, yīzhǔ.

2. Case in the text: A new patient comes to the respiratory medicine department with a high fever and suffers from a serious cough.

(1) Shíshíshēng xiàng, bìngren zuò zìwǒ jièshào.

(2) Bìngren de zhǔsù, jìwǎng bìngshǐ.

(3) Zhèngzhuàng hé tǐzhēng: Fārè, késou, duō tán, xiōngmèn, xiōngkǒu téng.

(4) Tǐgé jiǎnchá: Fèibù tīngzhěn.

(5) Fǔzhù jiǎnchá: Xuèchángguī, xiōngpiàn, CT jiǎnchá.

(6) Zhěnduàn jiéguǒ: Fèiyán.

(7) Zhìliáo fāng'àn: Yàowù zhìliáo (Kàngshēngsù).

3. Oral language task: Role-play.

4. Best wishes to the patients: Zhù nǐ zǎorì kāngfù! Nǐ yídìng huì hǎoqǐlái de! Jiāyóu!

Chapter 5　Asthma

1. Core target words: Xiàochuǎn, fāzuò, étóu, màolěnghàn, zuǐchún, shǒuzhǐ, fāgàn, píngwò, xiàomíngyīn, huīfù, nánshòu, jìxù, zhìliáo fāng'àn, yàowù zhìliáo, qìwùjì, jiànyì.

2. Case in the text: The young man who suffers from asthma is sent to the hospital.

(1) Bìngren de zhǔsù, jìwǎng bìngshǐ, xiànbìngshǐ.

(2) Zhèngzhuàng hé tǐzhēng: Hūxī jícù, màolěnghàn, chúnzhǐ fāgàn, bù néng píngwò.

(3) Tǐgé jiǎnchá: Fèibù tīngzhěn.

(4) Fǔzhù jiǎnchá: Xuèchángguī, tán jiǎncè, X shèxiàn jiǎnchá.

(5) Zhěnduàn jiéguǒ: Xiàochuǎn.

(6) Zhìliáo fāng'àn: Yàowù zhìliáo (Kàngguòmǐn).

(7) Qítā: Bìngren yào zhùyì yùfáng gǎnmào, fángzhǐ yānwù, huāfěn guòmǐn.

3. Oral language task: Retell the text.

4. Case record writing.

Chapter 6   Bronchiectasis

1. Core target words: Zhīqìguǎn, kuòzhāng, bìnglì(case), jiāshǔ, jìlù, fùfā, hūxīdào, gǎnrǎn, bìngshǐ, kǎxiě, diǎnxíng, zànshí, xiāoshī, chǔzhuàngzhǐ, zhīqìguǎn zàoyǐng, quèzhěn, guòmǐn.

2. Case in the text: The chief doctor introduces the new patient's condition to interns in Respiratory Medicine, and then they go to see the patient.

(1) Zhèngzhuàng hé tǐzhēng: Késou, duō tán, kǎxiě, chǔzhuàngzhǐ.

(2) Tǐgé jiǎnchá: Xiōngbù tīngzhěn.

(3) Fǔzhù jiǎnchá: Fèigōngnéng jiǎnchá, X shèxiàn jiǎnchá, zhī qìguǎn zàoyǐng.

(4) Zhěnduàn jiéguǒ: Zhīqìguǎn kuòzhāng.

(5) Zhìliáo fāng'àn: Yàowù zhìliáo.

(6) Qítā: Bìngren yào zhùyì bìmiǎn yānwù, huīchén, huāfěn yǐnqǐ de guòmǐn.

3. Oral language task: Design a dialogue between a doctor and a patient.

4. Extension writing task: The patient's revisit to hospital one month later.

Chapter 7   Gastroenteritis

1. Core target words: Chángwèiyán, jíxìng, xiāohuà, quánshēn wúlì, dùzi, fùxiè, shuǐyàngbiàn, ěxin, ǒutù, ànyā, dàbiàn chángguī, huàyàndān, yìcháng, shūyè, xiāoyán, hǎozhuǎn, yātòng.

2. Case in the text: The patient who has been suffered from serious abdominal pain is transferred to In-patient department of Gastroenterology from Emergency.

(1) Bìngren de zhǔsù.

(2) Zhèngzhuàng hé tǐzhēng: Ěxīn, ǒutù, dùzi téng, fùxiè, quánshēn wúlì.

(3) Tǐgé jiǎnchá: Chùzhěn.

(4) Fǔzhù jiǎnchá: Xuèchángguī, dàbiàn chángguī.

(5) Zhěnduàn jiéguǒ: Shíyòng guòliàng hǎixiān yǐnqǐ de jíxìng chángwèiyán.

(6) Zhìliáo fāng'àn: Yàowù zhìliáo.

3. Oral language task: Role-play.

4. Case record writing.

Chapter 8   Acute Pancreatitis

1. Core target words: Yíxiànyán, yíxiàn, línchuáng biǎoxiàn, zhǒngdà, pífū, zǐsèbān, fàngshè, yǐnqǐ, xuèqīng diànfěnméi, shēnggāo, gēnjù, chángqī, bàoyǐn bàoshí, báijiǔ.

2. Case in the text: A patient is sent to the hospital because of serious abdominal pain.

(1) Bìngren de zhǔsù, jìwǎng bìngshǐ, xiànbìngshǐ.

(2) Zhèngzhuàng hé tǐzhēng: Ěxīn, ǒutù, fùbù zhàngtòng.

(3) Tǐgé jiǎnchá: Chùzhěn.

(4) Fǔzhù jiǎnchá: Xuèchángguī, niàochángguī, CT jiǎnchá.

(5) Zhěnduàn jiéguǒ: Jíxìng yíxiànyán.

(6) Zhìliáo fāng'àn: Yàowù zhìliáo.

(7) Yīzhǔ: Jìnshí wǔ tiān.

(8) Qítā: Chūyuàn hòu, bìngren yào zhùyì shǎo chī gāo zhīfáng shípǐn.

3. Extension writing task: The patient's revisit to hospital two months later.

Chapter 9　Gall Stone

1. Core target words: Dǎnshízhèng, dǎnnángyán, shàngfùbù, yǐntòng, jùtòng, mòfēishìzhēng, xiǎobiàn, yángxìng, yīnxìng, B chāo, jiéshí, chūzhěn, kàngshēngsù, jiějìngyào, guānchá, yóunì.

2. Case in the text: In in-patient department of Gastroenterology, a patient is telling the doctor that he has been suffered from abdominal pain for a long time.

(1) Zhèngzhuàng hé tǐzhēng: fārè, fùbù jùtòng, xiǎobiàn shēnhuángsè, dǎnnáng zhǒngdà, Mòfēishìzhēng yángxìng.

(2) Tǐgé jiǎnchá: Chùzhěn, kòuzhěn.

(3) Fǔzhù jiǎnchá: B chāo, fùbù CT jiǎnchá.

(4) Zhěnduàn jiéguǒ: Dǎnnángyán, dǎnjiéshí.

(5) Zhìliáo fāng'àn: Yàowù zhìliáo.

(6) Qítā: Bìngren yào zhùyì shǎo chī yóunì de shíwù.

3. Oral language task: Retell the text.

4. Case record writing.

Chapter 10　Gastric Ulcer

1. Core target words: Wèikuìyáng, huànbìng, wèichūxuè, wèichuānkǒng, fùmóyán, wēixiǎn, qiánxuè, shīxuè, bànyǒu, wèijìng, bànlǐ, zhuǎnkē, shǒuxù, jiěshì, tóngyì, zhǔfù.

2. Case in the text: The patient who had been diagnosed as gastric hemorrhage in Emergency is transferred to In-patient department now.

(1) Bìngren de zhǔsù, jìwǎng bìngshǐ.

(2) Zhèngzhuàng hé tǐzhēng: Fùbù téngtòng, tùxiě.

(3) Gè xiàng jiǎnchá: Dàbiàn chángguī, xuèchángguī, wèijìng jiǎnchá.

(4) Zhěnduàn jiéguǒ: Wèikuìyáng yǐnqǐ de wèichūxuè.

(5) Zhìliáo fāng'àn: Yàowù zhìliáo, shǒushù zhìliáo.

(6) Yīzhǔ: Jìnshí sān tiān.

3. Case record writing.

Chapter 11　Coronary Artery Disease

1. Core target words: Guānxīnbìng, xīnjiǎotòng, xīnjī gěngsè, tóuyūn, màibó, xuèyā, háomǐ gǒngzhù(mmHg), bìnglǐxìng, záyīn, chūzhěn, fùzhàng, fǎntiàotòng, míngxiǎn, huáiyí, xīndiàntú, xià jiélùn.

2. Case in the text: An old man who has slipped into a cardiogenic coma is sent to

the hospital.

(1) Bìngren de zhǔsù, jìwǎng bìngshǐ, xiànbìngshǐ.

(2) Zhèngzhuàng hé tǐzhēng: Xiōngkǒu téng, tóuyūn, duōhàn, xīnjì (palpitation).

(3) Tǐgé jiǎnchá: Tīngzhěn.

(4) Fǔzhù jiǎnchá: Xuèchángguī, guānzhuàng dòngmài zàoyǐng, xīndiàntú.

(5) Zhěnduàn jiéguǒ: Xīnjī gěngsè.

(6) Zhìliáo fāng'àn: Yàowù zhìliáo.

(7) Qítā: Bìngren yào zhùyì ànshí chīyào, yào bǎochí qíngxù wěndìng, bù néng tài jīdòng.

3. Extension writing task: The patient's revisit to hospital one month later.

Chapter 12　Apoplexy

1. Core target words: Nǎozhòngfēng, éyè, dànǎo xuèzhǒng, nǎochūxuè, yāpò, shénjīng, tóutòng, hūnmí, tānhuàn, niàoshījìn, xīnlǜ, bìngqíng, wěndìng, chūyuàn, bǎonuǎn, jiàngyāyào, qíngxù, jiùhùchē.

2. Case in the text: A patient is sent to the hospital because of deep coma.

(1) Bìngren de zhǔsù, jìwǎng bìngshǐ.

(2) Zhèngzhuàng hé tǐzhēng: Tóutòng, ǒutù, zhītǐ yìcháng, niào shījìn.

(3) Fǔzhù jiǎnchá: Xuèchángguī, nǎobù CT jiǎnchá, nǎobù hécígòngzhèn (MRI).

(4) Zhěnduàn jiéguǒ: Nǎochūxuè.

(5) Zhìliáo fāng'àn: Yàowù zhìliáo.

(6) Qítā: Chūyuàn hòu, bìngren yào zhùyì shǎo chī gāo dànbái, gāo zhīfáng, gāo rèliàng de shípǐn.

3. Oral language task: Design a dialogue between a chief doctor and an intern.

4. Case record writing.

Chapter 13　Leukemia

1. Core target words: Báixuèbìng, xuèyèbìng, báixìbāo, hóngxìbāo, xuèhóng dànbái, xuèxiǎobǎn, pínxuè, gǔsuǐ túpiàn, línbāxìbāo, lèixíng, yízhí, xiàoguǒ, huàliáo, liáochéng, ānbiànxīlín, bìngdúzuò, gǎnrǎn, zhàogù, yǒuxìnxīn.

2. Case in the text: The hematology department accepted a young patient today.

(1) Bìngren de zhǔsù, jìwǎng bìngshǐ, xiànbìngshǐ.

(2) Zhèngzhuàng hé tǐzhēng: Liǎnsè cāngbái, quánshēn wúlì, tóuyūn, fārè, késou, pínxuè.

(3) Fǔzhù jiǎnchá: Xuèchángguī, gǔsuǐ túpiàn jiǎnchá.

(4) Zhěnduàn jiéguǒ: Jíxìng fēi línbāxìbāo báixuèbìng.

(5) Zhìliáo fāng'àn: Yàowù zhìliáo.

(6) Qítā: Yīshēng ānwèi bìngren, gǔlì tā pèihé yīyuàn de zhìliáo.

3. Oral language task: Retell the text.

4. Extension writing task: The patient's revisit to hospital two months later.

Chapter 14　Chronic Nephritis

1. Core target words: Shènyán, shènxiǎoqiú, shènbìngzōnghézhēng, fúzhǒng,

yǎnjiǎn, niàoliàng, pàomò, shìzhěn, wéichí, shēnghuà, gāngōngnéng, fálì, dìngliàng, kǒufú, qiángdísōng, gānluóyīn, xiàjiàng, xiāoshī.

2. Case in the text: A lady is admitted into the hospital for general edema.

(1) Bìngren de zhǔsù, jìwǎng bìngshǐ.

(2) Zhèngzhuàng hé tǐzhēng: Fúzhǒng, fálì, méi jīngshen, yāosuān, niàoliàng jiǎnshǎo, ěxīn, ǒutù, méiyǒu shíyù.

(3) Fǔzhù jiǎnchá: Niàochángguī, xuèchángguī, shèngōngnéng jiǎnchá, B chāo.

(4) Zhěnduàn jiéguǒ: Mànxìng shènxiǎoqiú shènyán, shèn gōngnéng bùquán.

(5) Zhìliáo fāng'àn: Yàowù zhìliáo.

(6) Qítā: Bìngren yào zhùyì shǎo chī xīnlà de shíwù, xūyào shìliàng bǔchōng wéishēngsù.

3. Case record writing.

Chapter 15　Rheumatoid Arthritis

1. Core target words: Lèifēngshīxìng guānjiéyán, jiāngyìng, yáncháng, jiāzhòng, shuìmián, bùluòfēn, xuèchén, C fǎnyìng dànbái, kàng O, lèifēngshī yīnzǐ, gǔzhì shūsōng, fēizāitǐ, kàngyányào, tángpízhì jīsù, zhèntòng, wèiniánmó, fùzuòyòng, huámó, yánzhèng, chángqī, nàixīn.

2. Case in the text: The patient visits the out-patient department with arthragia of the hands and feet.

(1) Bìngren de zhǔsù, jìwǎng bìngshǐ, xiànbìngshǐ.

(2) Zhèngzhuàng hé tǐzhēng: Guānjié hóngzhǒng, téngtòng, shǒujiǎo jiāngyìng.

(3) Fǔzhù jiǎnchá: Zhǒu guānjié X shèxiàn jiǎnchá, xīguānjié X shèxiàn jiǎnchá, xuèchángguī, kàng O jiǎnchá, xuèchén jiǎnchá, C fǎnyìng dànbái jiǎnchá.

(4) Zhěnduàn jiéguǒ: Lèifēngshīxìng guānjiéyán.

(5) Zhìliáo fāng'àn: Yàowù zhìliáo.

3. Oral language task: Retell the case.

4. Case record writing.

Chapter 16　Hyperthyroidism

1. Core target words: Jiǎkàng, nèifēnmì, yǎnqiú, tūchū, shīmián, xīnjì, xiōngmèn, tǐzhòng xiàjiàng, wèikǒu, shǒudǒu, dàohàn, jiǎnqīng, jiǎzhuàngxiàn, diǎn, jiǎkàngpíng, tābāzuò, xīndé'ān.

2. Case in the text: The patient has been suffered from hyperthyroidism for three years. She feels worse when she stopped taking pills.

(1) Bìngren de zhǔsù, jìwǎng bìngshǐ, xiànbìngshǐ.

(2) Zhèngzhuàng hé tǐzhēng: Yǎnqiú tūchū, shīmián, xīnjì, xiōngmèn, tǐzhòng xiàjiàng, méiyǒu wèikǒu, shǒudǒu, dàohàn.

(3) Fǔzhù jiǎnchá: Gāngōngnéng jiǎnchá, jiǎzhuàngxiàn gōngnéng jiǎnchá.

(4) Zhěnduàn jiéguǒ: Jiǎkàng.

(5) Zhìliáo fāng'àn: Yàowù zhìliáo.

(6) Qítā: Bìngren yào zhùyì shǎo chī hán diǎn de shíwù.

3. Oral language task: Design a dialogue between a doctor and a patient.

Chapter 17　Diabetes Mellitus

1. Core target words: Tángniàobìng, dīxuètáng, pútáotáng, jìngmài, zhùshè, jìliàng, yōujiàngtáng, jiàngtángyào, fǎnyìng, tànshuǐ huàhéwù, bǔchōng, qīngdù, qiàdàng, xiédài, xīnhuāng, kòngzhì.

2. Case in the text: A man is sent to hospital because of the coma of hypoglycemia.

(1) Bìngren de zhǔsù.

(2) Zhèngzhuàng hé tǐzhēng: Duōyǐn, duōniào, duōshí, pífá wúlì, xiāoshòu, fúzhǒng, dīxuètáng.

(3) Fǔzhù jiǎnchá: Kōngfù xuètáng jiǎnchá, pútáotáng nàiliàng jiǎncè, yídǎo gōngnéng jiǎnchá.

(4) Zhěnduàn jiéguǒ: Qīngdù Ⅱ xíng tángniàobìng.

(5) Zhìliáo fāng'àn: Yàowù zhìliáo, shíliáo, yùndòng liáofǎ.

3. Extension writing task: The patient's revisit to hospital two months later.

Chapter 18　Chronic Hepatitis

1. Core target words: Mànxìng gānyán, shíyù búzhèn, yǐntòng, yǐgān, gāngōngnéng, dàsānyáng, xiǎosānyáng, kàngyuán, kàngtǐ, biǎomiàn, héxīn, yīnxìng, yángxìng, dǎnhóngsù, liǎngduìbàn, zhōngdù, kàng bìngdú, kàng xiānwéihuà, zhǐbiāo, bìngdú xiédàizhě, chuánrǎn.

2. Case in the text: A patient who had been diagnosed as hepatitis in Out-patient department is transferred to the In-patient department of infectious disease.

(1) Bìngren de zhǔsù, jìwǎng bìngshǐ, xiànbìngshǐ.

(2) Zhèngzhuàng hé tǐzhēng: Fálì, shíyù búzhèn, ěxīn, fùzhàng, gānqū téngtòng.

(3) Fǔzhù jiǎnchá: Xuèchángguī, gāngōngnéng jiǎnchá, yǐgān jiǎncè.

(4) Zhěnduàn jiéguǒ: Mànxìng yǐ xíng gānyán.

(5) Zhìliáo fāng'àn: Yàowù zhìliáo (kàng bìngdú, kàng xiānwéihuà).

3. Oral language task: Retell the text.

4. Extension writing task: The patient's revisit to hospital three months later.

Chapter 19　Epilepsy

1. Core target words: Diānxián, chōuchù, tóngkǒng, báimò, fēnmì, zhìxī, qiǎngjiù, hùlǐ, hécígòngzhèn, shìjué, tīngjué, yìyùzhèng, jīngshén fēnliè, kǎmǎxīpíng, bǐngwùsuānnà, yàoxiào.

2. Case in the text: The patient's mother is introducing her son's case history in Neurosurgery.

(1) Bìngren de zhǔsù, jìwǎng bìngshǐ, xiànbìngshǐ.

(2) Zhèngzhuàng hé tǐzhēng: Zhītǐ chōuchù, tóngkǒng kuòzhāng, kǒu tù báimò.

(3) Fǔzhù jiǎnchá: Nǎobù CT jiǎnchá, nǎobù hécígòngzhèn (MRI).

(4) Zhěnduàn jiéguǒ: Diānxián.

(5) Zhìliáo fāng'àn: Yàowù zhìliáo, bìyào shí shǒushù zhìliáo.

(6) Qítā: Yīshēng gàojiè bìngren bù néng chénmíyú wǎngluò yóuxì, yào ànshí chīyào.

3. Case record writing.

Chapter 20　Malignant Tumor

1. Core target words: Fèi'ái, xiàn'ái, èxìng zhǒngliú, liángxìng zhǒngliú, wǎnqī, gǔzhuǎnyí, yuánfā bìngzào, zhuǎnyí bìngzào, xiōngzhuī, jiānjiǎgǔ, jiēduàn, fàngshè zhìliáo, fàngshèxiàn, shāsǐ, jìnyíbù.

2. Case in the text: An intern is telling the doctor about the patient's pathological report and CT report of lung biopsy.

(1) Bìngren de zhǔsù, jìwǎng bìngshǐ, xiànbìngshǐ.

(2) Línchuáng biǎoxiàn: Gǔtou téngtòng, ǒutù, shìlì xiàjiàng, xiāoshòu.

(3) Fǔzhù jiǎnchá: Xiōngbù X shèxiàn jiǎnchá, fèibù huójiǎn, CT jiǎnchá.

(4) Zhěnduàn jiéguǒ: Fèiái Ⅳ qī; dì sì, dì wǔ xiōngzhuī hé zuǒ jiānjiǎgǔ chūxiàn gǔzhuǎnyí.

(5) Zhìliáo fāng'àn: Huàliáo, fàngshè zhìliáo.

(6) Qítā: Yīshēng ānwèi bìngren, gǔlì tā pèihé yīyuàn de zhìliáo.

3. Oral language task: Retell the case.

4. Case record writing.

Chapter 21　Acute Appendicitis

1. Core target words: Lánwěiyán, lánwěi chuānkǒng, mángcháng, dùqí, zhōuwéi, xīshōu, kòuzhěn, màishìdiǎn, chángmíngyīn, qiēchú shǒushù, bìmiǎn, bìngfāzhèng, fángzhǐ, fùmóyán.

2. Case in the text: General surgery admitted a patient with abdominal pain.

(1) Bìngren de zhǔsù, jìwǎng bìngshǐ, xiànbìngshǐ.

(2) Zhèngzhuàng hé tǐzhēng: Fùbù téngtòng, ěxīn, ǒutù, fārè, yòuxiàfù yātòng, fǎntiàotòng, fùjī jǐnzhāng.

(3) Tǐgé jiǎnchá: Kòuzhěn, chùzhěn.

(4) Fǔzhù jiǎnchá: Xuèchángguī, niàochángguī, xuèqīng diànfěnméi jiǎnchá, B chāo.

(5) Zhěnduàn jiéguǒ: Jíxìng lánwěiyán.

(6) Zhìliáo fāng'àn: Shǒushù zhìliáo.

3. Case record writing.

Chapter 22　Hernia

1. Core target words: Shànqì, zhǒngliú, zhǒngkuài, zhàngtòng, biànmì, fùgǔgōu, qiánlièxiàn, chǔlǐ, ànyā, guānchá, hé……yǒuguān, kuòdà, xiānwéi, jiǔcài, tōngchàng, wànyī.

2. Case in the text: The patient's wife is talking to the doctor about the patient's situation in Hepatobiliary surgery.

(1) Zhèngzhuàng hé tǐzhēng: Fùzhàng, biànmì.

(2) Tǐgé jiǎnchá: Chùzhěn.

(3) Fǔzhù jiǎnchá: B chāo, CT jiǎnchá.

(4) Zhěnduàn jiéguǒ: Fùgǔgōu shànqì.

(5) Zhìliáo fāng'àn: Shǒushù zhìliáo.

(6) Qítā: Yīshēng jiànyì bìngren duō chī cūxiānwéi shíwù, shǐ páibiàn tōngchàng.

3. Oral language task: Design a dialogue to retell the case.

Chapter 23   Congenital Heart Disease

1. Core target words: Xiāntiānxìng xīnzàngbìng, xīnshì jiàngé quēsǔn, qìchuǎn, xuèshuān, xīnzàng cǎichāo, zǔsè, shǒushù xiūbǔ, qǐbóqì, qiēkǒu, zhìyù, rùyuàn zhèngmíng, juédìng, tóngyì, xiéyìshū, qiānzì.

2. Case in the text: The young patient looks thinner than others at his age.

(1) Bìngren de zhǔsù.

(2) Línchuáng biǎoxiàn: Qìchuǎn, fálì, xūruò, duōhàn.

(3) Fǔzhù jiǎnchá: Chāoshēng xīndòngtú jiǎnchá, xīndiàntú, xīnzàng cǎichāo, xuèguǎn zàoyǐng jiǎnchá.

(4) Zhěnduàn jiéguǒ: Xiāntiānxìng xīnzàngbìng shìjiàngé quēsǔn.

(5) Zhìliáo fāng'àn: Shǒushù zhìliáo, xiūbǔ xīnshì jiàngé quēsǔn.

3. Extension writing task: The patient's revisit to hospital three months later.

Chapter 24   Rupture of Spleen

1. Core target words: Pípòliè, zhuàngdào, shuāidǎo, chíxùxìng téngtòng, jiànxiēxìng téngtòng, shēnhūxī, quánmiàn jiǎnchá, xiōngtòu, shòushāng, chuāncì, níngjié, lèigǔ, xiōngqiāng, jīxiě, xiūkè.

2. Case in the text: A young man fell off the table when he was repairing the lamp and is sent to the hospital.

(1) Línchuáng biǎoxiàn: Miànsè cāngbái, fùbù zhǒngzhàng téngtòng, yātòng, fǎntiàotòng, jījǐnzhāng.

(2) Fǔzhù jiǎnchá: B chāo, CT jiǎnchá, xuǎnzéxìng fùqiāng dòngmài zàoyǐng jiǎnchá.

(3) Zhěnduàn jiéguǒ: Lèigǔ gǔzhé, pípòliè, fùqiāng jīxiě.

(4) Zhìliáo fāng'àn: Jǐnjí shǒushù zhìliáo.

3. Oral language task: Design a dialogue to retell the case.

4. Case record writing.

Chapter 25   Hepatic Carcinoma

1. Core target words: Gānnángzhǒng, jùdà, niánmó, biǎomiàn, gānqū, zēnghòu, fùzá, mázuì, nángbì, nángyè, chōngxǐ, yǐnliúshù, fǔzhù, fēngxiǎn, fāng'àn, zhèngchángzhí, biǎomíng, zhuǎnyí.

2. Case in the text: The doctor and the interns are discussing the patient's condition in Hepatobiliary surgery.

(1) Bìngren de zhǔsù, jìwǎng bìngshǐ, xiànbìngshǐ.

(2) Zhèngzhuàng hé tǐzhēng: Gānqū zhàngtòng, ěxīn, ǒutù, dīshāo.

(3) Fǔzhù jiǎnchá: B chāo, CT jiǎnchá, fùqiāngjìng jiǎnchá.

(4) Zhěnduàn jiéguǒ: Gān'ái.

(5) Zhìliáo fāng'àn: Cǎiyòng fùqiāngjìng shǒushù zhìliáo.

3. Oral language task: Retell the text.

Chapter 26   Humerus Fracture

1. Core target words: Gǔzhé, gōnggǔ, bāndòng, zhǒngdà, yìcháng, liè, cuòwèi, zhíchǐ jiǎnyàn, fùwèi, gùdìng, shígāo, bēngdài, juǎn, kāngfù zhìliáo, ruǎnzǔzhī, jīròu,

rèndài, xiāozhǒng, gài.

2. Case in the text: A young boy fell down when playing basketball, and he feels great pain in the right arm.

(1) Línchuáng biǎoxiàn: Jiānbǎng zhǒngzhàng, téngtòng, shàngzhī bù néng dòng.

(2) Fǔzhù jiǎnchá: X shèxiàn jiǎnchá.

(3) Zhěnduàn jiéguǒ: Gōnggǔ gǔzhé.

(4) Zhìliáo fāng'àn: Fùwèi, gùdìng, kāngfù zhìliáo.

3. Case record writing.

Chapter 27   Lumbar Disc Herniation

1. Core target words: Yāotuǐtòng, zhuījiānpán tūchū, qiānshètòng, fàngshètòng, fǎnshètòng, yāozhuī huátuō, zhèngcèwèipiàn, túxiàng, bìngbiàn, fànwéi, wòchuáng, huǎnjiě, qiānyǐn, fàngsōng, wānqū, wùlǐ zhìliáo.

2. Case in the text: A middle age patient is telling the doctor about his waist pain.

(1) Bìngren de zhǔsù, jìwǎng bìngshǐ, xiànbìngshǐ.

(2) Línchuáng biǎoxiàn: Yāotòng, xiàzhī fàngshètòng,

(3) Fǔzhù jiǎnchá: X shèxiàn jiǎnchá, CT jiǎnchá.

(4) Zhěnduàn jiéguǒ: Yāozhuījiānpán tūchū.

(5) Zhìliáo fāng'àn: Zhēnjiǔ liáofá, yàowù zhìliáo, qiānyǐn zhìliáo.

(6) Qítā: Yīshēng jiànyì bìngren shuì yìngbǎnchuáng.

3. Extension writing task: The patient's revisit to hospital two months later.

Chapter 28   Acute Cystitis

1. Core target words: Pángguāngyán, pángguāng jiéshí, niàopín, niàojí, páiniào kùnnán, xuèniào, pángguāng'ái, qǔshí shǒushù, jīguāng suìshí shǒushù, shēnglǐ yánshuǐ, jiāoguàn, zhíjìng, lǐmǐ, èrcì gǎnrǎn, chūxiàn.

2. Case in the text: A patient goes to hospital because of frequent urination, dysuria and hematuria.

(1) Bìngren de zhǔsù, jìwǎng bìngshǐ, xiànbìngshǐ.

(2) Línchuáng biǎoxiàn: Niàopín, niàojí, páiniào kùnnán, xuèniào.

(3) Tǐgé jiǎnchá: Chùzhěn.

(4) Fǔzhù jiǎnchá: Niàochángguī, xuèchángguī, B chāo jiǎnchá, pángguāngjìng jiǎnchá.

(5) Zhěnduàn jiéguǒ: Jíxìng pángguāngyán, pángguāng jiéshí.

(6) Zhìliáo fāng'àn: Jīguāng suìshí shǒushù.

3. Extension writing task: The patient's revisit to hospital two months later.

Chapter 29   Esophageal Cancer

1. Core target words: Shíguǎn'ái, tūnyàn gěngzǔ, xiōnggǔhòu téngtòng, yēzhù, fǎnsuān, shāoxīn, gānyìng, xīfàn, línbājié, shíguǎn bèicān jiǎnchá, wěnluàn, pòhuài, pínggū, jìnjì, xiōngqiāng bìshì yǐnliú, yìzhì, zhèntòngyào, jìnshí.

2. Case in the text: Mr. Wang goes to the thoracic surgery department to see the doctor because he has been suffered from swallow obstruction when eating for three

months.

(1) Línchuáng biǎoxiàn: Tūnyàn kùnnán, fǎnsuān, shāoxīn, ǒutù.

(2) Fǔzhù jiǎnchá: Shíguǎn zàoyǐng jiǎnchá, xiānwéi wèijìng jiǎnchá, xiōngbù CT jiǎnchá.

(3) Zhěnduàn jiéguǒ: Shíguǎn'ái zǎoqī.

(4) Zhìliáo fāng'àn: Shíguǎn'ái qiēchú, wèishíguǎn wěnhé shù.

3. Oral language task: Design a dialogue to retell the case.

Chapter 30   Burn Injury

1. Core target words: Shāoshāng, shuǐpào, chuāngmiàn, pòliè, chōngxǐ, chéngdù, qiǎndù, yùhén, bāhén, wújūn shǒutào, kàngshēngsù yóushā, miándiàn, qùchú, túcā, miánqiān, zhàn, bāozā, bǎohù.

2. Case in the text: A man got burn injury by gas stove when cooking outdoor, and he is sent to the hospital.

(1) Bìngren de zhǔsù.

(2) Línchuáng biǎoxiàn: Pífū hóngzhǒng, qǐ shuǐpào.

(3) Zhěnduàn jiéguǒ: Ⅱ dù shāoshāng.

(4) Zhìliáo fāng'àn: Fūyào (kàngshēngsù), bàolù liáofǎ.

(5) Qítā: Bìngren yào zhùyì bǎochí chuāngmiàn qīngjié, gānzào.

3. Oral language task : Design a dialogue to retell the case.

4. Case record writing.

Chapter 31   Pelvic Inflammatory Disease

1. Core target words: Pénqiāngyán, yīndàoyán, fēnmìwù, réngōng liúchǎn, tǎolùn, jiēshòu, zǐgōng, chūbù zhěnduàn, pénqiāng fùmóyán, búyù, jìnzhǐ, jiāochā gǎnrǎn, shìdàng.

2. Case in the text: The patient comes to the gynecological department because of pruritus of vulva and excessive vaginal discharge.

(1) Línchuáng biǎoxiàn: Fārè, fùbù téngtòng, yīndàonèi fēnmìwù guò duō.

(2) Fùkē jiǎnchá.

(3) Fǔzhù jiǎnchá: Xuèchángguī, fēnmìwù jiǎnyàn, fùbù chāoshēng jiǎnchá.

(4) Zhěnduàn jiéguǒ: Jíxìng pénqiāngyán.

(5) Zhìliáo fāng'àn: Shǒushù zhìliáo.

3. Case record writing.

Chapter 32   Menstrual Disorder

1. Core target words: Yuèjīng shītiáo, chíxùxìng, gōngnéng shītiáoxìng zǐgōng chūxuè, xiěkuài, gōngnèi jiéyùqì, zǐgōngjǐng, bāokuài, tuōxià, bìnglǐ jiǎnyàn, zhǐxuèyào, zhǔfù, xiángxì, guāchúshù, gǎishàn.

2. Case in the text: The patient comes to the gynecological department because of her irregular menstruation and continued vaginal bleeding.

(1) Línchuáng biǎoxiàn: Yuèjīng bù guīlǜ, chūxiàn bù guīzé yīndào liúxuè.

(2) Fùkē jiǎnchá.

(3) Fǔzhù jiǎnchá: B chāo, bìnglǐ jiǎnyàn.

(4) Zhěnduàn jiéguǒ: Gōngnéng shītiáoxìng zǐgōng chūxuè.

(5) Zhìliáo fāng'àn: Guāgōng shǒushù, yàowù zhìliáo.

3. Extension writing task: The patient's revisit to hospital two months later.

Chapter 33　Pregnancy and Labor

1. Core target words: Huáiyùn, chǎnfù, chǎnqián, yùnzhōu, yùchǎnqī, jiēduàn, yǐnchǎn, wújīrě shìyàn, tāidòng, gōngsuō, tāiwèi, cuīchǎnsù, chūshēng, yángshuǐ, pōufùchǎn, chǎnhòu, réngōng pòmóshù, yīng'ér.

2. Case in the text: The patient of 39 weeks' pregnancy complains ankle edema.

(1) Línchǎn xiānzhào: Jiǎlínchǎn, tāi'ér xiàjiàng gǎn, pòshuǐ, jiànhóng.

(2) Chǎnqián tǐgé jiǎnchá: Yùnfù xuèyā, tǐzhòng, xīnfèi, yīndào, gōngjǐng jiǎnchá; tāixīnyīn jiǎncè.

(3) Chǎnqián fǔzhù jiǎnchá: Xuèchángguī, niàochángguī, chāoshēng jiǎnchá, xīndiàntú jiǎnchá.

(4) Qítā: Chǎnhòu, yīshēng jiànyì mǔrǔ wèiyǎng.

3. Oral language task: Retell the text.

4. Case record writing.

Chapter 34　Ectopic Pregnancy

1. Core target words: Lìjià, yùnfù, rénliú shǒushù, xīgài, wānqū, niào rènshēn shìyàn, yìwèi rènshēn, gōngwàiyùn, shūluǎnguǎn, pēitāi, bìyùn, shībài, chénggōng, yìzhì, zīyǎng, zǔzhī, héchéng, rènshēnnáng, yíchú, bǎoliú, liúshí.

2. Case in the text: The patient arrives in the Emergency complaining of abdominal pain, amenorrhea and a little vaginal bleeding.

(1) Bìngren de zhǔsù, jìwǎng bìngshǐ.

(2) Zhèngzhuàng hé tǐzhēng: Tíngjīng, fùbù téngtòng, yīndào liúxuè.

(3) Fùkē jiǎnchá.

(4) Fǔzhù jiǎnchá: Niào rènshēn shìyàn, chāoshēng jiǎnchá, fùqiāngjìng jiǎnchá.

(5) Zhěnduàn jiéguǒ: Yìwèi rènshēn.

(6) Zhìliáo fāng'àn: Shǒushù zhìliáo.

3. Extension writing task: The patient's revisit to hospital one month later.

Chapter 35　Postpartum Complications

1. Core target words: Bìngfāzhèng, chǎnhòu chūxiě, gōngsuō fálì, tāipán, zìrán fēnmiǎn, gōngkǒu kāiquán, zǐgōng yāpò, ruǎnchǎndào, xuèzhǒng, shūxuè, zhàogù, sīliè, níngxuè, páichú, ànmó, suōgōngsù.

2. Case in the text: The puerpera who finished delivery suffers from postpartum hemorrhage.

(1) Línchuáng biǎoxiàn: Chǎnhòu yīndào liúxuè chāoguò 600 háoshēng.

(2) Fùkē jiǎnchá.

(3) Fǔzhù jiǎnchá: Xuèchángguī, níngxuè chángguī.

(4) Zhěnduàn jiéguǒ: Gōngsuō fálì, ruǎnchǎndào sǔnshāng.

(5) Zhìliáo fāng'àn: Jìngmài zhùshè suōgōngsù bāngzhù zhǐxuè, shūxuè.

(6) Qítā: Chǎnfù yào zhùyì fángzhǐ gǎnrǎn.

3. Case record writing.

Chapter 36   Uterine Tumor

1. Core target words: Zǐgōng jīliú, shēngzhí, xìbāo zēngshēng, tòngjīng, báidài zēngduō, gōngqiāngjìng jiǎnchá, xìngjīsù shuǐpíng jiǎncè, fùfā, chùmō, yāpò, búshì, fùzuòyòng, dǎozhì, zǐgōng nèimó'ái.

2. Case in the text: A post-menopausal women comes to hospital with vaginal bleeding.

(1) Bìngren de zhǔsù, jìwǎng bìngshǐ, xiànbìngshǐ.

(2) Línchuáng biǎoxiàn: Yuèjīngliàng zēngduō, fùbù yǒu bāokuài.

(3) Fùkē jiǎnchá.

(4) Fǔzhù jiǎnchá: Chāoshēng jiǎnchá, gōngqiāngjìng jiǎnchá, xìngjīsù shuǐpíng jiǎncè.

(5) Zhěnduàn jiéguǒ: Zǐgōng nèimó'ái.

(6) Zhìliáo fāng'àn: Shǒushù zhìliáo.

(7) Qítā:Yīshēng jiànyì shùhòu qián liǎngnián, bìngren měi gé 3-6 gè yuè lái yīyuàn fùzhěn.

3. Extension writing task: The patient's revisit to hospital three months later.

Chapter 37   Jaundice

1. Core target words: Róngxuèxìng huángdǎn, shēnglǐxìng huángdǎn, yòu'ér, xīnshēng'ér, zǎochǎn, xuèxíng, dǎnhóngsù, nóngdù, guāngliáo, hóngwàixiàn, zǐwàixiàn, bǐngzhǒng qiúdànbái, huànxuè.

2. Case in the text: The neonatal ICU has just received a baby patient.

(1) Zhèngzhuàng hé tǐzhēng: Gǒngmó huángrǎn, fūsè ànhuáng, fùzhàng, ǒutù.

(2) Tǐgé jiǎnchá: Chùzhěn.

(3) Fǔzhù jiǎnchá: Xuèchángguī.

(4) Zhěnduàn jiéguǒ: Xīnshēng'ér róngxuèxìng huángdǎn.

(5) Zhìliáo fāng'àn: Guāngliáo, yàowù zhìliáo.

3. Oral language task: Retell the case.

Chapter 38   Viral Myocarditis

1. Core target words: Bìngdúxìng xīnjīyán, pífá, xīnlǜ shīcháng, zǎobó, chāoshēng xīndòngtú, záyīn, xīngōngnéng bùquán, huǎnjiě, bìngdú gǎnrǎn, sǔnshāng, èhuà, xīnlì shuāijié, cùsǐ, xīnyuánxìng xiūkè, jǐnzǎo, xīnzàng fùhè.

2. Case in the text: A boy was taken to the out-patient department of pediatrics by his parents for fatigue, chest distress and heart pain.

(1) Bìngren de zhǔsù, jìwǎng bìngshǐ, xiànbìngshǐ.

(2) Zhèngzhuàng hé tǐzhēng: Xiōngmèn, qìduǎn, fálì, liǎnsè cāngbái.

(3) Fǔzhù jiǎnchá: Xiōngbù X shèxiàn jiǎnchá, chāoshēng xīndòngtú jiǎnchá, xīndiàntú jiǎnchá.

(4) Zhěnduàn jiéguǒ: Bìngdúxìng xīnjīyán, xīngōngnéng bùquán.

(5) Zhìliáo fāng'àn: Yàowù zhìliáo, bìyào shí shǒushù zhìliáo.

(6) Qítā: Bìngren xūyào wòchuáng xiūxi.

3. Oral language task : Design a dialogue to retell the case.

Chapter 39　　Nutritional Diseases

1. Core target words: Yíngyǎng bùliáng, zōnghézhēng, wéishēngsù, gōulóubìng, pínfán kūnào, jīxiōng, jìngluán, sàngshī yìshí, xīyǎng, diànjiězhì wěnluàn, pútáotáng suāngài, gǔgé jīxíng, yuánsùgài, jiǎoxíng.

2. Case in the text: A baby is taken to the Out-patient department of pediatrics by his parents because he always wakes up and cries easily.

(1) Bìngren de zhǔsù, jìwǎng bìngshǐ.

(2) Línchuáng biǎoxiàn: Shuìmián bù'ān, pínfán kūnào, tóushang duō hàn, gǔgé jīxíng.

(3) Fǔzhù jiǎnchá: Xuèyè jiǎncè, X shèxiàn jiǎnchá.

(4) Zhěnduàn jiéguǒ: Wéishēngsù D quēfáxìng gōulóubìng.

(5) Zhìliáo fāng'àn: Kǒufú bǔchōng wéishēngsù D, kǒufú bǔchōng yuánsùgài, bìyàoshí jiǎoxíng zhìliáo.

3. Extension writing task: The patient's revisit to hospital three months later.

Chapter 40　　Pertussis

1. Core target words: Bǎirìké, zǐgàn, zàntíng, dǎpēnti, jīluánsuō, bǎibáipò yìmiáo, jiēzhòng, yábāo gǎnjūn, hóngméisù, shènshàngxiàn pízhì jīsù, xiázhǎi, duījī, zhìxī, chuánrǎnxìng jíbìng, gélí, páichì.

2. Case in the text: A young boy whose skin turns into violaceous color is transferred to the In-patient department from Emergency.

(1) Zhèngzhuàng hé tǐzhēng: Késou, chōuchù, zǐgàn, hūxī zàntíng.

(2) Fǔzhù jiǎnchá: Tán jiǎnyàn, fèibù X shèxiàn jiǎnchá.

(3) Zhěnduàn jiéguǒ: Hūxīdào tán duījī yǐnqǐ de hūxī zàntíng, dànǎo quēyǎng.

(4) Zhìliáo fāng'àn: Yàowù zhìliáo (hóngméisù hé shènshàngxiàn pízhì jīsù).

(5) Qítā: Bìngren xūyào gélí.

3. Oral language task: Retell the case.

Chapter 41　Tympanitis

1. Core target words: Zhōng'ěryán, xiǎonǎo, huànóng, ějìng, fùfā, kuìlàn, yǎndǐ zàoyǐngjì, xiāoyányào, gēnchú, liúnóng, qīngméisù, jiǎxiāozuò, tóubāo, wánhǎo, fùzhěn.

2. Case in the text: The patient's father is telling the doctor about his son's situation.

(1) Bìngren de zhǔsù.

(2) Zhèngzhuàng hé tǐzhēng: Huànóng, tīnglì jiǎntuì.

(3) Fǔzhù jiǎnchá: Ějìng jiǎnchá, tīnglì jiǎnchá, X shèxiàn jiǎnchá.

(4) Zhěnduàn jiéguǒ: Mànxìng huànóngxìng zhōng'ěryán.

(5) Zhìliáo fāng'àn: Yàowù zhìliáo, shǒushù zhìliáo.

3. Oral language task: Retell the case.

Chapter 42   Exanthematous Diseases

1. Core target words: Pízhěn, qiūbānzhěn, guānjiétòng, yǎng, zhuānáo, yānyán, biǎntáotǐ, línbājié, gānpí zhǒngdà, gǔsuǐ chuāncì, dānhé xìbāo zēngduōzhèng, kàngbìngdú zhìliáo, jīsù zhìliáo, āmòxīlín, bàixiězhèng.

2. Case in the text: A sick child is taken to the pediatrics department by his mother because of fever and exanthema.

(1) Bìngren de zhǔsù, jìwǎng bìngshǐ, xiànbìngshǐ.

(2) Zhèngzhuàng hé tǐzhēng: Biǎntáotǐ hóngzhǒng, jǐngbù línbājié zhǒngdà, gānpí zhǒngdà, fārè.

(3) Fǔzhù jiǎnchá: Niàochángguī, xuèchángguī.

(4) Zhěnduàn jiéguǒ: Chuánrǎnxìng dānhé xìbāo zēngduōzhèng.

(5) Zhìliáo fāng'àn: Yàowù zhìliáo (kàngbìngdú, jīsù zhìliáo), bìyào shí shǒushù zhìliáo.

(6) Qítā: Yīshēng jiànyì bìngren bìmiǎn zuò jùliè yùndòng.

3. Oral language task : Retell the case.

Chapter 43   Senile Cataract

1. Core target words: Báinèizhàng, shìlì jiǎntuì, chéngshú jiēduàn, guāngdìngwèi, lièxìdēng jiǎnchá, húnzhuó, jīngtǐ nángwài zhāichúshù, réngōng jīngtǐ zhírùshù, pèidài, yǎnzhào, yǎnyàoshuǐ, yǎnjiǎomó, juānzèng, páichì.

2. Case in the text: The old patient who suffers from eye blind is sent to the department of ophthalmology.

(1) Bìngren de zhǔsù.

(2) Línchuáng biǎoxiàn: Pàguāng, shìlì jiǎntuì.

(3) Fǔzhù jiǎnchá: Shìjué mǐngǎndù jiǎncè, yǎnbù B chāo, lièxìdēng jiǎnchá.

(4) Zhěnduàn jiéguǒ: Xiāntiānxìng báinèizhàng.

(5) Zhìliáo fāng'àn: Shǒushù zhìliáo (jīngtǐ nángwài zhāichúshù, réngōng jīngtǐ zhírùshù).

(6) Qítā: Yīshēng zhǔfù bìngren yào jiānchí dī yǎnyàoshuǐ, wàichū shí pèidài yǎnzhào.

3. Extension writing task: The patient's revisit to hospital three months later.

LANGUAGE PRACTICAL

1. To visit the Emergency department in hospital.

2. To visit the Internal Medicine in hospital.

3. To visit the Surgery department in hospital.

4. To visit the Gynecology & Obstetrics in hospital.

5. To visit the Pediatrics in hospital.

6. Medical organization tour.

7. Pharmaceutical company tour.

8. Competition of role-play performance.

9. Competition of case record writing.

A SURVEY OF CHINA
中 国 概 况

Chief Editors（主编）
Deng Yongzhong（邓永忠） Jinan University（暨南大学）
Chen Jun（陈君） Southern Medical University（南方医科大学）

Deputy Chief Editors（副主编）
Yu Huifen（余惠芬） Jinan University（暨南大学）
Luo Hongbin（罗宏斌） Jinan University（暨南大学）

Editors（编委）（按姓氏拼音排序）
Chen Jun（陈君） Southern Medical University（南方医科大学）
Deng Yongzhong（邓永忠） Jinan University（暨南大学）
Luo Hongbin（罗宏斌） Jinan University（暨南大学）
Yu Huifen（余惠芬） Jinan University（暨南大学）

Course Description

A Survey of China is a compulsory course offered to international students coming to study in China. This course introduces general knowledge about China. Focusing on the major aspects of Chinese culture and civilization, it covers a broad range of topics, including China profile, history, philosophy, religion, literature, economy, language and characters, calligraphy and paintings. The aim of the course is to help students to gain a systemic and sound knowledge of China and prepare them for further study and research in the related fields.

Objectives

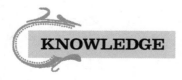

KNOWLEDGE

At the end of the course, students shall be able to:
1. Have a sound knowledge about China's natural conditions and hiotorical background;
2. Form an objective judgment on Chinese society and culture;
3. Develop intercultural communicative competence;

4. Promote cultural exchanges between China and foreign countries in the relevant aspects.

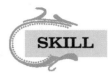

SKILL

At the end of the course, students shall be able to communicate with confidence about general topics related to China in social or academic occasions.

Teaching and Learning Methods

Theory: Presentations by instructor(s) through PowerPoints and videotapes along with students'classroom discussions.

Practical: A field trip to a local museum or traditional culture attraction.

Recommended Textbooks

Dong Xiaobo (董晓波). 2014. Introduction to Chinese History and Culture (English Version) [M]. Beijing: University of International Business and Economics Press.

Guo Peng (郭鹏), Cheng Long (程龙). 2012. China Panoram [M]. Beijing: Higher Education Press.

Liao Huaying (廖华英). 2015. A Glimpse of Chinese Culture (Revised Edition) [M]. Beijing: Foreign Language Teaching and Research Press.

Yu Huifen (余惠芬), et al. 2017. An Introduction to Chinese Culture [M]. 2nd ed. Gangzhou: Jinan University Press.

Schedule Table

Chapter	Contents	Hours	Chapter	Contents	Hours
1	Brief Introduction to China	4	6	Chinese Literature	4
2	Chinese History	8	7	Chinese Language and Characters	3
3	Chinese Philosophy	4	8	Chinese Calligraphy and Paintings	3
4	Chinese Religions	4	9	Field Trip	2
5	Chinese Economy	4		Total	36

Course Contents

Chapter 1　Overview of China

1. National symbols:　country name, national anthem, national emblem, national flower etc.

2. Geographical features: territory, mountains and rivers, topography and climate.

3. Administrative regions, population and language.

4. State structure and political system.

5. Famous historical and cultural cities and cultural heritages.

Chapter 2　Chinese History

1. Earliest period.

(1) Human origin in Chinese culture.

(2) Primal ancestors of Chinese: the Yellow Emperor and the Yan Emperor.

(3) Archaeological evidence to support some certainty of legends.

(4) Appearance of written language and recorded history.

2. The Zhou Dynasty (1066 BC-221 BC).

(1) The Western Zhou and Eastern Zhou.

(2) Mandate of Heaven.

3. The first empire: the Qin Dynasty (221 BC-206 BC）

(1) Appearance of the first centralized empire.

(2) The fall of the Qin Dynasty.

4. The consolidation of empire: the Han Dynasty (206 BC-220 AD).

(1) Western Han and Eastern Han.

(2) The Silk Road.

(3) The development of literary activities.

(4) The Huns and Wang Zhaojun.

5. The Three Kingdoms, Jin, North and South dynasties.

(1) The Three Kingdoms: Wei (220-265), Shu(221-263) and Wu (222-280).

(2) The Jin Dynasty (256-420).

(3) The South-North Dynasty (420-589).

6. The restoration of the empire: Sui & Tang dynasties.

(1) The Sui Dynasty (581-618).

(2) The Tang Dynasty (618-907).

(3) Tang Tai Zong: an enlightened emperor.

(4) The decline of the Tang Dynasty, Five Northern Dynasties and Ten Southern Kingdoms.

7. A weak empire: the Song Dynasty (960-1279).

(1) Northern Song (960-1127) and Southern Song (1127-1279).

(2) Developments of arts, science and technology in Song Dynasty.

(3) Social custom of foot-binding.

8. An empire with the largest territory: Yuan Dynasty (1279-1368).

(1) Cheng Ji Si Han and Mongolian Whirl Wave.

(2) External relations during the Yuan Dynasty.

9. The Ming Dynasty (1368-1644).

(1) The rise and fall of the Ming Dynasty.

(2) Zheng He and his naval expeditions.

10. The earlier period of the Qing Dynasty (1644-1840).

(1) The resurgence of the Manchus and its governance into China.

(2) The flourishing period under emperors of Kang Xi, Yong Zheng and Qian Long.

(3) The end of ancient Chinese history.

11. Modern period.

Chapter 3   Chinese Philosophy

1. Brief introduction.

(1) Origin of Chinese ancient philosophy.

(2) Historical development of Chinese philosophy.

2. Chinese philosophical thoughts.

(1) Confucianism: Confucius, spirit of Confucianism (benevolence, ritual propriety, doctrine of the Mean, Rectification of Names, Four Books and Five Classics).

(2) Taoism/Daoism (Lao Zi, Dao De Jing, the concepts of Dao & De, the principles of Dao, The wisdom of Laozi, the Dao of human life).

Chapter 4   Chinese Religions

1. Primitive and ancient religion: worship of nature, worship of totems and worship of ancestors.

2. Chinese religious beliefs.

(1) General introduction to Chinese religious belief.

(2) Brief introduction to the main religions in China.

3. Chinese Buddhism.

(1) Siddhartha Gautama, the founder (563 BC-480 BC).

(2) Basic doctrines of Chinese Buddhism.

(3) Influence of Buddhism on Chinese society and culture.

3. Religious Daoism.

(1) Lao Zi and Zhuang Zi.

(2) Daoist beliefs and influence on Chinese culture.

Chapter 5   Chinese Economy

1. Highlights of ancient Chinese economic thoughts and business culture.

2. China's opening-up policy.

3. China's economic outlook.

Chapter 6   Chinese Literature

1. The Book of Songs.

2. Chu Ci.

3. Yue Fu.

4. Tang Poetry.

5. Song Ci.

6. The Yuan Variety Play /The Zaju of the Yuan Dynasty.

7. Ming and Qing fictions.

Chapter 7　Chinese Language and Characters

1. Chinese language: speakers, dialects, Huanyu Pinyin and Mandarin.
2. Chinese characters.
(1) Origin and development of Chinese writing system.
(2) Structure of Chinese characters.
3. Influence of Chinese language and characters.

Chapter 8　Chinese Calligraphy and Paintings

1. Chinese calligraphy.
(1) Origin of Chinese calligraphy.
(2) Calligraphy Set—Four Treasures of the Study.
(3) How to appreciate Chinese calligraphy.
(4) Famous calligraphers in chinese History.
2. Chinese paintings.
(1) Origins of Chinese brush painting.
(2) General characteristics of Chinese brush painting.
(3) Symbolism in Chinese paintings.

MEDICAL INFORMATION RETRIEVAL
医学信息检索

Chief Editors（主编）

Zhou Jinyuan（周金元） Jiangsu University（江苏大学）

Wu Daili（吴代莉） Wenzhou Medical University（温州医科大学）

Deputy Chief Editors（副主编）

Liu Haijun（刘海军） Jiangsu University（江苏大学）

Zhang Ren（张壬） Jiangsu University（江苏大学）

Liu Guifeng（刘桂峰） Jiangsu University（江苏大学）

Chen Guijin（陈桂金） Wenzhou Medical University（温州医科大学）

Zhou Xiaozhen（周晓政） Nanjing Medical University（南京医科大学）

Editors（编委）（按姓氏拼音排序）

Chen Guijin（陈桂金） Wenzhou Medical University（温州医科大学）

Liu Guifeng（刘桂峰） Jiangsu University（江苏大学）

Liu Haijun（刘海军） Jiangsu University（江苏大学）

Wu Daili（吴代莉） Wenzhou Medical University（温州医科大学）

Zhang Ren（张壬） Jiangsu University（江苏大学）

Zhou Jinyuan（周金元） Jiangsu University（江苏大学）

Zhou Xiaozhen（周晓政） Nanjing Medical University（南京医科大学）

Course Description

Information retrieval (IR) is a broad area of Computer Science focused primarily on providing the users with easy access to information of their interest, as follows. Information retrieval deals with the representation, storage, organization of, and access to information items such as documents, Web pages, online catalogs, structured and semi-structured records, multimedia objects. There presentation and organization of the information items should be such as to provide the users with easy access to information of their interest. In terms of scope, the area has grown well beyond its early goals of indexing text and searching for useful documents in a collection. Nowadays, research in IR includes modeling, Web search, text classification, systems architecture, user interfaces, data visualization, filtering, languages.

In terms of research, the area may be studied from two rather distinct and complementary points of view: a computer-centered one and a human-centered one.

In the computer—centered view, IR consists mainly of building up efficient indexes, processing user queries with high performance, and developing ranking algorithms to improve the results. In the human-centered view, IR consists mainly of studying the behavior of the user, of understanding their main needs, and of determining how such under-standing affects the organization and operation of the retrieval system. In this book, we focus mainly on the computer—centered view of IR. which is dominant in academia and in the market place.

Objectives

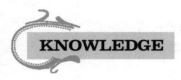

KNOWLEDGE

At the end of the course, the students shall be able to:

1. Know the importance of cultivating the sense of information.

2. Know how to find resources, selection of resources. Understanding and understanding of the various information sources related to the professional, can identify a variety of information resources.

3. Master retrieval skills, familiar with the basic principles of information retrieval, knowledge.

4. Get to know the way to get documents, know where to get the original document you want.

5. Learn how to evaluate and use information.

6. Enhance information security awareness.

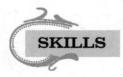

SKILLS

At the end of the course, the student shall be able to practice the following experiments:

1. Task Definition.

Define The Information Problem.

- What does this assignment require me to do?
- What will my product/project look like if I do a really good job?
- What problem needs to be solved?

2. Information Seeking Strategies.

Determine the range of possible sources (brainstorm).

This means that you need to make a list of all the possible sources of information that will help you answer the questions you wrote in Task Definition. Consider library books, encyclopedias, and web sites to which your library subscribes (ask your librarian!), people who are experts in your subject, observation of your subject, free web sites and survey.

Evaluate the different possible sources to determine priorities (select the best sources) Now, look carefully at your list. Which ones are actually available to you and are easy for you to use? Circle these. If there are some that you need help using, ask your teacher, librarian.

3. Location and Access.

Locate sources.

Figure out where you will get these sources. Beside each source, write its location. If it is a web site, list its web address. Try to use those that your teacher or librarian have linked or bookmarked. This will save you time. If your source is a person, figure out how you will contact him or her and make a note of this.

Now, you will actually get the sources. You may have to get and use them one at a time. If so, come back to this step to locate each source.

Find information within sources.

Now that you have the source in hand, how will you get to the information that you need? (Remember the questions you wrote in Task Definition?) This all depends on the source.

4. Use of Information.

Engage in the source (read, listen, view, touch).

Most likely you will need to read, listen or view your source. If you can't understand any of it, be sure to ask an adult to help you. It's OK not to understand, it's not OK not to ask for help. You are looking for the information you need. You may not need to read, listen to, or view all of your source. You may be able to skip around, finding subheadings and topic sentences (read the first sentences in each paragraph) that will take you to your information.

Take out the relevant information from a source.

It's time to take some notes.

5. Synthesis.

Organize information from different sources. Decide how you will put together your notes and add your ideas and insights.

You may:

Write a rough draft.

Build an outline.

Create a storyboard.

Draw a sketch.

Present the inform.

6. Evaluation.

Judge your product (effectiveness). Before turning in your assignment, compare it to your teacher's requirements.

Did you do and include everything that was required?

Did you give credit to all of your sources, and did you write it the way your teacher requested?

Is your work neat?

Is your work complete and does it include heading information (name, date, etc.).

Would you be proud for anyone to view this work?

Judge your information problem-solving process (efficiency).

Think about what you did to finish this assignment. You may have learned some skills to use anytime you need information to answer questions!

What skill(s) did you learn that you can use again?

How will you be able to use the skill(s) again?

What did you do well this time?

What would you do differently next time?

Which information sources were most useful? You may be able to use them again when you need information.

What information sources did you need but the library did not have? Talk to your librarian about the possibility of getting them.

Teaching And Learning Methods

Theory: Teaching medical information retrival to undergraduate medical student is provided with the help of lectures and tutorials that deal with the theory and principles of medical information retrival.

Practical: Practical training asks students to know the basic principles, methods and techniques, strategies, and skills for the medical information retrival.

Recommended Textbooks

Beze Yates, et al. 2011. Modern Information Retrieval English Version [M]. Beijing: Mechanical Industry Press.

Huang Xiaoli , et al. 2010. Medical Information Retrieval Bilingual Textbooks [M]. 6th ed. Beijing: People's Health Publishing House.

SCHEDULE TABLE

Chapter	Contents	Hours	Chapter	Contents	Hours
1、2、3	An overview of information literacy, An overview of information literacy cultivation, An overview of information resources	2	9	Information service organizations and service modes	2
4	An overview of information retrieval	2	10	Medical information analysis and medical research topic selection	2
5	Chinese information retrieval tools	4	11	Medical information investigation	4
6	English information retrieval tools	6	12	Medical papers writing	2
7	Network medical resources	2		Total	30
8	Patent literature retrieval	4			

Course Contents

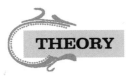

THEORY

Chapter 1　An overview of information literacy

1. Definition and composition of information literacy.
2. Characteristics of information literacy.
3. Information consciousness.
4. Information ability.
5. Information morality.
6. Information exchange and information literacy.

Chapter 2　An overview of information literacy cultivation

1. The necessity of information literacy cultivation.
2. The feasibility of information literacy cultivation.
3. Principles and requirements of information literacy cultivation.
4. Classification of information literacy cultivation.
5. Ways of information literacy cultivation.
6. Evaluation of information literacy.

Chapter 3　An overview of information resources

1. Related concepts about information.
2. Types and distribution of information resources.
3. Organization of network information resources.
4. Information retrieval language.
5. Information retrieval systems and tools.
6. Evaluation of network information resources.

Chapter 4　An overview of information retrieval

1. Principles of information retrieval.
2. Classification of information retrieval.
3. The Purpose and significance of information retrieval.
4. Information retrieval methods.
5. Information retrieval procedures.
6. The function and logic operation of information retrieval.
7. Evaluation of information retrieval and its influencing factors.

Chapter 5　Chinese information retrieval tools

1. China Academic Journals Full-text Database (CNKI).
2. Wanfang Database.
3. Chongqing Vip Database (CQVIP).
4. Database of reprinted papers by Renmin University of China.
5. Chinese Biomedical Literature Database (CBMdisc).
6. Chinese Biomedical Journal Database (CMCC).

Chapter 6　English information retrieval tools

1. Science Citation Index (SCI).
2. Springer Link.
3. Conference Proceedings Citation Index-Sciece (CPCI-S/former ISTP).
4. Chemical Abstracts (CA).
5. EBSCO.
6. ScienceDirect.
7. Medline/Pubmed.

Chapter 7　Network medical resources

1. Types and characteristics of network resources.
2. Web search engines.
3. Search of medical software.
4. Open access to medical information.

Chapter 8　Patent literature retrieval

1. Basic knowledge of patent.
2. Patent literature.
3. Chinese patent literature.
4. Chinese patent literature retrieval.
5. World patent literature retrieval.

Chapter 9　Information service organizations and service modes

1. Libraries.
2. Information institutions.
3. Archives.
4. Medical record room.

Chapter 10　Medical information analysis and medical research topic selection

1. An overview of information analysis.
2. Steps of information analysis.
3. Basic methods of information analysis.
4 Medical research topic selection.

Chapter 11 Medical information investigation

1. An overview of medical information investigation.
2. Material collection, identification and collation.
3. Intelligence analysis research and forecasting.
4. Science and technology novelty searching on medicine.

Chapter 12 Medical papers writing

1. An overview of medical research papers.
2. Basic formats and requirements of medical papers.
3. Methods and steps of writing medical papers.
4. How to write a medical review.
5. How to write a medical abstract.

COMPUTER APPLICATION
计算机应用基础

Chief Editor（主编）
  Wang Changda（王昌达） Jiangsu University（江苏大学）

Deputy Chief Editors（副主编）
  Ge Guiping（葛桂萍） Yangzhou University（扬州大学）
  Hua Jin（华进） Nantong University（南通大学）

Editors（编委）（按姓氏拼音排序）
  Ge Guiping（葛桂萍） Yangzhou University（扬州大学）
  Hua Jin（华进） Nantong University（南通大学）
  Wang Changda（王昌达） Jiangsu University（江苏大学）
  Wu Xiulin（吴秀琳） Jiangsu University（江苏大学）
  Yang Yang（杨洋） Jiangsu University（江苏大学）
  Zhang Xing（张星） Jiangsu University（江苏大学）

Course Description

The course introduces the essential concepts for computer as well as train students using the most popular office desktop applications nowadays.

The course is designed for the students who have finished the study of Foundations of Computer and/or Computer Science. The course focuses on Microsoft Windows operating system and Microsoft Office applications which include Word, Excel, PowerPoint, and Access, etc.

The course leads students to reach a variety of skills for Word that include but not limited to information retrieving, text editing, spell checking, graphic generating and layout designing. Excel is mainly taught with data manipulating, arithmetic calculating, data retrieving, formulas creating and data visualizing. As a substitution for flip charts and black or white boards, the course also shows students how to use PowerPoint as an auxiliary tool to prepare their presentations efficiently. Access was taught in the course as a lightweight database management system with the basic data operation and statistical analysis skills.

Windows 8 and Office 2013 are recommended as the show case in the course by far.

Objectives

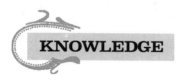

KNOWLEDGE

1. Create a PowerPoint presentation with a designated template and the available resources from the clip art, the images, the tables, the charts, the videos, the audios, the animations and the slide transition effects provided by Microsoft Office.

2. Create a Word document with the available resources from the clip art, the font sizes, the font types, the font styles as well as format the paragraphs.

3. Use Word to create multiple-page reports, posters as well as merge mails.

4. Create spreadsheet with different embedded functions of Excel. Furthermore, the fill handle using, the worksheet formatting, the absolute address referencing and the 3-D charts creating skills are recommended to be mastered.

5. Build a lightweight database management system with Access, which includes but not limited to the table creating, the records appending, the database querying, the customized report creating and the data redundancy eliminating.

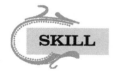

SKILL

At the end of the course, under the Windows Operating system, the students shall be able to use Microsoft Office to create presentations with PowerPoint; to write thesis with Word; to process data with Excel and Access.

Teaching and Learning Methods

We teach students through interaction method at a classroom which has desktop computers. The students follow the teacher's operation on their own computers. If some of them have the difficulty to repeat, the teacher can help them immediately. Furthermore, the practice classes are arranged independently for the students to achieve the objectives that the teacher has set according to the selected teaching objectives.

Recommended Textbooks

Help Document for Office 2013
Help Document for Windows 8
Microsoft Office Home and Student (1PC/1User) by Microsoft.
Microsoft Windows 8.1-Full Version Oct 18, 2013 by Microsoft.

Schedule Table

Chapter	Contents	Class Teaching	Practical
1	Essential Computer Concepts and Microsoft Windows	2	2
2	Microsoft Word	2	2
2	Microsoft Excel	4	2
3	Microsoft PowerPoint	4	2
4	Microsoft Access	4	2
5	Integrating the Office Suite	2	2
	Total	18	12

Course Evaluation and Grading

Grade Categories	Weight	Total Points	Grade Categories	Weight	Total Points
Assignment	40%	100	Teamwork	10%	100
Class Performance	25%	100	Total	100.00%	100
Quiz	25%	100			

Course Contents

Chapter 1　Essential Computer Concepts and Microsoft Windows

It is very important to know the basic terminologies that we are going to use in this chapter. To know about a computer, you have to understand the meanings of processor's speed, memory's capacity, as well as how does an operating system work and what are differences between Operating system, or system software, and application software.

In an extensive manner, you will study how to operate application software as well as manage the folders and the files in the secondary storages, no matter what kinds of Windows are involved, e.g., Windows XP, Vista, or 7, 8, 10.

Upon completion of this Chapter, we assumed that students are able to.

1. Create, search, copy, and move files effectively;

2. Tell the version of a Windows operating system;

3. Know the operations related to the folders and the files management;

4. Know about the attachment software of Windows operating system;

5. Know about the basic hardware for microcomputers;

6. Familiar with the performance measuring parameters for computer hardware as well as to buy a computer according to certain standards;

7. Use Internet to retrieve the latest information and/or specifications for computer hardware, architectures, and software, etc.;

8. Mange data with security concerns.

Chapter 2　Microsoft Word

You will learn the ways to generate a number of different documents, such as formal letters, articles, and even academic papers. How to complete a spreadsheet or database in Word are also discussed.

You are strongly recommended to get information through the Help Document, which not only contains the operating indications for users, but also provides the advanced features for Word in the latest version.

Upon completion of this Chapter, we assumed that students are able to.

1. Create well-designed letters and other type documents;

2. Use the Help Document to extend your knowledge which is not always found in textbooks;

3. Author different professional documents, e.g., invitation letter, data analysis report, and poster with a number of columns, etc.;

4. Familiar with the formatting features;

5. Familiar with the find, the replace, the copy, the cut, and the paste operations for the selected character strings;

6. Create and fill the table semi-automatically.

Chapter 3　Microsoft Excel

Excel, an example of spreadsheet, is a group of text and numbers organized as a grid or table. Spreadsheets are often used in business for balance budgeting and inventory managing because they can unite the text, the numbers, and the charts in a single document. The most important advantage of an electronic spreadsheet is that the data can be updated to reflect all the entries changes in a table by a click.

Upon completion of this Chapter, we assumed that students are able to.

1. Design and create a workbook, as well as navigate through a workbook and worksheet;

2. Input text, date, and numbers with correct format;

3. Insert and delete the selected rows, columns, and areas;

4. Format a workbook by changing the font size, the font style, and the font color;

5. Format data with the Format Painter; highlight cells with conditional formatting; set the printing area; insert page breaks; add print titles; create headers and footers; apply cell style and set page margins;

6. Insert formulas and functions that include but not limited to the data error values interpreting, the relative and absolute address referencing, the formulas and/or the data automatic filling;

7. Generate and edit charts.

Chapter 4　PowerPoint

Microsoft PowerPoint is a desktop application which helps you to prepare lecture notes, or a set of slides, which contain text, charts, pictures, sounds, footages, to name a few.

Upon completion of this Chapter, we assumed that students are able to.

1. Design the personalized lecture notes;

2. Apply a template to slides according to a certain requirement;

3. Edit and format the text; change the theme; edit the inserted photos, and make the speaker notes;

4. Print the slides, the handouts, and an outline of the presentation;

5. Apply a theme to a lecture notes; insert online pictures; insert and format the shapes; insert the tables; apply and modify the transitions and animations; add the videos; modify the playback options, and add the footers and headers for the lecture notes.

Chapter 5　Microsoft Access

Microsoft Access is a powerful relational database (DB) for microcomputers. All the popular databases nowadays are relational ones, for examples, Oracle, SQL server, to name a few. Such a DB consists of one or more related files that we refer them as tables. Each table consists of a number of rows which are denoted as records. Furthermore, each record has a series of fields. An example for the record used in Access could be a row for a person in your contacts, which includes ID, Name, Address, City, State, ZIP, Phone, and Department, etc., among which ID, Name and Address are all instances of fields.

Upon completion of this Chapter, we assumed that you are able to.

1. Know the correct ways to start, close, and stop a database in Access;

2. Familiar with Access environment, database related terminologies;

3. Create an Access table with Table Wizard;

4. Query the Access database;

5. Create data analysis report in Access;

6. View the table through datasheet and/or a form;

7. Open and close Access objects;

8. Modify a table's structure;

9. Merge two or more related tables;

10. Use the Access Help Document as a guidance for your operations.

Chapter 6　Integrating the Office Suite

In this Chapter, Word, PowerPoint, Excel, and Access are showed to work together by which to make an efficient paper work.

Upon completion of this Chapter, we assumed that you are able to.

1. Extract text and other objects from Microsoft Office documents as well as add them into Microsoft Office Clipboard;

2. Paste the chosen objects from Microsoft Office Clipboard into a Microsoft Office document;

3. Merge mails;

4. Import/Export data from a Microsoft Office document;

5. Import an Excel list from an Access database;

6. Export an Access query to a Word document.

MEDICAL CELL BIOLOGY
医学细胞生物学

Chief Editors（主编）

Li Guang（李光） Tianjin Medical University（天津医科大学）

Luo Yang（罗阳） China Medical University（中国医科大学）

Su Xiaobo（苏晓波） Guangzhou Medical University（广州医科大学）

Zhao Wenran（赵文然） Harbin Medical University（哈尔滨医科大学）

Deputy Chief Editors（副主编）

Liu Qi（刘琦） China Medical University（中国医科大学）

Wang Feng（王峰） Tianjin Medical University（天津医科大学）

Zhang Shujuan（张淑娟） Harbin Medical University （哈尔滨医科大学）

Editors（编委）（按姓氏拼音排序）

Cao Lihua（曹丽华） China Medical University（中国医科大学）

Gao Furong（高芙蓉） Tongji University（同济大学）

Li Guang（李光） Tianjin Medical University（天津医科大学）

Liu Qi（刘琦） China Medical University（中国医科大学）

Luo Yang（罗阳） China Medical University（中国医科大学）

Miao Xuhong（苗绪红） Tianjin Medical University（天津医科大学）

Su Xiaobo（苏晓波） Guangzhou Medical University（广州医科大学）

Wang Fang（王芳） Guangzhou Medical University（广州医科大学）

Wang Feng（王峰） Tianjin Medical University（天津医科大学）

Wo Xiaoman（沃晓嫚） Harbin Medical University（哈尔滨医科大学）

Zhang Lan（张岚） Guangzhou Medical University（广州医科大学）

Zhang Shujuan（张淑娟） Harbin Medical University （哈尔滨医科大学）

Zhao Wenran（赵文然） Harbin Medical University（哈尔滨医科大学）

Course Description

Cell biology is a scientific discipline that describes the structure and function of cells. This course will introduce students to the dynamic property and behaviour of cells such as proliferation, movement, signalling, differentiation, survival and death. Cell biology will give particular emphasis on the underlying molecular mechanisms that are required for the activity of eukaryotic cells. The format of this course consists of class lectures and practical (laboratory experiments).

Medial practice will increasingly benefit from the advance in basic science. The purpose of this course is to allow medical students to understand the fundamental principles of cell biology and to meet the demanding requirement for medical professionals to translate scientific discoveries to clinical applications.

Objectives

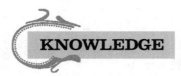

KNOWLEDGE

At the end of the course, students must be able to:
1. describe and understand the membrane structure and functions of the cell.
2. describe and understand the mechanism of protein synthesis and membrane trafficking.
3. understand the functions and the underlying molecular mechanism of cytoskeleton.
4. describe the structure of the nucleus and the packing of chromosomes.
5. understand the molecular mechanism of cell signaling.
6. understand the significance and mechanism of cell death.
7. understand the mechanism of cell proliferation.
8. understand the principles of cell differentiation.

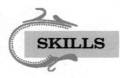

SKILLS

At the end of the course, students will be able to.
1. gain practical experience concerning the handing of laboratory instrument and procedures.
2. understand the strategies that are commonly used to resolve medical problems.
3. gain knowledge about the collection and analysis of data in the research of cell biology.

Teaching and Learning Methods

Theory: Teaching is provided by **class lectures** which are given in the form of power point presentations. The content of the lectures can be provided to students before or after each lecture according to the preference of the instructors. Other methodology such as in-class discussion, literature research, and reviews are highly encouraged.

Practical: Laboratory experiments introduce students to the fundamental strategies and techniques in the study of cell biology.

Examination Pattern and Mark Distribution

Examination is given in the form of final exam, in-class quizzes. Mark distribution can vary depending on the preference of the instructors. Course attendance of the students can also be considered as part of the total score, which accounts for around 10%. Practical (laboratory experiments), which is mandatory for students, can be scored separately or incorporated to the total score of this course.

Questions used in the examination may include single-choice questions, multiple-choice questions, term definition, short-answer questions, true-or-false questions, and analytical questions.

Recommended Textbooks

Bruce Alberts. 2014. The Molecular Biology of the Cell [M]. 6th ed. New York: Garland Science.

Bruce Alberts, Dennis Bray, Karen Hopkin, et al. 2013. Essential Cell Biology [M]. 4th ed. New York: Garland Science.

Gerald Karp, Janet Iwasa, Wallace Marshall. 2016. Cell and Molecular Biology: Concepts and Experiments [M]. 8th ed. New Yorks: Wiley.

Liu Jia（刘佳）, Xu Guoxiong（许国雄）, Liu Xiaoying（刘晓颖）. 2017. Cell Biology [M]. Beijing: People's Medical Publishing House.

The following textbooks are recommended, although other excellent textbooks aimed at undergraduate students are also acceptable.

Schedule Table

The table below provides information on the **class lectures**, which can be scheduled in 24 to 40 teaching hours.

Chapter	Contents	Hours	Chapter	Contents	Hours
1	Introduction to cell biology	1-2	12	Cell signaling	4-6
4	Membrane structure and function	1-4	13	Cell division and cell cycle	4-6
5	Cytoplasmic membrane system and membrane trafficking	2-6	15	Cell differentiation	2
7	Cytoskeleton and cell motility	2-6	16	Cell senescence and cell death	2-4
8	Chromosomes and nucleus	2-4			

Course Contents

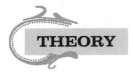

THEORY

Chapter 1   Introduction

1. Cell Biology: the concept and the scope in the study of cells.

2. The role of cell biology in life science and its connection with other disciplines.

3. The history of cell biology: the discovery of cells and the establishment of the cell theory; the application of microscopy and experimental approaches; the invention and application of electron microscope; the establishment and development of cell biology driven by the study of molecular biology.

4. Trends in the development of cell biology.

5. Cell biology and medicine: the link between cell biology and medicine; the medical significance of the studies of cell biology.

Chapter 2   Chemical and Physical Background of the Cell

1. The basic properties of cells: the concept of cell; molecular organization.

2. Two fundamentally different classes of cells: prokaryotic cell; eukaryotic cell; the sizes of cells and their components.

3. Viruses are noncellular pathogens; bacteria.

4. The origin of eukaryotic cell.

Chapter 3   Research Strategies

1. Light microscopy: light microscope; fluorescence microscopy.

2. Electron microscopy: transmission electron microscopy; scanning electron microscopy.

3. Cell culture: primary culture.

4. Cellular content fractionation: differential centrifugation; purification and fractionation of proteins/nucleic acids; measurement of protein and nucleic acid concentration.

5. Nucleic acid hybridization.

6. Recombinant DNA technology: restriction endonucleases; DNA cloning; gene transfer; PCR; DNA sequencing.

7. Antibody-related research methods.

Chapter 4   Membrane Structure and Function

1. The molecular structure of membrane: chemical composition of the membrane; membrane fluidity and asymmetry; fluid-mosaic model; lipid-raft model.

2. Membrane transport: passive transport; simple diffusion; facilitated diffusion; ion-channel; active transport; ion pump; co-transport.

3. Vesicular transport: endocytosis; exocytosis; receptor-mediated endocytosis.

Chapter 5   Cytoplasmic Membrane System and Membrane Trafficking

1. Endoplasmic reticulum: structure; types and function of endoplasmic reticulum; signal peptide; signal hypothesis.

2. Golgi complex: structure; polarity; function.

3. Lysosome: structure; function; the formation and maturation of lysosome.

4. Peroxisome: structure; function.

5. Vesicle and vesicular transport: types of vesicles; vesicle transport and

mechanism involved; membrane flow.

6. Endomembrane system and medicine.

Chapter 6   Mitochondria

1. The feature of mitochondria: structure; chemical composition; function.

2. The genetic materials of mitochondria: mitochondrial DNA.

3. The uptake of proteins into mitochondria: mitochondrion-targeting sequence; the role of molecular chaperones; TOM; TIM.

4. The origin of mitochondria.

5. The fission and fusion of mitochondria.

6. The machinery for ATP formation.

7. Mitochondria and diseases.

Chapter 7   Cytoskeleton and Cell Motility

1. Microtubule: structure; tubulin; microtubule associated protein; the assembly of microtubule; microtubule organizing center; the function of microtubule.

2. Microfilament: actin; microfilament associated protein; the assembly and function of microfilament.

3. Intermediate filament: the structure and types; the assembly and function.

4. Cell motility: microtubule and cell motility; microfilament and cell motility; molecular motors; kinesin; dynein; myosin; muscle contraction.

5. Cytoskeleton and diseases.

Chapter 8   Chromatin, Chromosomes, and the Nucleus

1. Components of the interphase nucleus: nuclear envelope, chromatin, nucleolus, nuclear matrix.

2. Nuclear envelope: structure and functions; nuclear pore complex: fish-trap; nuclear localization signals; importin; exportin.

3. Nuclear lamina: composition, structure; function.

4. Chromatin and chromosome: composition; the packing of chromosome; nucleosome.

5. Euchromatin and heterochromatin.

6. Structure of mitotic chromosome: telomere; kinetochore.

7. Nucleolus: structure and function.

8. Nuclear matrix.

Chapter 9   Genetic Information and Protein Synthesis

1. Gene, genome and central dogma.

2. Structure of prokaryotic and eukaryotic gene.

3. Basic principles of genetic information and translation.

4. Structure of ribosome.

5. Protein synthesis: initiation, elongation, and termination.

6. Post-translational modification of proteins: N-terminal modification, covalent

modification and hydrolysis.

7. Degradation of proteins: ubiquitin-proteasome system; role of lysosome.

8. The regulation of gene expression: temporal specificity; constitutive expression; spatial specificity; inducible gene; repressible gene; operon; cis-acting element; trans-acting element; enhancer; silencer; chromatin remodeling; sumoylation; histone code.

9. Genetic information and medicine.

Chapter 10　Cell Junction and Cell Adhesion

1. Cell junctions: occluding junction, anchoring junction, communication junction.

2. Tight junction: function.

3. Anchoring junctions: adhesion junction; desmosome; hemidemosome.

4. Gap junction and synapse.

5. Cell adhesion molecules: cadherin, selectin, immunogloblin superfamily, integrin.

Chapter 11　Extracellular Matrix

1. Composition of extracellular matrix: glycosaminoglycan, proteoglycan, collagen; fibronectin; laminin.

2. Collagen: types, distribution; synthesis and assembly; collagen and diseases.

3. Fibronectin: molecular structure; RGD sequence.

4. Basal lamina: composition and function.

5. Interaction between extracellular matrix and the cell.

Chapter 12　Signal Transduction

1. Extracellular signal (ligand): hormone, neurotransmitter, local mediator.

2. Receptor: cell surface receptor; ion channel-linked receptor; G protein-coupled receptor; receptor tyrosine kinase; intracellular receptor.

3. Second messenger and signaling pathway: cAMP; cGMP; IP3; DAG; protein kinase A; protein kinase C; protein kinase G; calmodulin and calcium.

4. Protein kinases in cell signaling: protein tyrosine kinase; serine/threonine kinase.

5. Other signaling pathways: MAPK (mitogen activated protein kinase) pathway; JAK-STAT (janus activated kinase-signal transducer and activator of transcription) pathway; Wnt signal pathway; TGF-β (transforming growth factor-β) pathway; NF-κB (nuclear factor-kappa B) pathway.

6. Signal transduction and diseases.

Chapter 13　Cell Division and Cell Cycle

1. Cell division: amitosis; mitosis; meiosis.

2. Mitosis: major events; cytokinesis; contractile ring.

3. Cell cycle: phases of cell cycle; major events; G_0

4. Control of cell cycle: cyclin; cyclin-dependent kinase (CDK); CDK inhibitor; MPF; anaphase promoting complex.

5. Cell cycle checkpoint.

6. Cell cycle and diseases: oncogene and tumor suppressor gene.

Chapter 14　Germ Cells and Fertilization

1. The development of germ cells: sperm and oocyte.

2. Fertilization and medicine.

3. The process of fertilization.

4. Assisted reproductive technology.

Chapter 15　Cell Differentiation

1. The concept of cell differentiation.

2. The potential of cell differentiation in development: totipotent cell; pluripotent cell; unipotent cell.

3. Cell determination.

4. Cell differentiation and cell plasticity: dedifferentiation; trans-differentiation; cellular reprogramming.

5. Temporal-spatial specificity of cell differentiation.

6. The molecular mechanism of cell differentiation: cytoplasmic factors of the oocyte; differential gene expression; the regulation of non-coding RNA; house-keeping gene; luxury gene.

7. Factors influencing cell differentiation: cell-cell interaction; embryonic induction; the effect of hormones; the influence of environment.

8. Cell differentiation and medicine.

Chapter 16　Cell Senescence and Cell Death

1. Cell senescence: manifestations; theories of cell senescence.

2. Cell senescence and diseases.

3. Types of cell death: necrosis; apoptosis.

4. Apoptosis: morphological changes; biochemical changes; anoikis.

5. Factors influencing apoptosis: inducing factors; inhibiting factors.

6. Molecular mechanisms of apoptosis: Bcl-2; Ced; ICE; p53; Fas/FasL; c-myc.

7. Apoptotic pathways: death receptor-mediated pathway; mitochondrion-mediated pathway.

8. Importance of apoptosis in human diseases.

9. Autophagy: macroautophagy; microautophagy; chaperone-mediated autophagy.

10. Processes and control of autophagy.

11. Autophagy and medicine.

Chapter 17　Stem Cells in Tissue Maintenance and Regeneration

1. Types of stem cells: embryonic stem cell; adult stem cell; totipotent stem cell, pluripotent stem cell and unipotent stem cell.

2. Morphological and biochemical characters of stem cells: morphologically similar with initial cells; activation of telomerase; expression of specific makers of stem cell (SSEA-1, AP); slow proliferation rate; self-renewal.

3. Cellular reprogramming and induced pluripotent stem cell (iPS).

4. Differentiation features of stem cells: lineage limitation; plasticity.

5. Niches of stem cells: secreted factors including Wnt, Hedgehog, PDGF, and BMP signaling pathways; integral membrane protein; integrin.

6. Biological features of embryonic stem cells.

7. Adult stem cells: hematopoietic stem cells; mesenchymal stem cells; neural stem cells; liver stem cells; spermatogonial stem cells.

8. Stem cell and medicine.

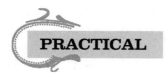

PRACTICAL

The laboratory work is designed to offer the students an opportunity to take a hands-on experimental approach towards understanding the important concepts and mechanisms of cell biology. The laboratory exercises can be also aimed to help students to learn the procedures involved in collection, documentation and analysis of scientific data. However, experiments designed to meet these purposes can vary according to the specific equipment of the laboratory or the preference of the instructors.

Attendance in lab is mandatory. Students are not given a make-up laboratory exercise under any circumstance. Students are required to complete a lab report in the end of each laboratory exercise. Score can be recorded for each laboratory exercise according to students'performance and the reports submitted. The score for laboratory work can be given separately or combined into the total course grade of cell biology.

Specific topics could include the following, while detailed experimental protocols can vary in distinct laboratories.

1. Microscopy.

2. Scientific units of measurement.

3. Micropipetting.

4. Use of the spectrophotometer and pH meter.

5. Cell culture.

6. Antibody-based assay (ELISA).

7. Density gradient centrifugation.

8. Reverse transcription-polymerase chain reaction (RT-PCR).

9. Mitochondrial function.

10. Cell signaling (e.g., action of hormones).

11. Bioinformatics.

MEDICAL ETHICS
医学伦理学

Chief Editors（主编）
Cao Yongfu（曹永福） Shandong University（山东大学）
Li yong（李勇） Nanjing Medical University（南京医科大学）

Deputy Chief Editors（副主编）
Wang Yunling（王云岭） Shandong University（山东大学）
Wu Xuesong（吴雪松） Harbin Medical University（哈尔滨医科大学）

Editors（编委）（按姓氏拼音排序）
Cao Yongfu（曹永福） Shandong University（山东大学）
Li yong（李勇） Nanjing Medical University（南京医科大学）
Sun Hongliang（孙宏亮） Dalian Medical University（大连医科大学）
Wang Yunling（王云岭） Shandong University（山东大学）
Wu Xuesong（吴雪松） Harbin Medical University（哈尔滨医科大学）
Zheng Linjuan（郑林娟） Shandong University（山东大学）

Secretary（秘书）
Zheng Linjuan（郑林娟） Shandong University（山东大学）

Course Description

Medical ethics is a professional curriculum in the specialties of clinical medicine in China.

Medical ethics course focuses on the social, ethical and legal issues in the bio-medical research and medical profession. These issues include the codes and guidelines of medical ethics, the bio-med-ethical principles, the virtues of the health professions, the theories of medical ethics such as teleology, deontology and virtue ethics. The course involves many bio-medical ethical issues such as ethical decision-making, the relationship between doctor and patient, institutional review board(IRB), informed consent, privacy and confidentiality, the beginning of life, the death and dying(euthanasia and hospice care) and so on.

Therefore, medical ethics is an essential course in the clinical medical curriculum.

Objectives

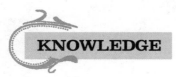

KNOWLEDGE

At the end of the course, the MBBS students shall be able to:
1. To know well the foundation knowledge of bio-medical ethics.
2. To develop their moral personality and medical professionalism.

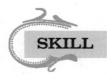

SKILL

At the end of the course, the student shall be able to have the ability of medical ethical decision-making and revalue their medical ethical behavior.

Teaching and Learning Methods

1. Teaching theories.
2. Class discussion.
3. To watch audio-visual materials.

Recommended Textbooks

Albert R. Jonsen. 1998. The Birth of Bioethics[M]. New York: Oxford University Press.

Mark Timmons. 2010. Disputed Moral Issues: A Reader[M]. 2th ed. New York: Oxford University Press.

Tom L. Beauchamp, James F. Childress. 2001. Principles of Biomedical Ethics[M]. 5th ed. New York: Oxford University Press.

Schedule Table

Chapter	Contents	Hours	Chapter	Contents	Hours
1	Introduction	4	5	Medical Professionalism	2
2	Ethical Theories	2	6	The Ethics of Procreation and Eugenics	2
3	Principles of Bio-medicine Ethics	2	7	Assisted Reproductive Technology and Medical Ethics	2
4	Doctor-patient Relationship	2	8	The Morality of Abortion	2

Continued

Chapter	Contents	Hours	Chapter	Contents	Hours
9	The Ethics of Death and Hospice	2	13	The Ethics of Bio-medical Research Involving Human Subjects	2
10	Euthanasia	2	14	The Ethics of Public Health	2
11	The Ethics of Human Organ Transplantation	2	15	Medical Ethics Committee	2
12	The Ethical Treatment of Animals	2		Total	32

Course Contents

Chapter 1　Introduction

1. Ethics and medical ethics.
(1) Definition and types of ethics.
(2) Definition of medical ethics.
(3) The relationship between medical ethics and medicine.
2. The three development phases of medical ethics.
(1) Ancient medical morals.
(2) Modern medical ethics.
(3) Bioethics.
3. What does medical ethics research?
(1) What is morality?
(2) What is ethic?
(3) The research object of medical ethics.
4. Why and how to learn medical ethics?

Chapter 2　Ethical Theories

1. Consequentialism.
(1) Definition of consequentialism.
(2) Essential features of consequentialism.
(3) Utilitarianism.
The principle of utility; hedonistic utilitarianism; perfectionist utilitarianism.
2. Kantian moral theory.
(1) Golden rule.
(2) The humanity formulation (ends and means).
(3) The universal law formulation.
3. Virtue ethics.
(1) Definition of virtue ethics.
(2) A short list of moral virtues and their corresponding vices.
4. Natural law theory.
(1) Introduction of natural law theory.
(2) Theory of Intrinsic value (according to Aquinas's version).
(3) The basic principle of natural law theory.

5. Rights-based moral theory.

(1) Rights: some basic elements.

(2) Categories of rights.

(3) Rights and moral theory.

Chapter 3　Principles of Bio-medicine Ethics

1. The background of the principles of bio-medical ethics.

2. The principle of respect.

(1) Autonomy of the patients.

(2) Dignity of the patients.

(3) Privacy and confidentiality of the patients.

3. The principle of nonmaleficence.

(1) What is nonmaleficence?

(2) Rules supported by the principle of nonmaleficence.

4. The principle of beneficence.

(1) four elements (according to William Frankena).

(2) The doctrine of Double Effect.

(3) Conflicts between autonomy and beneficence.

5. The principle of justice.

(1) The formal principle of justice (Aristotle).

(2) The material principle of justice.

Chapter 4　Doctor-patient relationship

1. Nature of the doctor-patient relationship.

2. The type of doctor-patient relationship.

3. The moral character of the physician-patient relationship.

(1) The both sides of the doctor and the patient have the coherence of the benefits.

(2) The trait of imbalance and asymmetry.

(3) Conclusion.

4. Physicians'right and their obligation.

5. Patients'right and their obligation.

(1) *Patient's bill of rights* (American Hospital Association).

(2) *Declaration of Lisbon on the Rights of the Patient* (World Medical Association).

(3) Some important rights and obligations of patients.

6. How to build a harmonious doctor-patient relationship?

Chapter 5　Medical Professionalism

1. Professionalism and Medical Professionalism.

2. Ways to teach professionalism.

(1) To setting expectations.

(2) To performing assessments.

(3) To remediating inappropriate behaviors.

(4) To preventing inappropriate behaviors.

(5) To implementing a cultural change.

3. Medical Professionalism in the New Millennium: A Physician Charter.

(1) Fundamental principles.

(2) A set of professional responsibilities.

4. Declaration on Chinese physician.

5. Why should we promote medical professionalism?

(1) professional commitment.

(2) self-regulation of the medical doctor association.

Chapter 6   The Ethics of Procreation and Healthy Birth

1. Planned parenthood(birth control) and family planning.

(1) two typical population theories.

(2) Procreation's characteristics.

(3) Possibility of population control.

(4) Chinese policy of planned parenthood and other countries'policy.

2. Healthy birth.

(1) Definition and Types of healthy birth.

(2) Some lessons from Eugenics.

(3) Some moral principles of healthy birth.

Chapter 7   Assisted Reproductive Technology and Medical Ethics

1. Definition of assisted reproductive technology (ART).

2. Types of ART.

(1) Artificial insemination.

(2) In vitro fertilization and embryo transfer (IVF, test tube baby).

(3) Sperm bank, egg bank, embryo bank and surrogate mother.

3. The ethical problems of ART.

(1) ART is unnatural.

(2) ART causes confusion of human ethical relations. Such as "who is mother?"

(3) IVF damages the marital relationship.

(4) Can we buy or sell sperm\ovum freely?

(5) Can a single female have right to use ART?

4. Ethical principles of ART.

Chapter 8   The Morality of Abortion

1. The Definition of Abortion.

2. The moral status of the embryo.

3. Should embryos be used in medical research?

4. Reasons for seeking an abortion.

(1) Therapeutic reasons.

(2) Healthy birth reasons.

(3) Humanitarian reasons: incest or rape.

(4) Social and economic reasons of Abortion debate: Is abortion ever morally

permissible?

5. The legality of abortion: the 1973 U.S. Supreme Court decision in Roe v. Wade.

Chapter 9　The Ethics of Death and Hospice

1. Determination of death.

(1) Traditional criteria of death.

(2) The new criteria of death—brain death.

(3) Persistent Vegetative State.

(4) The ethics on determination of death.

2. Death education.

(1) Life and death is a natural law.

(2) Religious explanation of death.

(3) Confucian attitude of death.

(4) Why and how to stady death education?

3. Hospice care.

(1) Definition of hospice care.

(2) Psychological characteristics of dying people.

(3) History and actuality of hospice care.

(4) The ethical values of hospice care.

Chapter 10　Euthanasia

1. Definition of euthanasia.

2. Types of euthanasia.

(1) Active Euthanasia and Passive Euthanasia.

(2) Voluntary Euthanasia, Non-voluntary Euthanasia and Involuntary　Euthanasia (murder).

(3) Physician-assisted suicide and advance directives.

3. The case of Terri Schiavo.

4. Arguments supporting the morality of euthanasia.

(1) Mercy.

(2) Gold rule: Do unto others as you would have them do unto you.

(3) Human dignity.

(4) Human rights.

5. Arguments opposing the morality of euthanasia.

(1) The sacred life.

(2) We can't really judge that a patient's condition is hopeless.

6. Legislation of Euthanasia.

Chapter 11　The Ethics of Human Organ Transplantation

1. Definition and types of the human organ transplantation.

2. History and actuality of the human organ transplantation.

3. Problems of human organ transplantation.

(1) which circumstance could a volunteer donor be considered free from undue

influence?

(2) Dose the law permit operation which mutilate the donor for the advantage of another person?

(3) What special protection must be given to minors, people of low intelligence, or prisoners in regard to clinical trials or donation of tissue?

(4) To what extent must a community underwrite the cost, however great, of the latest means of sustaining life?

(5) The organ shortage.

3. The source\supply of organs.

(1) Voluntary donation (which includes deceased-donor and living-donor).

(2) Presumed Consent.

(3) Marketing of organs or buying and selling them for compensation.

(4) Fetal organ.

(5) Animal organs.

(6) The artificial organs.

4. Selection of patients for a scarce resource.

(1) "God committee": a Medical Advisory Committee; an Admissions and Policy Committee.

(2) Medical standard (the most appropriate donor-recipient match, urgency, etc.).

(3) Donors'will.

(4) The order of registration.

(5) Other consideration: relative likelihood of success, life-expectancy, family role, potential future contribution to society, past services rendered to society, etc.

5. The ethical principles of human organ transplantation.

(1) The patients health first.

(2) The only choice.

(3) Voluntary, free and prohibition of commercialization.

(4) Informed consent.

(5) Respect for and protection of the donor.

(6) Keeping confideutiality.

(7) Justice.

(8) Ethical review.

Chapter 12　The Ethical Treatment of Animals

1. Definition of animal experiment.

2. The History of animal experiment.

3. Types of experiment.

4. Views on animal experiment.

(1) The miserable torture of vivisection places the body in an unnatural state.

(2) Does the benefit to humans justify the harm to animals?

(3) Animals are inferior to humans and so different that results from animals can't be applied to humans.

(4) Experiments on animals are necessary to advance medical and biological

knowledge.

(5) Experiments causes suffering to animals.

(6) Do animals have rights?

5. Ethics on animal Welfare.

(1) The Three Rs (reduction, refinement and replacement).

(2) Institutional Animal Care and Use Committees (IACUCs).

(3) Animals welfare(five freedoms).

Chapter 13　The Ethics of Bio-medical Research Involving Human Subjects

1. Definition of bio-medical research involving human subjects.

2. Types.

(1) Physician self-experimentation.

(2) Voluntary participation (Patients and the healthy volunteer).

(3) Deceptive human trials.

(4) Compulsive\forced human trials.

3. History and lessons of bio-medical research Involving human subjects.

(1) Yellow fever—20th century.

(2) The Nazi experiments—World War II.

(3) Tuskegee syphilis experiment.

4. Ethical principles of bio-medical research involving human subjects.

(1) *Nuremberg Code*.

(2) *The Helsinki Declaration*.

(3) *The Belmont Report*.

(4) Rights of human subjects.

(5) *International Ethical Guidelines for Biomedical Research Involving Human Subjects 2016*.

(6) Some moral principles of bio-medical research involving human subjects.

Chapter 14　the Ethics of Public Health

1. The concepts and definitions.

(1) Definition of public health.

(2) Definition of public health ethics.

(3) the difference between public health ethics and bioethics.

2. History of public health ethics.

(1) History of public health ethics in USA.

(2) History of public health ethics in China.

3. Public health ethical principles.

(1) Ethical guidelines from the Public Health Leadership Society and adopted by the American Public Health Association.

(2) *The Public Health Professional's Oath*.

4. Ethics in the prevention and control of diseases.

(1) Ethical issues on the prevention and control of infectious disease.

(2) Ethical issues on the prevention and control of chronic disease.

5. Ethics in public health emergencies.

6. Ethics in Health Care Reform.

(1) Ethics in US health care reform.

(2) Ethics in Chinese health care reform.

Chapter 15　Medical Ethics Committee

1. What is medical ethics committee (MEC)?

(1) Hospital ethics committee.

(2) Institutional review board (IRB).

(3) National Commission for the Protection of Human Subjects of Bio-medical and Behavioral Research.

2. The historical background of formation of MEC.

3. The function of MEC.

(1) Clinical ethics consultation.

(2) Ethics education.

(3) Ethical review.

4. Reflection and questions.

(1) May a clinical investigator be an IRB member?

(2) Does the IRB have diversity of members?

(3) Why should we set up IRB or MEC?

5. Procedure of IRB.

To applicate; to review; to approve or not.

MEDICAL PSYCHOLOGY

医学心理学

Chief Editors（主编）
Pan Fang（潘芳） Shandong University（山东大学）
Zhao Xudong（赵旭东） Tongji University（同济大学）

Deputy Chief Editors（副主编）
Wang Wei（王伟） Zhejiang University（浙江大学）
Qian Ming（钱明） Tianjin Medical University（天津医科大学）

Editors（编委）（按姓氏拼音排序）
Di Min（狄敏） Tianjin Medical University（天津医科大学）
Liu Dexiang（刘德祥） Shandong University（山东大学）
Lu Yanxia（鲁燕霞） Zhejiang University（浙江大学）
Pan Fang（潘芳） Shandong University（山东大学）
Qian Ming（钱明） Tianjin Medical University（天津医科大学）
Wang Wei（王伟） Zhejiang University（浙江大学）
Zhang Hongjing（张红静） Shandong University（山东大学）
Zhang Qian（张茜） Shandong University（山东大学）
Zhao Xudong（赵旭东） Tongji University（同济大学）
Zhou Shiyu（周世昱） Dalian Medical University（大连医科大学）

Course Description

Medical psychology is a subject which studies the psychological problems arising in the practice of medicine. Medical psychology focuses on the psychological aspects of medicine such as pain, terminal illness, bereavement, disability, and reactions to medical advice. The research field of medical psychology includes the interactions between mental factors and health / disease. Medical psychology addresses the behaviors are important factors in onset, diagnosis, treatment and prevention of psycho-somatic diseases and mental disorders. The theories of medical psychology include psychoanalysis, behaviorism theory, cognition theory and humanistic theory. It uses the observation method, survey method, experiment method, mental test and other methods to study psychological activities.

The purposes for medical psychology study are to master the basic theory of medical psychology and skills including psychological diagnosis, psychological intervention and health promotion, as well as patients-doctor communication and to provide theoretical basis for clinical practice.

Objectives

At the end of the course, the MBBS students shall be able to:

1. To master the basic principles of medical psychology.

2. To master the basic knowledge of medical psychological theories, study methods, psychological evaluation and psychological intervention.

3. To understand the process and mechanism of stress and disease.

4. To master the basic knowledge and methods of health promotion.

5. To master the knowledge and skills of communication between patients and doctors.

Teaching and Learning Methods

Teaching medical psychology to medical students is provided with the help of lectures and tutorials that deal with the principles of mental tests, psychological intervention and communication. Group discussion and presentation are used in learning.

Recommended Textbooks

Bruce E. Compas, Ian H. Gotlib. 2002. Introduction to Clinical Psychology [M]. New York: McGraw-Hill Higher Education.

Lewis R. Aiken, Gary Groth-Marnat. 2005. Psychological testing and assessment. 12th ed. Boston: Allyn and Bacon.

Marvin R. Goldfried, Gerald C. Davison. 1994. Cilnical Behavior Therapy [M]. New York: John Wiley and Sons.

Richard R. Bootain, Joan Ross Acocella, Lauren B. Alloy. 1993. Abnormal Psychology Current Perspectives [M]. 6th ed. New York: McGraw-Hill.

Robert S. Feldman. 2003. Essentials of Understanding Psychology [M]. 5th ed. New York: McGraw-Hill Higher Education.

Schedule Table

Chapter	Contents	Hours	Chapter	Contents	Hours
1	Introduction	2	7	Clinical psychological evaluation	4
2	The theories of medical psychology	2	8	Psychological therapy	4
3	Basic psychology	8	9	Psychological counseling	2
4	Stress and health	4	10	The relationship between patients and doctor, patients role	4
5	Psychosomatic disease	2	11	Mental health	2
6	Psychological disorders	2		Total	36

Course Contents

Chapter 1　Introduction

1. Concept of medical psychology and its role in medicine.

(1) Concept of medical psychology.

(2) Medical model and the role of medical psychology in medicine.

2. Objectives, tasks and subfields of medical psychology.

(1) Objectives of medical psychology.

(2) Tasks of medical psychology.

(3) Subfields and relative fields of medical psychology.

3. Research methods of medical psychology.

(1) Experimental research.

(2) Psychological testing.

(3) Survey.

(4) Observational study.

(5) Prospective, retrospective longitudinal, cross-sectional study.

Chapter 2　Theories of Medical Psychology

1. Psychoanalysis.

2. Behaviorism.

3. Physiological psychology.

4. Humanistic psychology.

5. Cognitive psychology.

Chapter 3　Basic Psychology

1. The science of psychology.

(1) The concept and fields of psychology.

(2) The concept and classifications of mental activities.

(3) The essentials of mental activities (biology and culture establish both the possibilities and the constraints within which people think, feel, and act.).

2. The cognitive process.

(1) Sensation and perception.

(2) Learning and memory.

(3) Thinking.

3. Emotion.

(1) The concept of emotion, the basic emotions.

(2) The biological basis of emotion.

(3) Communicating emotion such as voice quality, facial expression, body language, personal space and gestures.

(4) The theories of emotion.

4. Willed Process.

(1) The concept and characteristics of will.

(2) Bad will characteristics.

5. Need, motive, frustration and defense mechanisms.

(1) The concept of need and a hierarchy of needs.

(2) The concept of motive and perspectives on motive.

(3) The motive conflicts and frustration.

(4) The defense mechanisms.

6. Mental ability and intelligence.

(1) The concept and classifications of mental ability.

(2) Theories of mental ability.

7. Personality.

(1) The concept and characteristics of personality.

(2) Temperament.

(3) Character.

(4) Theories of personality.

Chapter 4　Stress and Health

Psychological Stress.

(1) The concept of psychological stress.

(2) The theory of Stress.

(3) Stress and Health.

Chapter 5　Psychosomatic Diseases

1. The concept of psychosomatic diseases.

2. The opinions of modern medicine on the relationship between mind and body.

3. Pathogenic theory of psychosomatic diseases.

4. Common psychosomatic diseases.

Chapter 6　Psychological Disorders

1. Introduction of psychological disorders.

(1) Definition of psychological disorders.

(2) Basic standards on identifying abnormal behavior.

(3) Perspectives on psychological disorders.

2. Major psychological disorders.

(1) Depressive disorders.

(2) Anxiety disorders.

(3) Somatic symptom and related disorders.

(4) Personality disorders.

(5) Obsessive-compulsive and related disorders.

(6) Trauma and stressor-related disorders.

Chapter 7　Clinical Psychological Evaluation

1. Introduction to clinical psychological evaluation.

(1) An overview of psychological evaluation.

(2) The methods for clinical psychological evaluation.

2. Psychological test.

(1) The concept of psychological test.

(2) Classifications of commonly used psychological tests.

(3) The basic characteristics of standardized psychological test.

(4) The selection of psychological tests.

3. Commonly used psychological tests and rating scales.

(1) Intelligence tests.

(2) Personality tests.

(3) Rating scales.

Chapter 8　Psychotherapy

1. Introduction of psychotherapy.

(1) Definition of psychotherapy.

(2) Psychotherapy applicable.

2. Psychoanalysis.

(1) Psychoanalysis.

(2) Development of psychoanalysis.

3. Behavior therapies.

(1) Basic principles of behavior modification.

(2) Behavior therapies.

4. Cognitive therapies.

(1) Rational-emotive therapy.

(2) Beck's cognitive therapy.

5. Humanistic therapy.

(1) Basic concept of client-centered therapy.

(2) Client-centered therapy.

6. Other therapies.

(1) Meditation and hypnosis.

(2) Morita therapy.

(3) Biofeedback therapy.

Chapter 9　Psychological Counseling

1. The basics of psychological counseling.

(1) The concept of psychological counseling.

(2) The scope of psychological counseling.

(3) The goals of psychological counseling.

(4) The principles of psychological counseling.

2. The targets and ways of psychological counseling.

(1) The targets and content of psychological counseling.

(2) The ways of psychological counseling.

3. The techniques of psychological counseling.

(1) Involvement techniques (listening).

(2) Influencing techniques.

(3) Non-verbal techniques.

Chapter 10　The Relationship between Doctor and Patient, Patients Role

1. Doctor-patient relationship.

(1) The concept of doctor-patient relationship.

(2) The three modes of doctor -patient relationship.

(3) The forms and levels of doctor -patient communication.

(4) The compliance of patients and affecting factors.

(5) The problems in doctor -patient communication.

2. The roles and behaviors of patients.

(1) The characteristics of patients'roles.

(2) Adaptation of patients'roles.

(3) Seeking behaviors of medical services.

(4) Psychological problems and needs of patients.

Chapter 11　Mental Health

1. Introduction.

(1) The concept and implications of mental health.

(2) The responsibilities of mental health practice.

(3) The research methods and scientific approaches of mental health.

2. Mental health of childhood.

3. Mental health of adolescence and youth.

4. Mental health of middle-aged adults.

5. Mental health of old-aged adults.

SYSTEMIC ANATOMY

系统解剖学

Chief Editors（主编）

Sun Chenyou（孙臣友） Wenzhou Medical University（温州医科大学）

Lü Guangming（吕广明） Nantong University（南通大学）

Zhang Ping（张平） Tianjin Medical University（天津医科大学）

Deputy Chief Editors（副主编）

Cui Huairui（崔怀瑞） Wenzhou Medical University（温州医科大学）

He Guiqiong（贺桂琼） Chongqing Medical University（重庆医科大学）

Editors（编委）（按姓氏拼音排序）

Cui Huairui（崔怀瑞） Wenzhou Medical University（温州医科大学）

Ding Maochao（丁茂超） Wenzhou Medical University（温州医科大学）

Ding Yuqiang（丁玉强） Tongji University（同济大学）

He Guiqiong（贺桂琼） Chongqing Medical University（重庆医科大学）

Lü Guangming（吕广明） Nantong University（南通大学）

Mao Yihua（毛以华） Wenzhou Medical University（温州医科大学）

Sun Chenyou（孙臣友） Wenzhou Medical University（温州医科大学）

Zhang Ping（张平） Tianjin Medical University（天津医科大学）

Zhang Jianse（张建色） Wenzhou Medical University（温州医科大学）

Zhou Peng（周鹏） Wenzhou Medical University（温州医科大学）

Course Description

Systemic anatomy is the subject which describes the normal organ morphology and structures, their physiological function, and growth and development of human body mainly according to the body's organ function system such as the motor system, digestive system, respiratory system, urinary system, reproductive system, vascular system, sensory organs, nervous system and endocrine system, etc. Systemic anatomy is one of the important, indispensable, professional and compulsory basic courses for medical students. The purpose of learning systemic anatomy is to enable medical students to master the normal structure of the organs in each system of human body and their adjacent relationship, and the rules of growth and development and their functional significance. The most important task of systemic anatomy is to lay a solid foundation for learning other medical courses. On the basis of grasping the normal morphology and structures of human organs, medical students can correctly identify their normal and abnormal conditions, understand their physiological phenomena and pathological changes, and finally make the correct prevention, diagnosis and treatment for diseases. There are one third of the medical terms which are derived from anatomy, so anatomy is an important cornerstone to learn various disciplines.

Like other basic disciplines, systemic anatomy also makes obvious progress with the times advancing. With the innovation of the scientific and technical methods, promotion of adjacent disciplines with each other, it makes ancient systemic anatomy expand continuously in the research scope, deepen in the research level, and produce many marginal disciplines.

Objectives

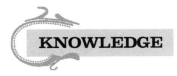

KNOWLEDGE

At the end of the course, the MBBS students shall be able.

1. To master the terms about describing directions and anatomical planes that are associated with the human body.

2. To master the composition (bones, joints and muscles) and describe the names, locations and structures of the bones, joints and principal skeletal muscles of the human body.

3. To understand the composition of alimentary system and be familiar with the division of alimentary canal and the composition of alimentary gland; grasp the composition and function of lingual papillae and muscles, and the classification and structure of the teeth, and the composition of salivary glands and the opening of large salivary glands; be familiar with the division and function of the mouth, the composition and structure of palate, the dental formula and the division and structure of tongue; understand the structure of the lips and cheeks, and the composition of the peridontium; grasp the position, portion and structure of pharynx, and the composition and function of the pharyngeal lymphatic ring; grasp the position, portion, narrow and structure of esophagus; grasp the formation and portion of the stomach, and be familiar with the position, relation and structure of the stomach; be familiar with the composition of small intestine, and the portion, flexure and structure of duodenum; understand the position and structural feature of jejunum and ileum; grasp three structural features of cecum and colon; be familiar with the composition of large intestine, the position and surface projection of vermiform appendix, the portion and structural feature of colon, and the structural feature of rectum and anal canal; grasp the formation and lobulation of the liver; be familiar with the position and relation of the liver; understand the composition of intrahepatic duct and segmentation of the liver; grasp the composition of the extrahepatic biliary duct, the portion and structure of gallbladder, and surface projection

of the fundus of gallbladder; be familiar with the bile elimination pathway; be familiar with the position, portion and structure of the pancreas.

4. To understand the composition and function of respiratory system; be familiar with the composition of the upper and lower respiratory tract; grasp the position, portion and structure of the nasal cavity, and the composition, position, structural feature and opening of the paranasal sinuses; understand the portion of the nose and the formation of the external nose; grasp the composition and structure of laryngeal cartilage, and the portion and structure of laryngeal cavity; be familiar with the connections (joint, conus elasticus, ligament and membrane) of the larynx; understand the position and composition of the larynx, and the composition and function of laryngeal muscles; grasp the structural feature of the right and left principal bronchus; understand the position and portion of trachea; be familiar with the position, formation and structure of the lung; grasp the division of pleura and the pleural recess; be familiar with the surface projection of the pleurae and lungs, and the concept and structural feature of the pleura and pleural cavity; be familiar with the concept and division of mediastinum.

5. To name and locate the organs that compose urinary system; explain what the terms including renal hilum, renal pedicle, renal sinus and renal region refer to; locate the renal capsule, renal cortex, renal medulla, renal pyramids, minor calyces, major calyces, renal sinus, renal pelvis and ureter; describe the anatomy of the ureters, urinary bladder and urethra and discuss the differences between male and female urethras.

6. To grasp the composition and function of male or female reproductive system; grasp the position, structure and function of testes; grasp the position and function of epididymis; grasp the conducting ducts of spermatic fluid; understand the position and function of scrotum; understand the composition and function of penis; grasp the shape, position and fixing device of ovaries; grasp the position, shape and subdivision of uterine tube and understand the place of tubal sterilization and fertilization; grasp the position, shape, subdivision and fixing device of uterus; grasp the shape and position vagina, understand the relationship between posterior fornix of vagina and rectouterine pouch and know about its clinical significance; grasp the structure of the mammary glands and track the flow of milk from the alveoli to the nipple; grasp the definition of perineum and describe its sub-regions; grasp the position of ischiorectal fossa and know its clinical significance; know about the composition and function of urogenital diaphragm and pelvic diaphragm.

7. To grasp the definition of peritoneum and peritoneal cavity and know about the functions of peritoneum; grasp the relationship between the abdominopelvic viscera and peritoneum; grasp the position and formation of lesser omentum and greater omentum; grasp the position of omental bursa and omental foramen; know about the name and position of the attachment of mesentery and the ligaments of liver, spleen and stomach; know about the peritoneal recesses and folds; grasp the name and position of peritoneal pouches.

8. To grasp the composition of cardiovascular system and the circulative routes

of blood; be familiar with the structural characteristics of blood vessels and the anastomoses of blood vessels; grasp the location, size, orientation, the external and internal structures of the heart, and the conduction system of the heart, and the vessels of the heart; be familiar with the fibrous skeleton of the heart, the wall of the heart and the pericardium of the heart; name the branches of the ascending aorta, aortic arch, thoracic aorta, and abdominal aorta, and denote what body region they supply with blood; list the differences between the venous circuit and the arterial circuit; name the longest vein in the body and the venipuncture site; grasp the main tributaries of superior vena cava, inferior vena cava and hepatic portal vein; name and locate the organs that compose the lymphatic system on a diagram; explain what the terms lymphatic vessels, regional lymph node, cisterna chili, thoracic duct and right lymphatic duct refer to; describe the anatomy of the spleen, axillary lymph nodes and inguinal lymph nodes.

9. To define the term "sensory organ", and classify and distinguish the three kinds of receptors; explain what the terms walls of eyeball including fibrous tunic, vascular tunic and retina, and explain the contents of the eyeball including chamber of eye, lens and vitreous body, and locate the lacrimal gland and lacrimal passages; understand the roles of lens and extraocular muscles; explain the terms including tympanic membrane, walls of the tympanic cavity, auditory tube, bony and membranous labyrinths, and understand and master the roles of spiral organ (Organ of Corti), macula utriculi, macula sacculi and ampullary crests.

10. To grasp the name, location, morphology and structure of endocrine organs such as hypophysis, thyroid gland, parathyroid gland, suprarenal gland, thymus and pancreas; understand main function of these endocrine organs.

11. To master the terminology of nervous system, and name the two major divisions of the nervous system, and understand the basic components of reflex arc and the function the nervous system; grasp the external structure of the spinal cord in terms of its length, start, end, number of segments and enlarged areas; name the terminal point of the spinal cord; fully understand the cross-sectional anatomy of the spinal cord; compare and contrast ascending and descending tracts, and discuss the general characteristics of nerve tracts; grasp the important structures in the three major parts of the brain stem, and name of cranial nerves attached to the brainstem; and the names of nuclei of cranial nerves and their functions and fiber connections in the brain stem; understand the important non-cranial nerve nuclei of brain stem; grasp the characters of important long ascending and descending tracts in the brain stem; understand three important parts in the cerebellum and their main functions; understand major compositions of diencephalon and their main functions; grasp the main sulci and gyri on the superolateral and medial surfaces of the cerebrum; name the five lobes of cerebrum; understand the limbic lobe and limbic system; grasp the important function organization of the cerebral cortex; understand the main composition of basal nuclei, and grasp the paleostriatum and neostriatum; grasp the three parts of internal capsule and their fibers projection; understand the four parts of lateral ventricles; understand the characteristics of spinal nerves in terms

of number and composition; grasp the areas that anterior braches of the thoracic nerves innervate, and the main branches of four major nerve plexuses and their innervations; grasp the name of the twelve pairs of cranial nerves, and innervations of motor and mixed cranial nerve; understand the fiber components of each cranial nerve and their courses; designate them by Roman numeral, and designate them as sensory, motor, or mixed cranial nerves; grasp the comparison of the characteristics of the somatic and visceral motor nerves, and sympathetic and parasympathetic division of the autonomic nervous system (ANS); grasp the names and locations of three or four orders of neurons and their fibers or fiber decussation in main sensory pathways; master the pyramidal systems in motor pathways; understand the symptoms after injury of the nervous pathways; master the names of meninges of brain and spinal cord, and understand their functions; master the main arteries supplying the brain, and understand the blood vessels of spinal cord; master the circulation route of cerebrospinal fluid (CSF).

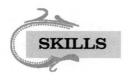

SKILLS

At the end of the course, the student shall be able to grasp the following skills by using the atlas, models and specimen in the practical class:

1. To palpate the important bony landmarks in the living body: 7th cervical vertebra; spinous process of the thoracic and lumbar vertebra; jugular notch; sternal angle; costal arch; xiphoid process; sacral hiatus; sacral horns; promontory of sacrum; spine of scapula; inferior angle of scapula; acromion of scapula; clavicle; greater tubercle of humerus; medial and lateral epicondyle of humerus; head of radius; olecranon of ulna; styloid process of radius and ulna; pisiform bone; head of metacarpal bone; iliac crest; anterior superior iliac spine; tubercle of iliac crest; posterior superior iliac crest; ischial tuberosity; greater trochanter; patella; tibial tuberosity; fibular head; medial and lateral malleolus; calcaneal tuberosity; external occipital protuberance; mastoid process; zygomatic arch; superciliary arch; angle of mandible; hyoid.

2. To identify the structures of main direct and indirect articulations in each part of the body.

3. To palpate the muscular marks in the living body: masseter; temporalis; sternocleidomastoid; trapezius; erector spinae; pectoralis major; rectus abdominis; deltoid; biceps brachii; tendon of the flexor carpi radialis, palmaris longus, flexor carpi ulnaris, abductor pollicis longus, extensor pollicis brevis, extensor pollicis longus; quadriceps femoris; patellar ligament; gastrocnemius; soleus.

4. To identify the composition of upper and lower digestive tract; the formation, portion and structure of the mouth (lips, cheeks, palate, tongue, teeth and salivary glands), the pharynx, the esophagus, the stomach, the small intestine, the large intestine, the liver, the extra-hepatic biliary ducts and pancreas.

5. To identify the formation and structure of upper respiratory tract (nose, pharynx and larynx), lower respiratory tract (trachea and bronchi), lungs, pleura and mediastinum.

6. To identify the renal hilum, renal capsule, adipose capsule, renal fascia, renal cortex, renal medulla (renal pyramids, renal papilla), renal columns, minor calyx (plural is calyces), major calyx, renal pelvis; identify three parts and three narrow places of ureters; identify the trigone, ureteric orifices and internal urethral orifice of urinary bladder; identify the external urethral orifice, female urethra and male urethra.

7. To observe the testes, scrotum, epididymis, vas (ductus) deferens, seminal vesicle, ejaculatory duct, prostate gland, bulbourethral glands, urethra, and penis; identify the position of female internal genital organs and their relationships; identify the fixing device of ovaries and uterus; identify the subdivision of uterine tube and uterus; observe the female external genital organs; identify the position and structures of mammary glands; identify the boundaries and regions of the perineum.

8. To identify lesser and greater omentum; explore the omental bursa and omental foramen; observe the mesenteries and ligaments of all kinds of organs; explore the hepatorenal recess, rectovesical pouch in male and rectouterine pouch, vesicouterine pouch in female.

9. To observe the models of heart, and identify the external and internal structures of heart; dissect a bovine heart and identify its structures with the instruction of teacher; observe the origin, course and parts of the aorta, and observe the carotid sinus and identify the branches of common carotid artery, subclavian artery and upper limb artery, and observe the arteries of thorax and abdomen, especially celiac trunk, superior mesenteric artery and inferior mesenteric artery, and observe internal iliac artery and its branches, and observe lower limb with arteries, and observe the superior vena and inferior vena cava and their tributaries, especially the hepatic portal vein in the specimen; identify the lymphatic capillaries, afferent lymphatic vessels, efferent lymphatic vessels, lymphatic trunks, lymphatic ducts, lymph nodes, spleen, etc.

10. To identify the cornea, sclera, sinus venosus sclera, chamber of eye, iris, ciliary body, choroid, retina, blind part, blind spot, aqueous humor, lens; identify the auditory and vestibular apparatuses, tympanic cavity, auditory tube, bony and membranous labyrinths, organs of balance and hearing.

11. To identify the endocrine organs such as hypophysis, thyroid gland, parathyroid gland, suprarenal gland, thymus and pancreas.

12. To observe the models of spinal cord and brain, and identify the external and internal main structures of spinal cord; the important structures of three part of brain stem and nuclei of cranial nerves; the external feature of cerebellum and main structures; identify dorsal thalamus, metathalamus, epithalamus and hypothalamus on brain models; identify the main sulci and gyri on the superolateral and medial surfaces of the cerebrum, and five lobes of cerebrum; identify the location of important function organization of the cerebral cortex; identify the basal nuclei and internal capsule on the model of horizontal sections of

cerebrum; observe the models of spinal nerves and cranial nerves, and identify the main spinal nerves and cranial nerves and their important branches; trace the origin, course, termination and their innervations of main spinal nerves such as phrenic nerve, median nerve, ulnar nerve, musculocutaneuous nerve, radial nerve, femoral nerve and sciatic nerve with its two divisions (tibial nerve and common peroneal nerve) in the specimen; observe the fissures, foramens or canals in the internal surface of skull and match the cranial nerves and passages of the skull; by the model, identify the comparisons between the sympathetic and parasympathetic division of the ANS; observe the models of nervous pathways, and identify the name and location of three orders of neurons and their neural fibers in the following nervous pathways: conscious proprioceptive and fine touch pathway of trunk and limbs; pain, temperature and crude touch pathway of trunk and limbs; pain, temperature and crude touch pathway of head and face; visual pathway; pyramidal system; identify the meninges of spinal cord and brain, and cerebral falx, cerebellar tentorium and dural sinuses; identify the main arteries of brain and the composition of Willis circle; show the students the circulation of CSF by model.

Teaching and Learning Methods

With regard to the methodology of teaching and learning, it varies depending on the individual teacher.

Theory: The lectures in the systemic anatomy are carried out with the aid of multimedia lectures. Some important structures in each system are discussed in detail by using power point (PPT) containing the diagrams or pictures, the animation or flash, the video demo, etc.

Practical: Many strategies are used including the atlas, models, specimens and video tapes to show the student important structures of each organ. In addition, the teachers demonstrate the surface markings of important organs to the students on their own bodies.

Recommended Textbooks

Frank H. Netter. 2015. Netter's Atlas of Human Anatomy[M]. Beijing: People's Health Publishing House.

George L. Romanes. 1996. Cunningham's Manual of Practical Anatomy[M]. Vols. I, II & III. 15th ed. London: Oxford University Press.

Keith L. Moore, Anne M R. Agur. 2002. Essential Clinical Anatomy[M]. 2nd ed. Baltimore: Lippincott Williams & Wilkins.

Liu Zhiyu (刘执玉), Ying Dajun (应大君). 2008. Textbook of Systemic Anatomy[M]. 2nd ed. Beijing: Science Press.

Richard Drake, A. Wayne Vogl, Mitchell Adam. 2013. Gray's Basic Anatomy[M]. Beijing: Peking University Medial Press.

Susan Standring. 2004. Gray's Anatomy[M]. 39th ed. London: Churchill Livingstone.

Wang Huaijing (王怀经). 1996. Human Anatomy[M]. 2nd ed. Changchun: Jilin Science and Technology Press.

Schedule Table

Chapter & systems	Contents	Hours	
		Lecture	Practical
1. Introduction	Introduction	2	0
2. Locomotor System	Osteology	1	12
	Arthrology	3	1.5
	Myology	6	1.5
3-9. Splanchnology	Introduction of splanchnology	0.5	3
	Alimentary system	5	
	Respiratory system including mediastinum	4	
	Urinary system	2	
	Reproductive system including mammary gland and perineum	5	
	Peritoneum	2	
10. Cardiovascular System & Lymphatic System	Introduction of angiology	1	2.5
	Heart	3	
	Arteries	3	
	Veins	2	
	Lymphatic system	1.5	
11. Sensory Organs	Introduction of sensory organs	0.5	0.5
	Eyeball	2.5	
	Accessory organ of eye	0.5	
	Vestibulocochlear organ	2	
12-13. Endocrine System & Nervous System	Endocrine system	1	6
	Introduction of nervous system	1.5	
	Spinal cord	3	
	Brain stem	5	
	Cerebellum and diencephalon	3	
	Telencephalon	4	
	Spinal nerve	5	
	Cranial nerve	6	
	Autonomic nervous system	2	
	Nervous pathway	3.5	
	Meanings, blood supply of brain and spinal cord, CSF	3.5	
	Total	84	27

Course Contents

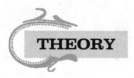

THEORY

Chapter 1　An Introduction to the Anatomy

1. The levels of structural organization: atom, molecule, cell, tissue, organ, system, organism.

2. The anatomical terminology: anatomical position.

3. The anatomical planes or sections: sagital plane, mid-sagital plane, frontal or coronal plane, transverse or horizontal plane, etc.

Chapter 2　Locomotor System

Part Ⅰ. Osteology.

1. The shape, structure, function, chemical compositions and physical properties of bones.

2. The general features and each region of main characteristics in the vertebrae.

3. The formation, general shape and parts of the ribs.

4. The shape and parts of the sternum and sternal angle.

5. The composition, parts, arrangement, position and main shape of the bones of upper limb.

6. The composition, parts, arrangement, position and the main shape of the bones of lower limb.

7. The position, parts and function of skull; the name and the position of each cerebral cranium and facial cranium; the internal surface of the calvaria; the superior, posterior, lateral and anterior view of the cranium; the main structures of the internal and external surfaces of the cranial base; the formation, shape, holes and fissures of orbit; the formation of the bony nasal cavity and the names; the positions and the opening of each paranasal sinuses; the characters of skull at birth and its change after birth.

Part Ⅱ. Arthrology.

1. The classification of articulation; the essential structures and the functions of fibrous joints, cartilaginous joints and synostosis; the essential and accessory structures and their functions of synovial joints; the classification of synovial articulation and the basic movements of joints.

2. The connections of vertebral bodies; the position, shape, structure, function and clinical significance of the intervertebral discs; the connections of vertebral arch; the position and function of the anterior and posterior longitudinal ligaments and the ligaments flava; the lumbosacral joints; the vertebral column as a whole and its movements.

3. The joints between the ribs and the vertebral column, and between the cartilages and the sternum; the costal arch; the composition, form and function of the thorax.

4. The structures and movements of the joints of the girdle of upper limb; the formation, characteristics and movements of main joints of free upper limb.

5. The connection of the girdle of lower limb; the formation and the parts of the bony pelvis; the formation, characteristics and movements of main joints of free lower limb.

6. The main connections of the bones of skull; the structures and movements of the temporomandibular joint.

Part III. Myology.

1. The shape, structure, origin and insertion of skeletal muscle; the relationship among muscle groups; the nomenclature of muscles and supplementary structures of muscles.

2. The names, locations and actions of muscles of head and face.

3. The names, locations and actions of muscles of neck.

4. The names, locations and actions of muscles of trunk; the location, form, action and hiatuses of diaphragm.

5. The names, locations and actions of muscles of upper and lower limbs.

Chapter 3　Splanchnology and Alimentary System

Part I. General description of splanchnology.

1. The general structure of viscera: tubular organ and parenchymatous organ.

2. The reference lines and abdominal regions: reference lines of the thorax, and abdominal regions.

Part II. Alimentary system.

1. Mouth.

(1) The regions of the mouth: oral vestibule and oral cavity proper.

(2) The Lips and cheeks.

(3) The palate: hard palate and soft palate, isthmus of the fauces.

(4) The tongue: surface formation of tongue, papillae of tongue, lingual muscles.

(5) The teeth: structure of teeth, type of teeth, dental formula.

(6) The salivary glands: parotid glands, submandibular glands and sublingual glands.

2. Pharynx.

(1) The nasopharynx.

(2) The oropharynx.

(3) The laryngopharynx.

(4) The pharyngeal structure.

3. Esophagus.

(1) The three parts: cervical part, thoracic part and abdominal part.

(2) The three narrows: superior, middle and inferior narrows.

4. Stomach.

(1) The formation: cardia, pylorus, lesser curvature and greater curvature.

(2) The portions: cardiac, fundus, body and pyloric part, pyloric antrum, pyloric canal, pyloric sphincter.

(3) The position and relations.

(4) The gastric microstructure.

5. Small intestine.

(1) The duodenum: four parts, three flexures, two duodenal papillae, one suspensory ligament.

(2) The jejunum.

(3) The ileum.

6. Large intestine.

(1) The cecum.

(2) The vermiform appendix.

(3) The colon: four parts (ascending colon, transverse colon, descending colon and sigmoid colon), two flexures.

(4) The rectum: two flexures, one rectal ampulla.

(5) The anal canal: anal columns, anus, internal anal sphincter and external anal sphincter.

7. Liver.

(1) The formation: superior and inferior surface; H-shaped fissures (left and right longitudinal fissure, transverse fissure, and porta hepatis).

(2) The lobulation: right lobe, left lobe, quadrate lobe and caudate lobe.

(3) The position and relations.

(4) The hepatic segments: Glisson system and hepatic venous system.

8. Extrahepatic biliary ducts.

(1) The gallbladder: fundus, body, neck and cystic duct.

(2) The biliary ducts: right and left hepatic ducts, common hepatic duct, cystic duct, common bile duct, hepatopancreatic ampulla or ampulla of Vater, sphincter of the hepatopancreatic ampulla or sphincter of Oddi.

9. Pancreas.

(1) The portion: head, neck, body, tail.

(2) The pancreatic duct: main and accessory pancreatic duct.

Chapter 4   Respiratory System and Mediastinum

Part Ⅰ. Respiratory tract.

1. Nose.

(1) The external nose.

(2) The nasal cavity: nasal septum, nasal vestibule and proper nasal cavity, respiratory region and olfactory region, lateral wall of nasal cavity.

(3) The paranasal sinuses: frontal, ethmoidal, sphenoidal and maxillary sinuses.

2. Pharynx.

(1) The nasopharynx: pharyngeal tonsil.

(2) The oropharynx: fauces, palatine and lingual tonsils.

(3) The laryngopharynx or hypopharynx.

3. Larynx.

(1) The cartilages: thyroid cartilage (Adam's apple), epiglottis (glottis), cricoid cartilage, arytenoid cartilages.

(2) The connections: joint, conus elasticus, ligament and membrane.

(3) The muscles.

(4) The ventricular folds or false vocal cords; the vocal folds or true vocal cords.

(5) The laryngeal cavity.

4. Trachea.

(1) The cervical part and thoracic part.

(2) The carina of trachea.

5. Bronchus (plural is bronchi).

(1) The right and left primary bronchi, secondary bronchi or lobar bronchi, tertiary bronchi or segmental bronchi, bronchioles, terminal bronchioles.

(2) The bronchial tree.

Part II. Lungs.

1. The formation: base and apex of lung, costal surface, mediastinal surface or medial surface, hilum, root, cardiac notch, fissures (oblique fissure in both lungs and horizontal fissure in right lung), lobes (superior and inferior lobes in both lungs, middle lobe in right lung).

2. The bronchial tree and segment: bronchopulmonary segments, lobules, respiratory bronchioles, alveolar ducts alveolus (plural is alveoli) and blood supply to lungs.

Part III. Pleura.

1. The concepts: thoracic cavity, pleural membrane (parietal pleura, visceral pleura and pleural cavity).

2. The surface projection of pleurae and lungs.

Part IV. Mediastinum.

1. The concept and borders.

2. The divisions and contains: superior and inferior (anterior, middle and posterior).

Chapter 5　Urinary System

1. Kidney.

(1) The features, the shape of renal hilum, the renal pedicle and the renal sinus.

(2) The location.

(3) The structures: renal cortex (outer portion of kidney); renal medulla (inner portion of kidney); renal pyramids (cone shaped masses of tissue in renal medulla); renal pelvis; major calyces; minor calyces.

2. Ureters.

(1) The features.

(2) The location.

3. Urinary bladder.

(1) The features and the location.

(2) The structures: trigon of urinary bladder.

4. Urethra.

Chapter 6　Male Reproductive System

Part Ⅰ. The internal genital organs of male.

1. Testis.

(1) The shape: It is ovoid structures that held within the scrotum.

(2) The internal structure of testis: Each testis is divided into lobules; each lobule contains seminiferous tubules (production of sperm cells) which are separated by interstitial cells (production of male sex hormones); the seminiferous tubules unite and give rise to the epididymis on the outer surface of the testis.

(3) The testis can produce sperm and male sex hormones.

2. Epididymis: It is highly coiled tube leading to vas deferens and a site of storage of sperm cells.

3. Vas (Ductus) deferens: It is muscular tube which passes upward from testis, passes through parietal peritoneum (inguinal canal) and into abdominal cavity. It passes upward within the inguinal canal and composes the spermatic cord along with a testicular artery, autonomic nerves, testicular veins, lymphatic vessels and the cremaster muscle. It fuses with duct from seminal vesicle to form ejaculatory duct (within prostate gland). The funicular pocnt is place for site of vasectomy.

4. Seminal vesicle: It is a sac-like structure attached to vas deferens and secretes an alkaline fluid that is rich in nutrients.

5. Prostate gland: It surrounds urethra below bladder and secretes a milky, alkaline fluid which enhances sperm motility.

6. Bulbourethral glands: They are two small structures beneath prostate and can secrete lubricant for penis.

Part Ⅱ. The external genital organs of male.

1. Scrotum: It has a pouch of skin and a subcutaneous tissue that encloses the testes. Its cremaster muscle is an extension of the internal oblique abdominis that elevates the scrotum during sexual arousal and on exposure to cold.

2. Penis.

(1) It is male excitatory organ and is specialized to become erect for insertion into vagina during sexual intercourse. Its cylindrical body composes of three columns of erectile tissue. It completely surrounds urethra.

(2) The structures: It has a pair of dorsally located corpora cavernosa. It has a single corpus spongiosum which extends at its distal end to form the enlarged glans penis. Each column is surrounded by a tough capsule of white fibrous connective tissue called tunica albuginea. A loose fold of skin called the prepuce covers the glans as a sheath.

Chapter 7　Female Reproductive System

Part Ⅰ. General description of female reproductive systems.

1. The composition of female reproductive system: the internal reproductive organs

include ovaries, uterine tubes, uterus, vagina; the external reproductive organs include vulva.

2. The function of female reproductive system: produce and transport egg cells; secret female hormones; promote the development of sexual organs; stimulate and maintain the secondary sexual features.

Part Ⅱ. Female internal genital organs.

1. Ovaries.

(1) The function: primary female sex organs which produce ova (eggs) and female sex hormones.

(2) The position: solid ovoid structures located (one on each side) on the posterior wall of the pelvic cavity.

(3) The shape: olive shape.

(4) The fixing device: suspensory ligament and proper ligament.

2. Uterine tube.

(1) The position: tubes which pass medially from ovaries to uterus.

(2) The subdivision (from medial to lateral): the uterine part (connect with the uterus); the isthmus part (the place of tubo sterilization); the ampulla (the place of fertilization); the infundibulum (connect with the ovary).

3. Uterus.

(1) The function: a muscular organ that receives embryo and sustains its life during development.

(2) The position: located in the middle of lesser pelvic cavity.

(3) The shape and subdivision: inverted pear-shape; consist of fundus, body, isthmus and cervix; cavity of uterus and cervical canal.

(4) The structure: endometrium (inner lining); myometrium (bundles of smooth muscle); bulk of uterus; perimetrium (visceral covering).

(5) The fixing device: broad, round, cardinal and uterosacral ligments.

4. Vagina.

(1) The function: To serve to receive the erect penis during coitus, to convey menses to the outside during menstruation, and to transport the fetus during parturition.

(2) The position: The vagina is situated at the center of the pelvis between the urinary bladder and the rectum. It is continuous with the canal of cervix of uterus.

(3) The definition of fornix and the clinical significant of posterior fornix of vagina.

5. Greater vestibular glands: They are the pea-size and lies in both sides of the vaginal orifice, posterior to the bulb of vestibule.

6. Female external genital organs: mons pubis, greater lip of pudendum, lesser lip of pudendum, clitoris, vaginal vestibule, hymen and so on.

Chapter 8　Mammary Glands and Perineum

1. Mammary glands.

(1) The location and features: It is located in the superficial fascia of breast and anterior to the pectoralis major. It is developed and can secrete the milk to nourish the newborn baby.

(2) The structure of mammary glands: It consists of 15-20 lobes separated by adipose tissue. Within the lobes, there are smaller units called glandular lobule which contain glandular alveoli that produce milk when a woman is lactating. The lobule has an excretory duct, called the lactiferous ducts which are arranged radically.

(3) The production/flow of milk: glandular alveoli → secondary tubules → mammary ducts → lactiferous sinuses → lactiferous ducts → nipple.

2. Perineum.

(1) The definition of perineum: In broad sense, the perineum is the diamond-shaped region of the inferior orifice of the small pelvis. In narrow sense, the perineum is the soft tissue structure between anus and the posterior end of the perineal cleft.

(2) The boundaries and regions of the perineum: anterior margin, (the inferior border of pubic symphysis); posterior margin (the apex of coccyx); lateral sides (ischial tuberosities). The perineum may be divided into two parts: the anterior urogenital triangle and the posterior anal triangle by a transverse line drawing between two ischial tuberosities.

(3) The urogenital triangle: The superior and inferior fasciae of urogenital diaphragm, the deep transverse muscle of perineum, and the urethral sphincter muscle form the urogenital diaphragm which encloses the urogenital triangle and supports the pelvic organs.

(4) The anal triangle: The levator ani and coccygeus together with the superior and inferior fascia of pelvic diaphragm form the pelvic diaphragm which encloses the anal triangle and can also support the pelvic organs.

Chapter 9　Peritoneum

Part Ⅰ. Description of peritoneum.

1. The definition of peritoneum: It lines the wall of abdominal and pelvic cavities, and covers the abdominal and pelvic viscera.

2. The subdivision of peritoneum: parietal peritoneum (lining the wall of abdominal and pelvic cavities); visceral peritoneum (covering the viscera); peritoneal cavity (the potential space between the parietal and visceral peritoneum). The male peritoneal cavity is closed, while female peritoneal cavity is connected with the outside by female internal genital organs.

3. The functions of peritoneum: secrete a small amount of serous fluid; absorb fluid and air in the abdominal cavity; support and fix the organs; defense and repair the injured tissue.

4. The relationship between the abdominopelvic viscera and peritoneum: intraperitoneal organs (almost completely surrounds with peritoneum); interperitoneal organs (covered by peritoneum on their three aspects); retroperitoneal organs (only the anterior part is covered by the peritoneum).

Part Ⅱ. Structures formed by the peritoneum.

1. Omentum.

(1) It is double-layered fold of peritoneum that connects the greater curvature or lesser curvature of the stomach.

(2) The lesser omentum (hepatogastric ligament and hepatoduodenal ligament); greater omentum, gastrocolic ligament.

(3) The omental bursa and omental foramen: The omental bursa is a potential, narrow space between the lesser omentum, the posterior wall of the stomach and the posterior wall of the abdomen, which is called omental bursa or lesser peritoneal cavity. The omental foramen is located posterior to the hepatoduodenal ligament, by which the omental bursa communicates with the peritoneal cavity.

2. Mesenteries and mesocolons.

3. Ligaments.

4. Peritoneal recesses, pouches and folds.

(1) The peritoneal recesses: hepatorenal recess—it is the lowest place in peritoneal cavity while lie on one's back.

(2) The peritoneal pouches: male (rectovesical pouch); female (the rectouterine pouch or Douglas pouch and the vesicouterine pouch). The rectovesical pouch in male and rectouterine pouch in female are the lowest place in peritoneal cavity while erecting or sitting.

(3) The peritoneal folds and fossa.

Chapter 10　Cardiovascular System and Lymphatic System

Part Ⅰ. General description of the cardiovascular system.

1. The composition of cardiovascular system: heart, arteries, capillaries and veins.

2. The circulative routes of blood: systemic (greater) circulation and pulmonary (lesser) circulation.

3. The characteristic and function of the vessels anastomoses: anastomoses between arteries, anastomoses between veins and anastomoses between arteries and veins.

Part Ⅱ. Heart.

1. The location and borders of the heart.

2. The external features of the heart: apex, base, two surface (sternocostal surface and diaphragmatic surface), three borders (right border, left border and inferior border), four grooves (coronary groove, anterior interventricular groove, posterior interventricular groove and interatrial groove), sulcus terminalis.

3. The internal features of the heart.

(1) Right atrium.

1) The atrium proper.

2) The sinus venarum cavarum: orifice of the superior vena cava, orifice of the inferior vena cava, orifice of the coronary sinus, fossa ovalis, right atrioventricular orifice.

(2) Right ventricle.

1) The supraventricular crest.

2) The sinous part: chordae tendineae, trabeculae carneae, papillary muscle, septomarginal trabecula and tricuspid complex (right atrioventricular orifice).

3) The infundibular part: conus arteriosus, pulmonary orifice, pulmonary valve (three semilunar leaflets).

(3) Left atrium.

1) To constitute the most part of the base of the heart.

2) The four pulmonary veins open into the upper posterolateral surfaces of the left atrium.

3) The pectinate muscles: fewer and smaller.

(4) Left Ventricle.

1) The sinous part (inflow tract): mitral complex (left atrioventricular orifice), chordae tendineae, papillary muscle and bicuspid valve.

2) The aortic vestibule (outflow tract): aortic orifice (aortic valve), aortic sinuses origination of (coronary arteries).

4. The structures of the heart.

(1) The fibrous skeleton of the heart.

(2) The wall of the heart: endocardium (smooth inner lining of heart chambers and valves); myocardium (cardiac muscle tissue); epicardium (visceral pericardium).

5. The conduction system of the heart.

(1) The sinoatrial node: It initiates each cardiac cycle, and sets a basic pace for the heart rate.

(2) The atrioventricular node.

(3) The atrioventricular bundle (His bundle).

(4) The Purkinje fibers.

6. The vessels of the heart.

(1) The arteries of the heart: right coronary artery and left coronary artery.

(2) The veins of the heart: coronary sinus, anterior cardiac veins, smallest cardiac veins.

7. Pericardium.

(1) The fibrous pericardium.

(2) The serous pericardium: visceral layer and parietal layer.

Part Ⅲ. Arteries.

1. Pulmonary circuits.

(1) The location and function of arterial ligament.

(2) The routes of pulmonary artery and vein.

2. Systemic circuits.

(1) The routes and branches of the ascending aorta and aortic arch.

(2) The origins, courses of left and right common carotid artery, locations and function of internal carotid sinus and arterial glomerulus, and the main branches of external carotid artery, and the courses and distribution of superior thyroid artery, facial artery, superficial temporal artery.

(3) The origins, courses of the subclavian artery, axillary artery, brachial artery, radial artery, ulnar artery and palmar arches.

(4) The origins, courses and distribution of thoracic aorta and its branches (intercostals, superior phrenics, bronchial artery and esophageal artery).

(5) The branches of abdominal aorta: inferior phrenics; celiac trunk (common hepatic artery, left gastric artery and splenic artery); superior mesenteric artery (arteries of small intestine, cecum, ascending, transverse colon, pancreas); suprarenal arteries; renal arteries; gonadal (ovarian/testicular) arteries; inferior mesenteric artery (arteries of

descending, sigmoid colon, rectum).

(6) The branches of common iliac arteries: external iliac arteries (femoral artery, popliteal artery, posterior tibial artery, plantar artery, anterior tibial artery and dorsalis pedis artery) and internal iliac arteries.

Part Ⅳ. Veins.

1. The jugular veins: external jugular vein and internal jugular vein.

2. The median cubital vein: venipuncture site.

3. The brachiocephalic veins: They are formed by the union of the subclavian and jugular veins on each side.

4. The superior vena cava: It is formed by the union of the left and right brachiocephalic veins.

5. The coronary sinus (cardiac veins).

6. The hepatic vein.

7. The hepatic portal vein: gastric vein, mesenteric vein and splenic vein.

Part Ⅴ. Lymphatic system.

1. Composition of the lymphatic system.

(1) Lymphatic vessels.

1) The lymphatic capillaries: microscopic closed-ended tubes that extend into interstitial spaces; receive lymph through their thin walls.

2) The lymphatic vessels: be formed by the merging of lymphatic capillaries; have walls similar to veins and possess valves that prevent backflow of lymph; lead to lymph nodes as "afferent" LVs, leave lymph nodes as "efferent" LVs, and then merge into lymphatic trunks.

3) The lymphatic trunks.

4) The lymphatic ducts.

The right lymphatic duct: It receives right bronchomediastinal, right subclavian, and right jugular trunks, and drains the right upper body (25% of total body).

The thoracic (left lymphatic) duct: It is largest lymphatic vessel, and begins cisterna chili, and receives left and right lumbar, intestinal, left bronchomediastinal, left subclavian and left jugular trunks, and drains the remaining 75% of the body's lymph.

(2) Lymphatic tissues: diffuse lymphatic tissue and lymphatic nodule.

(3) Lymphatic organs.

1) The lymph nodes.

2) The thymus.

3) The spleen.

2. Lymphatic nodes and lymph drainage of whole body.

(1) The lymphatic nodes of head and neck.

(2) The lympatic nodes of upper limb: cubital lymphatic nodes, infraclavicular lymphatic nodes, axillary lymphatic nodes (pectoral, lateral, subscapular, central and apical lymphatic nodes).

(3) The lymphatic nodes of thorax.

(4) The lymphatic nodes of lower limb: popliteal, inguinal lymphatic nodes (superficial inguinal lymphatic nodes: upper group are located below inguinal ligament

and lower group are located around the terminal part of great saphenous vein; deep inguinal lymphatic nodes: they are located along femoral vein and lie in femoral canal).

(5) The lymphatic nodes of pelvis.

(6) The lymphatic nodes of abdomen.

Chapter 11　Sensory Organs

Part Ⅰ. Visual organ.

1. Walls of eyeball.

(1) The outer (fibrous) tunic.

1) The cornea: anterior portion, transparent, highly curved, numerous sensory nerve terminals.

2) The sclera: posterior portion, white, protection and attachment of eye muscles, sinus venosus sclera.

(2) Middle (vascular) tunic.

1) The iris: anterior colored ring around pupil; it separates the anterior cavity of the eye into an anterior chamber and posterior chamber; the entire anterior cavity is filled with aqueous humor; sphincter pupillae is innervated by parasympathetic nerve and decreases the pupil in size; dilator pupillae is innervated by sympathetic nerve and dilates the pupil.

2) The ciliary body: middle part of the vascular tunic; it is composed of ciliary processes and ciliary ring; ciliary muscles control the shape of the lens; suspensory ligaments extend from the ciliary processes to the lens.

3) The choroid membrane: It is joined loosely to sclera containing many blood vessels to nourish the tissues of the eye.

(3) The inner tunic (retina).

1) The three parts: iridial part, ciliary part and optic part. The first two parts are known as the blind part.

2) The optic disk: It is the location on the retina where nerve fibers leave the eye and join with the optic nerve; the central artery and vein also pass through this disk; no photoreceptors are present in the area of the optic disk (blind spot).

3) The macula lutea: It is near the center of the posterior part of the retina. It contains the fovea centralis, where visual acuity is highest.

4) There are two types of visual receptors (photoreceptors) in the retina: cones—photoreceptors for color vision and produce sharp images; rods—photoreceptors for night vision and produce silhouettes of images.

2. Contents of eyeball.

(1) The aqueous humor: colorless, transparent, and it is produced by ciliary body.

(2) The lens: transparent, elastic, biconvex body.

(3) The vitreous body: colorless, transparent, jelly-like body.

3. Accessory organs of eye.

(1) The eyelids: protective shield for the eyeball.

(2) The conjunctiva: inner lining of eyelid and anterior surface of the eyeball.

(3) The lacrimal apparatus: tear secretion and distribution.

1) The lacrimal gland: tear secretion.

2) The lacrimal passages: lacrimal puncta; lacrimal ductuli; lacrimal sac; nasolacrimal duct which carries tears into nasal cavity.

(4) The extraocular muscles: superior rectus muscle, inferior rectus muscle, lateral rectus muscle, medial rectus muscle, inferior oblique muscle, superior oblique muscle, levator palpebrae superior muscle.

(5) The connective tissue in the orbit.

4. Blood vessels and nerves of eye.

(1) The arteries: central artery of retina, short posterior ciliary arteries and long posterior ciliary arteries.

(2) The veins: ophthalmic veins and central vein of retina.

(3) The nerves: optic nerve, oculomotor nerve, trochlear nerve, abducent nerve, ophthalmic nerve, sympathetic nerve and parasympathetic nerve.

Part Ⅱ. Vestibulocochlear organ.

1. External ear.

(1) The auricle: Its function is collection of sound waves.

(2) The external acoustic meatus: Its function is to start vibrations of sound waves and directs them toward tympanic membrane.

(3) The tympanic membrane (eardrum).

2. Middle ear.

(1) Tympanic cavity.

1) The auditory ossicles: malleus, incus and stapes.

2) The oval window: the entrance to inner ear.

(2) Auditory tube.

1) The passageway: connect middle ear to nasopharynx.

2) The function: equalize the pressure on both sides of the tympanic membrane.

3. Inner ear.

(1) Bony labyrinth.

1) The cochlea: scala vestibule, scala tympani, cochlear duct.

2) The vestibule.

3) The semi-circular canals.

(2) Membranous labyrinth.

1) The cochlear duct: The spiral organ (Organ of Corti) is located on the basilar membrane, which is responsible for the sense of hearing.

2) The utricle and saccule: Macula utriculi and macula sacculi are the organs of static balance. They may be stimulated not only by the changes of the position of the head, but also by the linear movements on acceleration or deceleration of the head.

3) The semicircular duct: The ampullary crests are the organs of kinetic balance, which respond to rotational acceleration of the head.

Chapter 12   Endocrine System

1. The hypophysis (pituitary gland): It lies in the sella turcica at the base of brain. It is connected with the hypothalamus by the pituitary stalk. It consists of an anterior lobe

(adenohypophysis) and a posterior lobe (neurohypophysis).

2. The thyroid gland: It is the largest of the endocrine organs. It is located in the neck and consists of two lobes joined by the isthmus. It is supplied by the two pairs of blood vessels, namely, the superior and inferior thyroid arteries.

3. The parathyroid glands: It is located near the thyroid glands and has 4 tiny pea-shaped organs.

4. The suprarenal glands: They are located above the kidneys. Each has 2 parts: an outer covering (the adrenal cortex) and an inner core (the adrenal medulla). Each suprarenal gland is supplied by the superior suprarenal arteries (from the inferior phrenic artery), middle suprarenal arteries (from the aorta) and inferior suprarenal arteries (from the renal artery).

5. The thymus: It consists of two elongated lobes and is located in the upper mediastinum posterior to the sternum. It is quite large in infancy, but it atrophies after puberty.

6. The pancreas: It is a gland of having both exocrine and endocrine functions. It is attached to the second and third portion of the duodenum on the right. Endocrine function is performed by pancreatic island.

Chapter 13　Nervous System

Part Ⅰ. General description of nervous system.

1. The composition of nervous system.

(1) The central nervous system (CNS): brain and spinal cord.

(2) The peripheral nervous system (PNS): nerves that extend from the brain (cranial nerves) and spinal cord (spinal nerves).

2. The structures of nervous system.

(1) The neuron: the structural and functional unit of the nervous system; a nerve cell.

1) The cell body: central portion of neuron; contain usual organelles.

2) The neuron processes/nerve fibers: extensions from cell body.

The dendrites: many per neuron; short and process; receptive portion of a neuron; carry impulses toward cell body.

The axons: one per neuron; long, thin process; carry impulses away from cell body; note terminations of axon branch.

(2) The myelinated nerve fiber and unmyelinated nerve fibers: myelinated nerve fibers are the large axons that are surrounded by a myelin sheath; unmyelinated nerve fibers are small axons that do not have a myelin sheath.

(3) The grey matter and white matter: grey matter is a bundle of cell bodies or unmyelinated nerve fibers; white matter is a bundle of myelinated nerve fibers.

(4) The neural ganglion and nucleus.

(5) The neural tracts and nerves.

(6) The neuroglial cells: accessory cells of nervous system form supporting network for neurons.

1) The PNS: Schwann cells produces myelin.

2) The CNS: oligodendrocyte; astrocyte; microglia; ependymal cells.

3. Classification of neurons.

(1) Functional classification.

1) The sensory neurons: PNS; afferent neurons; carry sensory impulses from sensory receptors to CNS; input information to CNS; location of receptors (skin and sense organs).

2) The interneurons (association): CNS; link other neurons together (i.e. sensory neuron to interneuron to motor neuron).

3) The motor neurons: PNS; efferent neurons; carry motor impulses away from CNS and to effectors; output information from CNS; effectors (muscles and glands).

(2) Structural classification.

1) The multipolar neurons: many extensions; many dendrites lead toward cell body, one axon leads away from cell body.

2) The bipolar neurons: two extensions; one fused dendrite leads toward cell body, one axon leads away from cell body.

3) The unipolar neurons: one process from cell body; form central and peripheral processes; only distal ends are dendrite.

Part Ⅱ. Central nervous system.

Spinal cord.

1. Gross structure of spinal cord.

(1) The length: about 17 inches; start at the foramen magnum; it tapers to point (conus medullaris) and terminates near the intervertebral disc that lies the 1st-2nd lumbar (L1-L2) vertebra.

(2) It contains 31 segments (and therefore gives rise to 31 pairs of spinal nerves).

(3) The cervical and lumbar enlargements.

(4) The cauda equina: the lower lumbar and sacral nerves that travel downward.

(5) The filum terminale.

2. Cross-sectional anatomy of spinal cord.

(1) The gray matter: bundles of (interneuron) cell bodies; posterior (dorsal) horns; lateral horns; anterior (ventral) horns; central canal; gray commissure; anterior median fissure; posterior median sulcus.

(2) The white matter: myelinated (interneuron) axons; posterior (dorsal) funiculi; lateral funiculi; anterior (ventral) funiculi.

(3) Nerve tracts.

1) The ascending tracts: be located in the posterior (dorsal) funiculi; conduct sensory (afferent) impulses from body parts to brain.

2) The descending tracts: be located in the anterior (ventral) funiculi; conduct motor (efferent) impulses from brain to effectors.

3) The general characteristics of nerve tracts: most cross over; most consist of 2-3 successive neurons; most exhibit somatotopic organization; all pathways are paired (right and left).

3. Reflex of spinal cord and its reflex arc.

Brain stem.

1. Gross structure of brain stem.

(1) The medulla oblongata: anterior median fissure; pyramid; decussation of the pyramids; olives (inferior olivary nuclei); inferior cerebellar peduncles; gracile tubercle; cuneate tubercle; glossopharyngeal nerve; vagus nerve; accessory nerve; hypoglossal nerve.

(2) The pons: middle cerebellar peduncles; basilar groove; trigeminal nerve; abducent nerve; facial nerve; vestibulocochlear nerve.

(3) The midbrain: crus cerebri; interpeduncular fossa; cerebral aqueduct; quadrigeminal bodies (superior colliculus and inferior colliculus); oculomotor nerve; trochlear nerve.

(4) The rhomboid fossa: striae medullares; medial eminence; sulcus limitans; locus ceruleus; facial colliculus (nucleus of the abducent nerve); area vestibule (vestibular nuclei); auditory tubercle (dorsal cochlear nucleus); hypoglossal triangle (hypoglossal nucleus); vagal triangle (dorsal nucleus of vagus nerve).

2. Internal structure of brain stem.

(1) Nuclei of cranial nerves.

1) The somatic motor nuclei: oculomotor nucleus; trochlear nucleus; abducent nucleus; hypoglossal nucleus.

2) The special visceral motor nuclei: motor nucleus of trigeminal nerve; nucleus of facial nerve; nucleus ambiguous; accessory nucleus.

3) The general visceral motor nuclei: accessory oculomotor nucleus; superior salivatory nucleus; inferior salivatory nucleus; dorsal nucleus of vagus nerve.

4) The general and special visceral sensory nucleus: nucleus of solitary tract.

5) The general somatic sensory nuclei: spinal nucleus of trigeminal nerve; pontine nucleus of trigeminal nerve; mesencephalic nucleus of trigeminal nerve.

6) The special somatic sensory nuclei: cochlear nucleus; vestibular nucleus.

(2) Non-cranial nerve nuclei: gracile and cuneate nuclei; inferior olivary nuclear complex; pontine nuclei; nucleus of inferior colliculus; nucleus of superior colliculus; red nucleus; substantia nigra; pretectal nucleus area.

(3) Long ascending and descending tracts.

1) The long ascending tracts: medial lemniscus; spinothalamic lemniscus; trigeminal lemniscus; lateral lemniscus.

2) The long descending tracts: corticospinal tract; corticonuclear tract.

3. Transverse sections of brain stem.

Cerebellum.

1. The gross appearance of the cerebellum: cerebellar hemispheres; vermis; nodule; pyramid of vermis; tuber of vermis; flocculonodular lobe (archicerebellum or vestibulocerebellum); anterior lobe (paleocerebellum or spinocerebellum); posterior lobe (neocerebellum or cerebrocerebellum); tonsil of cerebellum.

2. The internal structures: cerebellar cortex; cerebellar nuclei (fastigial nucleus, emboliform nucleus, globose nucleus and dentate nucleus); white matter (inferior cerebellar peduncle, middle cerebellar peduncle and superior cerebellar peduncle).

3. The connections and functions of the cerebellum: coordinate all voluntary muscle movements (subconsciously); skilled movements, posture and equilibrium.

Diencephalon.

1. Dorsal thalamus.

(1) The ventral posteromedial nucleus (VPM) and ventral posterolateral nucleus (VPL).

(2) The central relay station for incoming sensory impulses (except smell) that directs the impulse to the appropriate area of the cerebral cortex for interpretation.

2. Metathalamus.

(1) The medial geniculate body and lateral geniculate body.

(2) Form part of the auditory and visual pathways.

3. Epithalamus: thalamic medullary stria, habenular trigone, pineal body.

4. Hypothalamus.

(1) The optic chiasma, tuber cinereum, infundibulum, mamillary bodies.

(2) The supraoptic nucleus, paraventricular nucleus, mamillary nucleus.

(3) The main visceral control center of the body; body temperature; water and electrolyte balance; control of hunger, body weight, digestive movements and secretions; regulation of sleep-wake cycles.

5. Third ventricle.

Telencephalon.

1. External features of cerebrum.

(1) It is divided into two cerebral hemispheres; hemispheres are connected by a deep bridge of nerve fibers called the corpus callosum; each hemisphere is divided into frontal, parietal, temporal, occipital and insular lobes.

(2) The main sulci and gyri of cerebrum: central sulcus (frontal/parietal); precentral and postcentral sulci; lateral sulcus (temporal/others); longitudinal fissure separates the two cerebral hemispheres; transverse fissure (cerebrum/cerebellum); parietooccipital sulcus; calcarine sulcus; cingulated sulcus; precentral and postcentral gyri; paracentral lobule; superior, middle and inferior gyri; supramarginal gyrus; angular gyrus; superior, middle and inferior temporal gyri; transverse temporal gyri; cingulated gyrus; cuneus; lingual gyrus; parahippocampal gyrus.

2. The limbic lobe and limbic system: It also includes structures in the frontal and temporal cortex, basal nuclei, and deep nuclei; It is involved in emotional response and sense of smell.

3. The cerebral cortex: It is composed of gray matters and bundles of neuron cell bodies. It is responsible for all conscious behavior mainly containing sensory, motor and language areas.

(1) The primary somatosensory cortex: It receives information from general receptors (i.e. temperature, touch, pressure, & pain) and is located in postcentral gyrus of parietal cortex and the posterior part of the paracentral lobule.

(2) The primary motor cortex: It initiates all voluntary muscle movements and is located in the gyrus just anterior to the central sulcus (precentral gyrus) and anterior part of the paracentral lobule.

(3) The visual cortex: It receives incoming information from vision receptors (in eye) and is located around the calcarine sulcus of occipital cortex.

(4) The auditory cortex: It receives incoming information from hearing reiceptors (in ear) and is located in the transverse temporal gyri of temporal cortex.

(5) Language areas.

1) The auditory (sensory) language areas: It is located the posterior part of the superior temporal gyrus and involved in high-order auditory discrimination and comprehension.

2) The visual speech area (reading area): It is located in the angular gyrus and involved in the visual word-images.

3) The motor speech area: It occupies the posterior portion of the inferior frontal gyrus and is essential for the appropriate and coordinated action of the muscles in speech.

4) The writing area: It lies in the posterior portion of the middle frontal gyrus and is involved in expressing their ideas by writing.

4. Internal structure of cerebrum.

(1) The basal nuclei: They are masses of gray matter, located deep within the white matter of the cerebral hemispheres, and include the corpus striatum (caudate nucleus and lentiform nucleus), claustrum and amygdaloid nucleus. They serve as relay stations for outgoing motor impulses from the brain.

(2) The medullary: association fibers (arcuate fibers; superior longitudinal fasciculus, uncinate fasciculus); commissural fibers (corpus callosum, fornical commissure and anterior commissure); projection fibers or internal capsule including anterior limb (anterior thalamic radiation); genu (corticonuclear tracts) and posterior limb (middle thalamic radiation, optic radiation, acoustic radiation and corticospinal tracts).

(3) The lateral ventricles: each includes central part, anterior horn, posterior horn and inferior horn.

Part Ⅲ. Peripheral nervous system.

Spinal nerves.

1. The introduction of spinal nerve: a spinal nerve is formed from the fusion of a dorsal and ventral root; spinal nerve passes through its intervertebral foramen; spinal nerves are associated with the spinal cord and are named for the region of the spinal cord from which they arise.

2. The general characteristics: 31 pairs (C1 - C8; T1 - T12; L1 - L5; S1 - S5; Co).

3. The composition: all mixed nerves.

4. The distribution of spinal nerves: At short distance after passing through its intervertebral foramen, a spinal nerve branches into several branches: posterior branch (i.e. dorsal ramus) and a large anterior branch.

5. The main branches of nerve plexuses

(1) The cervical plexus: superficial branches (lesser occipital nerve, great auricular nerve, transverse nerve of neck and supraclavicular nerve); deep branch (phrenic nerve).

(2) The brachial plexus: long thoracic nerve; median nerve; ulnar nerve; musculocutaneuous nerve; radial nerve; axillary nerve; thoracodorsal nerve; lateral and medial pectoral nerves.

(3) The lumbar plexus: iliohypogastric nerve; ilioinguinal nerve; lateral femoral cutaneous nerve; femoral nerve; obturator nerve.

(4) The sacral plexus: sciatic nerve (tibial nerve and common peroneal nerve-deep peroneal nerve and superficial peroneal nerve); posterior femoral cutaneous nerve; pudendal nerve.

Cranial nerves.

1. The introduction of cranial nerve: 12 pairs; 2 pairs to/from forebrain and 10 pairs to/from brain stem; sensory nerves (I, II and VIII); motor nerves (III, IV, VI, IX and XII); mixed nerves (V, VII, IX and X); contain seven fiber components.

2. Twelve pairs of cranial nerves and their function.

(1) The olfactory nerve: sense of smell.

(2) The optic nerve: sense of vision.

(3) The oculomotor nerve: innervate all extraocular muscles except for superior obliquus and lateral rectus, and changes in size of pupil and shape of lens.

(4) The trochlear nerve: innervate superior obliquus.

(5) The trigeminal nerve: largest; sensory from face; motor to chewing muscles.

(6) The abducent nerve: innervate lateral rectus.

(7) The facial nerve: carry nerve impulses associated with taste of anterior 2/3 of the tongue; secretion of lacrimal gland, submandibular gland and sublingual gland; muscles of facial expression.

(8) The vestibulocochlear nerve: carry nerve impulses associated with hearing and equilibrium.

(9) The glossopharyngeal nerve: carry nerve impulses associated with swallowing; secretion of parotid gland; taste of posterior 1/3 of the tongue.

(10) The vagus nerve: carry nerve impulses to and from many organs in the thoracic and abdominal cavities and innervates visceral smooth muscle.

(11) The accessory nerve: control head and shoulder muscles.

(12) The hypoglossal nerve: control tongue muscles.

Autonomic nervous system (ANS).

1. Introduction: It regulates the action of smooth muscles, cardiac muscle, and some glands. There are two major divisions of the ANS: the parasympathetic division functions under normal conditions (maintain homeostasis), and the sympathetic division of the ANS functions under stress.

2. The somatic vs. autonomic pathways.

(1) The Somatic pathways: one motor neuron; no ganglia; effectors (skeletal muscles).

(2) The ANS pathways: two motor neurons; synapse between neurons occur within a ganglion; effectors (smooth muscle, cardiac muscle and glands).

3. Two Divisions:

(1) The parasympathetic nerve: The 1st neuron (preganglionic) is long and the 2nd neuron (postganglionic) is short; parasympathetic ganglia are located at or near the effectors; parasympathetic nerves arise from the craniosacral regions of the brain & spinal cord; distribution is much narrower.

(2) The sympathetic nerve: The 1st neuron (preganglionic) is short and the 2nd neuron (postganglionic) is long; sympathetic ganglia are located on either side of the spinal cord (chain ganglia; sympathetic trunk) or in front of vertebral column (prevertebral ganglia), and are far from their effectors; sympathetic nerves arise from the thoracolumbar regions of the spinal cord; distribution is much wider.

Part Ⅳ. Nervous pathways.

1. Sensory pathways.

(1) The conscious proprioceptive and fine touch pathway of trunk and limbs: receptors (muscles, tendons, joins, ligaments); the first order of neurons and their fibers (spinal ganglion; fasciculus gracilis and fasciculus cuneatus); the second order of neurons and their fibers (gracile and cuneate nuclei; medial lemniscus and its decussation); the third order of neurons (VPL; central thalamic radiation); central area (superior and middle part of postcentral gyrus; posterior part of paracentral lobule).

(2) The pain, temperature and crude touch pathway of trunk and limbs: receptors (skin of trunk and limbs); the first order of neurons and their fibers (spinal ganglion and their central processes); the second order of neurons and their fibers (Lamina I, IV~VII of spinal cord; fibers decussation and then forming lateral spinothalamic tract for pain and temperature in lateral funiculus, and anterior spinothalamic tract for crude touch and pressure in anterior funiculus); the third order of neurons (VPL; central thalamic radiation); central area (superior and middle part of postcentral gyrus; posterior part of paracentral lobule).

(3) The pain, temperature and crude touch pathway of head and face: receptors (skin, mucosa of head and face); the first order of neurons and their fibers (trigeminal ganglion and their central processes); the second order of neurons and their fibers (pontine nucleus of trigeminal nerve for tactile and spinal nucleus of trigeminal nerve for pain and temperature; trigeminal leminiscus and their decussation); the third order of neurons (VPM; central thalamic radiation); central area (inferior part of postcentral gyrus).

(4) The visual pathway: receptors (rod and cone cells); the first order of neurons and their fibers (bipolar cells and their central processes); the second order of neurons and their fibers (ganglion cells; optic chiasma and optic tract); the third order of neurons (lateral geniculate body; optic radiation); visual area (calcarine cortex).

(5) The auditory pathway: receptors (spiral organ); the first order of neurons and their fibers (cochlear ganglion and their central processes); the second order of neurons and their fibers (cochlear nuclei, trapezoid body and lateral lemniscus); the third order of neurons and their fibers (inferior colliculus; brachium of inferior colliculus); the fourth order of neurons and their fibers (medial geniculate body; acoustic radiation); acoustic area (transverse temporal gyrus).

2. Motor pathways.

(1) Corticospinal tract.

1) The upper motor neuron: pyramidal cells of superior and middle parts of precentral gyrus cerebri, and anterior part of paracentral lobule.

2) The corticospinal tract: via posterior limb of internal capsule, lateral part of middle

3/5 of crus cerebri, basilar part of pons and pyramid of medulla oblongata; 75%-90% of fibers cross forming decussation of pyramid (lateral corticospinal tract) and 10%-25% of fibers uncross (anterior corticospinal tract).

3) The lower motor neuron: motor neurons in the anterior horn of spinal cord.

(2) Corticonuclear tract.

1) The upper motor neuron: pyramidal cells of inferior part of precentral gyrus cerebri.

2) The corticonuclear tract: via genu of internal capsule, medial part of middle 3/5 of crus cerebri.

3) The lower motor neuron: bilateral oculomotor, trochlear, trigeminal motor, abducens, superior part of facial, ambiguus and accessory nuclei; contralateral inferior part of facial and hypoglossal nuclei.

Part Ⅴ. The meninges and blood vessels of brain and spinal cord, and the CSF.

Meninges of brain and spinal cord.

(1) The meninges of spinal cord.

1) The spinal dura mater and epidural space.

2) The spinal arachnoid mater.

3) The spinal pia mater and subarachnoid space.

(2) The meninges of brain.

1) The cerebral dura mater (cerebral falx and cerebellar tentorium) and dural sinuses (superior sagital sinus, straight sinus, sigmoid sinus, transverse sinus, confluence of sinuses, cavernous sinus).

2) The cerebral arachnoid mater and subarachnoid space.

3) The cerebral pia mater.

Blood vessels of brain and spinal cord.

1. Arteries of brain.

(1) The vertebral-basilar arteries: send the anterior and posterior spinal arteries, posterior inferior cerebellar artery, anterior inferior cerebellar artery, pontine arteries and posterior cerebral artery.

(2) The internal carotid artery.

1) The anterior cerebral artery: form anterior communicating artery.

2) The middle cerebral artery.

3) The anterior choroidal artery.

4) The posterior communicating artery.

(3) The cerebral arterial circle (Willis circle): be formed by the anterior cerebral arteries and their anterior communicating, branches of the internal carotid artery, posterior cerebral arteries and their communicating.

2. The veins of brain: superficial cerebral vein and deep cerebral vein.

3. The arteries of spinal cord.

4. The veins of spinal cord.

Circulation of the CSF.

1. The ventricles: they are continuous with central canal of spinal cord; they are filled with CSF; they are lined by ependymal cells.

2. The secretion and circulation of CSF

(1) The CSF is secreted by specialized capillaries in choroid plexuses into the lateral ventricles.

(2) The CSF circulates down into the 3rd & then 4th ventricle and then into either the central canal of spinal cord or the subarachnoid space of meninges.

(3) The CSF is reabsorbed back into the bloodstream through arachnoid granulations that project into dural sinuses.

3. The functions of CSF: mechanical protection and chemical protection.

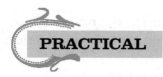

PRACTICAL

By a combination of lecture, tutorials and practical training, the student is able to grasp the gross morphology, shapes, location and structures of the organ systems, identify the organs in the human various systems, comprehend the normal dispositions and inter-relationships of the various organs or parts in each system, localize the surface markings of important organs, demonstrate the muscle testing, joints movements, pulsation of a particular artery, sites for lumbar puncture and the subcutaneous positions of large vein, etc., and gain an insight into the correlation between structures and functions. Having finished the course of systemic anatomy, it will provide the student with an understanding of the anatomical basis for the health and disease.

REGIONAL ANATOMY
局部解剖学

Chief Editors（主编）

He Guiqiong（贺桂琼）　Chongqing Medical University（重庆医科大学）

Lü Guangming（吕广明）　Nantong University（南通大学）

Deputy Chief Editors（副主编）

Shao Heng（邵珩）　Tianjin Medical University（天津医科大学）

Ran Jianhua（冉建华）　Chongqing Medical University（重庆医科大学）

Liu Shangqing（刘尚清）　North Sichuan Medical University（川北医学院）

Liu Chengxing（刘承杏）　Kunming Medical University（昆明医科大学）

Liu Haiyan（刘海岩）　Jilin University（吉林大学）

Editors（编委）（按姓氏拼音排序）

He Guiqiong（贺桂琼）　Chongqing Medical University（重庆医科大学）

Liu Chengxing（刘承杏）　Kunming Medical University（昆明医科大学）

Liu Haiyan（刘海岩）　Jilin University（吉林大学）

Liu Shangqing（刘尚清）　North Sichuan Medical University（川北医学院）

Lü Guangming（吕广明）　Nantong University（南通大学）

Ran Jianhua（冉建华）　Chongqing Medical University（重庆医科大学）

Shao Heng（邵珩）　Tianjin Medical University（天津医科大学）

Xu Jin（徐进）　Chongqing Medical University（重庆医科大学）

Yang Mei（杨美）　Chongqing Medical University（重庆医科大学）

Course Description

Regional Anatomy is the science which deals with the forms, positions, relationships, and related clinical applications of the structures of the human body in a given region just based on the knowledge of systematic human anatomy. To describe each location, the position of each organ, each layer, the related courses and their interrelationships in human body. The human body should be divided into eight parts: the head and face, the neck, the thorax, the abdomen, the pelvis and perineum, the vertebral region, the upper limb and the lower limb. Furthermore, by practically anatomical operations during class time, the clinical students or other ones in related domains must be cultivated to possess the capabilities of observation, analysis, thought and operation which can provide necessarily morphological basis of the study for future curriculum or clinical applications.

The technique of human dissection is acquired only by practice. Fortunately, the students will develop an adequate technique in a relatively short time. The technique of human dissection often requires patience rather than great skill. The method of dissecting the body is a regional one, in which the design is to see everything that is to be seen in a single area of the body at one time. In approaching any region of the body, the students firsthy identify the surface landmarks, then reflect the skin from that region. The structure to be exposed and studied after the skin is fascia. The dissection consists to a very great extent in removing the fascia without injuring the structures it contains. This process—the cleaning of the embedded muscles, nerves, arteries and other structures—is a tedious business. After finishing the dissection, the students should take time to review and study the structures as they appear in the body. A definite plan of study should be followed for each structure dissected. This plan should include the plane or part of the body in which it is located; the form, size, and shape of the structure; its origin, course, and distribution; and its function.

This subject is for clinical major. The assignment of learning hours is 108 (theory 28, practice 80). This lesson applies theory to the practice and operation. The ratio of theory to the practice and operation is nearly 1:3, which ensure enough time for operation.

Objectives

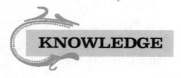

KNOWLEDGE

At the end of the course, the MBBS students shall be able to:

1. Describe the layer's structures and the relationship between layers in terms of each region in the body. 2. Comprehend the normal disposition, inter-relationships, gross, form, blood supply, nerve innervations, functional and applied anatomy of the various structures in the body.

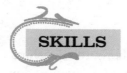

SKILLS

At the end of the course, the student shall be able to:

1. Grasp the basic skills of human dissection.

2. Demonstrate surface markings of important organs.

3. Localize important pulsation and the structures against which pressure can be applied in case of bleeding from a particular artery.

4. Locate the subcutaneous positions of large veins, Locate veins for venae puncture.

5. Locate the positions of nerves in each region.

Teaching and Learning Methods

Theory: Teaching human anatomy to undergraduate medical student is provided with the help of lectures and tutorials, so that they will gain the ability to comprehend the normal disposition, gross, functional and applied anatomy of the various structures in the body as a prerequisite for solving clinical problems.

Practical: Learning objectives are given to students before each session. Dissection is done by students on the cadavers and is being assisted/supervised by a team of teachers. Video tapes of some dissections are also shown on TV after the completion of dissection of the part/region to recaptulate the details of the part/region dissected.

Recommended Textbooks

Drake R, Vogl AW, Mitchell AWM. 2014. Gray's anatomy for students [M]. 2nd ed. Oxford: Elsevier Health Sciences.

Romanes GJ. 1986. Cunningham's Manual of Practical Anatomy, Vol. 2: Thorax and Abdomen [M]. 15th ed. Oxford: Oxford University Press.

Wang Huaijing (王怀经), Liu Yong (刘勇). 2009. Regional Anatomy [M]. 5th ed. Jilin: Jilin Science and Technology Publishing House.

Schedule Table

Chapter	Contents	Hours	Chapter	Contents	Hours
1	Head	Theory: 1 Practical: 3	6	Vertebral region	Theory: 1 Practical: 3
2	Neck	Theory: 4 Practical: 12	7	Upper limb	Theory: 6 Practical: 18
3	Thorax	Theory: 2 Practical: 6	8	Lower limb	Theory: 6 Practical: 18
4	Abdomen	Theory: 6 Practical: 18		Total	108 (Theory 28, Practical:80)
5	Pelvis and perineum	Theory: 2 Practical: 2			

Course Contents

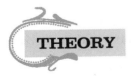

THEORY

Chapter 1　Head

1. The boundaries, parts and landmarks of the head.

2. The name of the facial muscles. The composition and function of masticatory muscles.

3. The origin, course and distribution of facial artery. The origin, branches and distribution of maxillary artery. The origin and distribution of superficial temporal artery.

4. The facial vein connections with cavernous sinus. The position of the "Danger triangle of the face".

5. The name, position and area drainage of the lymph nodes of the head. The position of submandibular lymph nodes.

6. The intracranial and intrapetrous course of the facial nerve and the relationships of its major branches to the middle ear in relation to damage of the nerve within the facial canal.

7. The branches of trigeminal nerve in face.

8. The structures vertical and transversal passing through the parotid gland. The relations of the parotid gland.

9. The boundaries and layers of the frontoparietooccipital region.

10. The boundaries and layers of the temporal region.

Chapter 2　Neck

1. The surface landmarks and projections of the neck. The parts, regions and triangles of the neck.

2. The name and arrangement of muscles of the neck. The origin, insertion, action and nerve supply of sternocleidomastoid, platysma and scalenus anterior.

3. The superficial fascia and the platysma. The deep fascial layers: investing layer, pretracheal layer, prevertebral layer and carotid sheath. The contents of carotid sheath.

4. The boundaries and contents of posterior and anterior triangles of the neck.

5. In the anterior triangle: the carotid triangle-the common, internal and external carotid arteries, the internal jugular vein, vagus nerve and its branches; the muscular triangle-the cervical part of trachea and esophagus, thyroid cartilage, larynx, thyroid and parathyroid glands; the submental triangle; the submandibular triangle-facial artery, mylohyoid, duct of submandibular gland and lingual nerve, hypoglossal nerve, superior root of ansa cervicalis, lingual artery. The Explain their clinical significance in relation to carotid insufficiency, central venous line insertion and emergency airway management.

6. In the posterior triangle: the occipital triangle-the accessory nerve, the cutaneous branches of cervical plexus, the roots and trunks of the brachial plexus, the lateral cervical lymph nodes; the supraclavicular trangle (greater supraclavicular fossa)-the phrenic nerve, the external jugular vein, the brachial plexus, the subclavian vessels in relation to penetrating neck trauma; the root of the neck – the terminal end of thoracic duct, the vagus nerve and right recurrent laryngeal nerve, the supraclavicular lymph nodes, the vertebral artery, the internal thoracic artery, the subclavian artery, the cervical sympathetic trunk.

7. The beginning, ending of the common carotid artery; the position and function

of carotid sinus, carotid glomus; the branches and distribution of the external carotid artery and locate the carotid pulse.

8. The beginning, ending, branches and distribution of the subclavian artery.

9. The position of external jugular vein. The beginning, ending and tributaries of the internal jugular vein. The beginning and ending of the subclavian vein. The concept and lymphatic duct drainage of venous angle.

10. The position and anatomy of the thyroid and parathyroid glands, their blood supply and the significance of the courses of the laryngeal nerves.

11. The formation, position and main branches of the cervical plexus. The formation and course of phrenic nerve in the neck.

12. The formation of the ansa cervicalis. The course of the hypoglossal nerve in neck. The distribution of the accessory nerve.

13. The course and branches of the vagus nerve in the neck. The branches and distribution of superior laryngeal nerve. The relationship between the external branch of superior laryngeal nerve and superior thyroid artery. The origin, course and distribution of recurrent laryngeal nerve. The relationship between the recurrent laryngeal nerve and inferior thyroid artery.

14. The position of cervical part of the sympathetic trunk.

15. The main lymph nodes of the neck. Master the position and area drainage of the superficial and deep lateral cervical lymph nodes.

Chapter 3　Thorax

1. Thoracic wall.

(1) The boundary and divisions of the thorax. The surface landmarks and the orientational lines on the thoracic wall.

(2) The structure and contents of intercostals spaces. The layers of thoracic wall. The arteries, veins, and nerves supplying thoracic wall.

(3) The position, origin, insertion and action of the external and internal intercostals muscles.

(4) The attachments and relations of the diaphragm and the structures that pass through and behind it. The movements of the diaphragm, its motor and sensory innervation and pleural and peritoneal coverings.

(5) The concept of dermatomes.

2. Thoracic cavity.

(1) The concept of the pleura and pleural cavities. The parts of parietal pleura, the positions of the pleural recesses. The surface markings of lower border of the lung and pleura.

(2) The structure of the tracheobronchial tree. The position and structure characteristics of trachea and principal bronchi.

(3) The shape, location and structures of lung. The concept of the bronchopulmonary segments for each lung. The lymph drainage of the lungs.

(4) The concept of mediastinum. The subdivisions and contents of the mediastinum. The visible structures of the right and left side of mediastinum.

(5) The position and shape of the thymus.

(6) The concept of pericardium. The position of pericardial sinuses.

(7) The location, surfaces of the heart. The principle features of four chambers of heart. The composition and location of conduction system of the heart. The structure of the heart. The principle features of interatrial and interventricular septums. The origin, course, main branches and distribution of right and left coronary artery. The venous drainage of the heart. The structures of the cardiac walls. The surface marking of the heart.

(8) The beginning, ending and parts of aorta. The beginning, ending and branches of ascending aorta. The beginning, ending and branches of the aortic arch. The beginning, ending and branches of the thoracic aorta.

(9) The pulmonary trunk, left and right pulmonary artery. The location of ligamentum arteriosum. The beginning, ending, and drainage of the superior vena cava. The beginning, ending, and drainage of the left and right brachiocephalic vein. The beginning, ending, and drainage of the azygos vein.

(10) The lymph nodes and vessels of the thorax. The beginning, course, opening, and areas of drainage of thoracic duct and right lymphatic duct.

(11) The formation, courses and function of vagus nerve and branches in thorax.

(12) The formation, courses and function of phrenic nerve.

(13) The he basic anatomy of the thoracic part of sympathetic trunk.

(14) The course, major relations and neurovascular supply of the esophagus within the thorax.

(15) The anatomy of the breast including its neurovascular supply. The lymphatic drainage of the breast and its clinical relevance to metastatic spread.

Chapter 4　Abdomen

1. Abdominal wall.

(1) The bony and cartilaginous landmarks visible or palpable on abdominal examination and explain their clinical significance.

(2) The surface projections of the abdominal organs onto the four quadrants and nine descriptive regions of the abdomen.

(3) The layers of anterior abdominal wall. The arrangements of the muscles of the anterior abdominal wall. The formation and features of sheath of rectus abdominis. The blood supply and innervations of the anterior abdominal wall.

(4) The position, formation of inguinal canal. The structures passing through the inguinal canal. Master the boundaries of inguinal triangle.

(5) The composition of spermatic cord. The features and structures of scrotum. The location, shape and function of testis and epididymis.

2. Abdominal cavity.

(1) The concept of peritoneum and peritoneal cavity. The relationship of various organs to their peritoneal covering. The structures formed by peritoneum. The location of lesser omentum, greater omentum, mesentery, mesoappendix, transverse mesocolon, sigmoid mesocolon, ligaments of liver, omental bursa, omental foramen,

and pouches.

(2) The position of: supracolic and infracolic compartments, paracolic gutters, lesser sac, hepatorenal pouch, subphrenic spaces.

(3) The location, shape and parts of stomach. The relations of the stomach. The blood supply of the stomach. The lymph drainage and nerve supply of the stomach.

(4) The disposition of the small intestine. The location, parts and structures of duodenum. The relations of the duodenum. The differences between jejunum and ileum.

(5) The disposition and surface features of large intestine. The location and structures of the caecum. The location of the vermiform appendix. The surface marking of the root of vermiform appendix. The disposition of the colon. The blood supply of the large intestine.

(6) The position and functional anatomy of the liver, its lobes, segments and their key anatomical relations. The peritoneal reflections of the liver and its movement during ventilation. Summarize the functional anatomy of the portal vein, the portal venous system, porto-systemic anastomosesand their significance in portal hypertension.

(7) The position, functional anatomy and vasculature of the gall bladder and biliary tree; explain their relations in the abdomen and the clinical significance of inflammation of the biliary system and biliary (gall) stones.

(8) The position and form of the pancreas and its relations to other abdominal organs. The significance of these relations to pancreatitis and biliary stone disease.

(9) The location, shape and surface marking of the spleen. The relations of the spleen. The peritoneal ligament of the spleen.

(10) The position and functional anatomy of the kidneys and ureters. Demonstrate their relations to other abdominal and pelvic structures. The clinical significance of renal and ureteric anatomy in relation to urinary stones.

(11) The location and general features of suprarenal glands.

(12) The origins, courses and major branches of the abdominal aorta, coeliac trunk, superior and inferior mesenteric, renal and gonadal arteries.

(13) The location and main tributaries of inferior vena cava.

(14) The lymph nodes of the abdomen. The formations of nine lymphatic trunks.

(15) The formation, position and main branches of the lumber plexuses.

(16) The branches of the vagus nerve in the abdomen. Know the locations of lumber sympathetic trunks.

Chapter 5　Pelvis and Perineum

1. Pelvic wall.

(1) The skeletal and ligamentous components of the pelvis, the anatomy of the pelvic inlet and outlet and recognize their normal orientation. Sexual differences in pelvic skeletal anatomy. The palpable anatomical landmarks of the ilium, ischium and pubis.

(2) The anatomy and functional importance of the pelvic diaphragm, its midline raphe, perineal body, attachment points and the structures passing through it in males and females, the disposition of the pelvic fascia, the clinical significance of the pelvic

diaphragm, e.g. in relation to continence, prolapse and episiotomy.

2. Pelvic cavity.

(1) The anatomy of the bladder, its base and ureteric openings and its relationship to the overlying peritoneum. The innervation of the bladder, its sphincters and the mechanism of micturition.

(2) The anatomy of the scrotum, testis and epididymis and their normal features on clinical examination. Explain the significance of the vascular supply of the testis in relation to torsion and varicocele and the lymphatic drainage in relation to tumour spread.

(3) The structure and course of the spermatic cord and ductus (vas) deferens.

(4) The anatomy and relations of the prostate gland and seminal vesicles. The normal form of the prostate when examined per rectum and how this changes in relation to hypertrophy and malignancy.

(5) The anatomy and relations of the ovary, uterine tubes, uterus, cervix and vagina, including their peritoneal coverings. Describe the changes that occur in the uterus and cervix with pregnancy.

(6) The origin, course and relations of the ovarian, uterine, vaginal and testicular arteries.

(7) The anatomy, relations and peritoneal coverings of the sigmoid colon, rectum and anal canal. The functional anatomy of puborectalis, the anal sphincters and their role in faecal continence.

(8) The blood supply and venous drainage of the distal bowel; the supply from superior rectal (from inferior mesenteric), middle rectal (from internal iliac) and inferior rectal arteries (from internal pudendal to anal canal only), and portosystemic venous anastomoses. The clinical significance of the blood supply and venous drainage of the distal bowel, e.g. in continence, haemorrhoids and anal fissures.

(9) The lymphatic drainage of the pelvic and perineal organs.

3. Perineum.

(1) The concept, boundary and parts of perineum.

(2) The location, boundaries and contents of ischiorectal fossa.

(3) The composition of male and female external genital organs. The general features of the urethra in the male and female.

(4) The disposition of the fascia of urogenital region. The formation of pelvic diaphragm. The location and contents of superficial and deep perineal spaces.

(5) The course and branches of the pudendal nerve and internal pudendal artery.

Chapter 6　Vertebral Region

1. The main anatomical features of typical and atypical vertebrae. Identify the atlas, axis, other cervical, thoracic, lumbar, sacral, and coccygeal vertebrae and recognize their characteristic features.

2. The anatomy of intervertebral joints. Explain the role of intervertebral discs in weight-bearing, give examples of common disc lesions and how they may compress adjacent neurological structures.

3. The regions and functions of the vertebral column. Describe the range of movement of the entire vertebral column and its individual regions. Explain the anatomical bases of common spinal injuries.

4. The principal muscles, ligaments and surface features of the vertebral column. Discuss their functional roles in stability and movement of the vertebral column.

5. The anatomical relationships of the meninges to the spinal cord and dorsal and ventral nerve roots, particularly in relation to root compression and the placement of epidural and spinal injections. Describe the anatomy relevant to performing a lumbar puncture.

6. The anatomy of a typical spinal nerve, including its origin from dorsal and ventral spinal roots, its main motor and cutaneous branches and any autonomic component.

Chapter 7   Upper Limb

1. The boundaries and divisions of the upper limbs.

2. The surface anatomy and the main landmarks of the clavicle, scapula, humerus, radius and ulna. The bones of the wrist and hand and their relative positions, identify those bones that are commonly injured, e.g. scaphoid.

3. The neurovascular structures lying in close relation to the bones and joints of the upper limb which are at risk of injury following fracture or dislocation.

4. The origin, course and distribution of the major arteries and their branches that supply the shoulder, arm, forearm and hand in relation to common sites of injury.

5. The importance of anastomoses between the branches. Identify those sites where neurovascular structures are at particular risk of damage from musculoskeletal injuries.

6. The sites at which pulses of the brachial, radial and ulnar arteries may be located.

7. The course of the main veins of the upper limb and contrast the functions of the deep and superficial veins. The common sites of venous access and describe their key anatomical relations.

8. The anatomy of the brachial plexus from its origin in the neck to its terminal branches. Recognize brachial plexus injuries and explain their clinical presentation.

9. The origin, course and function of the axillary, radial, musculocutaneous, median and ulnar nerves in the upper limb.

10. The major muscles and muscle groups that the axillary, radial, musculocutaneous, median and ulnar nerves supply, together with their sensory distribution.

11. The anatomy of the pectoral girdle, explain the movements of the pectoral girdle, the muscles and joints responsible for these movements. The main attachments and nerve supply of these muscles.

12. The boundaries and contents of the axilla, including the major vessels and relevant parts of the brachial plexus.

13. The name, position, action and nerve supply of muscles connecting the upper limb to the thoracic wall. The name, position, action and nerve supply of muscles connecting the scapula to the humerus. The origin, insertion, action and nerve supply of pectoralis major, trapezius, latissimus dorsi, and deltoid muscles.

14. The beginning, ending and branches of the axillary artery.

15. The anatomy of the axillary lymph nodes and explain their importance in the lymphatic drainage of the breast and skin of the trunk and upper limb and in the spread of tumors.

16. The contents of anterior and posterior fascial compartment of the arm.

17. The origin, insertion, action and nerve supply of biceps brachii and triceps.

18. The anatomy of the elbow joint. Identify the muscles responsible for these movements. Name the main attachments and nerve supply of these muscles.

19. The boundaries and contents of the cubital fossa.

20. The contents of anterior and posterior fascial compartment of the forearm.

21. The anatomy of the wrist. Describe and demonstrate movements at the wrist joints and name and identify the muscle groups responsible for the movements. The relative positions of the tendons, vessels and nerves in the region of the wrist in relation to injuries.

22. The boundaries and contents of the anatomical "snuff box".

23. The composition and contents of the carpal tunnel. The position and function of the retinacula of the wrist and the tendon sheaths of the wrist and hand in order to explain carpal tunnel syndrome and the spread of infection in the tendon sheaths.

24. The innervation of the muscles and skin of the hand. The formation and location of the superficial and deep palmar arches. The position of the fascial spaces of the palm.

25. The pulp space of the fingers. The nerves and arteries of fingers. The tendons and tendinous sheath of the fingers.

Chapter 8 Lower Limb

1. The boundaries and divisions of the lower limbs.

2. The osteology and surface landmarks of the pelvis, femur, tibia, fibula and foot.

3. The origin, course and branches of the major arteries that supply the gluteal region, hip, thigh, knee, leg, ankle and foot. The functional significance of anastomoses between branches of these arteries at the hip and knee.

4. The locations at which the femoral, popliteal, posterior tibial and dorsalis pedis arterial pulses can be palpated.

5. The course of the principal veins of the lower limb. The role of the perforator veins between the superficial and deep veins and the function of the 'muscle pump' for venous return to the heart. The surface landmarks for sites of venous access that can be used for "cut down" procedures in emergencies.

6. The origin of the lumbosacral plexus and the formation of its major branches.

7. The origin, course and function of the femoral, obturator, sciatic, tibial, common fibular (peroneal), sural and saphenous nerves and summarize the muscles and muscle groups that each supplies, as well as their sensory distribution.

8. The anatomical characteristics of the gluteal region. The structures exit the greater and lesser sciatic foramen. The origin, course and distribution of the sciatic nerve.

9. The lymphatic drainage of the lower limb and its relationship to infection and tumor spread.

10. The anatomical properties and movements of the hip joint. Summarize the

muscles responsible for these movements, their innervation and attachments.

11. The contents of anterior, medial and posterior osteofascial compartment of the thigh.

12. The structures formed by the deep fascia of the thigh.

13. The boundaries and contents of the femoral triangle with particular regard to arterial blood sampling and catheter placement. The composition and contents of the femoral sheath. The boundaries of the femoral ring. The beginning, ending and branches of the femoral artery. The origin, branches and distribution of the femoral nerve. The position and area drainage of the deep inguinal lymph nodes.

14. The boundaries, contents and openings of the adductor canal.

15. The anatomical properties and movements of the knee joint. Summarize the muscles responsible for these movements, their innervation and main attachments.

16. The boundaries and contents of the popliteal fossa.

17. The course and bifurcations of the popliteal artery.

18. The close relations of the knee joint, including major bursae and explain which of these structures may be injured by trauma.

19. The contents of anterior, lateral and posterior fascial compartment of leg.

20. The origin, insertion, action and nerve supply of tibialis anterior, gastrocnemius and soleus, and tibialis posterior.

21. The beginning, ending and branches of the anterior and posterior tibial arteries.

22. The distributions of the tibial, superficial and deep peroneal nerves.

23. The innervation of the muscles of the leg.

24. The beginning, ending and branches of the dorsalis pedis artery.

25. The structures that pass behind the medial malleolus beneath the flexor retinaculum from medial to lateral.

26. The anatomical properties of the ankle and subtalar joints. The movements of plantar flexion, dorsiflexion, inversion and eversion. Summarize the innervation and attachments of the muscles responsible for these movements.

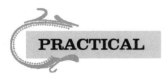

PRACTICAL

1. Head.

Dissection: Superficial and deep dissection of face. The Frontoparietooccipital region, temporal and infratemporal fossa, cranial cavity, naso and oropharyngeal regions.

2. Neck.

Dissection: Superficial and deep dissection of neck. The submandibular triangle, carotid triangle, the muscular triangle, the occipital triangle and the greater supraclavicular fossa. The root of neck.

3. Thorax.

Dissection: Chest wall, mediastinum, pleura, lungs, heart.

4. Abdomen.

Dissection: Anterior abdominal wall and inguinal region, external genitalia. The peritoneum, viscera and retroperitoneal space.

5. Pelvis and Perineum.

Dissection: Pelvic viscera, blood vessels and nerves. Prosected Parts: Perineum including ischio-rectal fossa.

6. Vertebral Region.

Dissection: Superficial and deep dissection of vertebral region.

7. Upper Limb.

Dissection: Pectoral region and axilla, anterior and posterior regions of arm, elbow, forearm and hand.

8. Lower Limb.

Dissection: Gluteal region, anterior, medial and posterior compartment of thigh, popliteal fossa, anterior, lateral and posterior compartment of the leg, malleolar canal and dorsum of foot.

HISTOLOGY AND EMBRYOLOGY
组织学与胚胎学

Chief Editors（主编）
Cao Bo（曹博） Harbin Medical University（哈尔滨医科大学）
Lei Lei（雷蕾） Harbin Medical University（哈尔滨医科大学）
Wang Junyan（王俊艳） Tianjin Medical University（天津医科大学）

Deputy Chief Editors（副主编）
ZhaoHui（赵惠） Jilin University（吉林大学）
Wang Shie（王世鄂） Fujian Medical University（福建医科大学）

Editors（编委）（按姓氏拼音排序）
Cao Bo（曹博） Harbin Medical University（哈尔滨医科大学）
Lei Lei（雷蕾） Harbin Medical University（哈尔滨医科大学）
Li Dongmei（李冬梅） Zhejiang University（浙江大学）
Liu Xiangqian（刘向前） Huazhong University of science and Technology
（华中科技大学）
Meng Xiaoting（孟晓婷） Jilin University（吉林大学）
SongYang（宋阳） DalianMedical University（大连医科大学）
Wang Junyan（王俊艳） Tianjin Medical University（天津医科大学）
Wang Shie（王世鄂） Fujian Medical University（福建医科大学）
ZhaoHui（赵惠） Jilin University（吉林大学）

Course Description

Histology and embryology course consists of two subjects. Histology is the study of the tissues and of how the tissues are arranged to constitute organs, which provides students with understanding of the structural and functional organization of the human body at the cellular and subcellular levels. Embryology is a subject that studies the normal development as well as the birth defects of a human being in the maternal uterus. The emphasis will be on the morphological changes and congenital anomalies that take place during development. The teaching purposes of these subjects are to guide the students acquiring the basic theories and knowledge of histology and embryology and gaining related basic skill training. Upon completion of this course, students will be able to know the general and specific features of tissues and organs, understand the early development of human embryo, and establish a solid basis for learning other basic and clinical medical courses.

Objectives

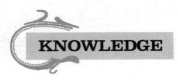

KNOWLEDGE

At the end of the course, the students shall be able to:

1. Comprehend the structure, functions and characteristics of four basic tissues.

2. Understand the structural and functional organization of the human body at the cellular and subcellular levels as a prerequisite for understanding the altered state in various disease processes.

3. Gain a systemic knowledge about the early development of the human embryo and the development of the main organs.

4. Explain developmental basis of the occurrence of major variations, abnormalities and congenital anomalies.

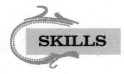

SKILLS

At the end of the course, the students shall be able to:

1. Know the principles of microscope and operate light microscope correctly.

2. Understand the preparation of tissue sections.

3. Describe and draw morphologic structure features of cells, tissues and organs observed under the microscope.

4. Comprehend the brief principle of electron microscopy and interpretation of ultra structure features.

Teaching and Learning Methods

Theory: The course is delivered by a variety of teaching methods to enhance and optimize student learning and understanding the microstructure of the human body as well as main processes of development of the embryo. Regular class lectures, group tutorials and review scientific frontiers throughout the taught part of the course provide means for students to consolidate their understanding of course content.

Practical: Lab lesson asks students to know common investigation methods of histology and to master how to use the light microscope. During practical training, students should obtain the ability to identify the cells, tissues and organs by observing histological sections or electron micrographs, and understand main processes of development of the embryo. Through the practical course, students should achieve these ends: linking the theory with the exercise; linking the structure with the function;

building a three-dimensional structure from a two-dimensional image; establishing a dynamical development sense.

Recommended Textbooks

Abraham L Kierszenbaum, Laura L Tres. 2016. Histology and Cell Biology: An Introduction to Pathology [M]. 4th ed. Philadelphia: Elsevier Saunders.

Anthony L Mescher. 2016. Junqueira's Basic Histology: Text and Atlas [M]. 14th ed. New York: McGraw-Hill Education.

Barbara Young, Geraldine O'Dowd, Phillip Woodford. 2014. Wheater's Functional Histology: A Text and Colour Atlas [M]. 6th ed. Philadelphia: Elsevier Churchill Livingstone.

Bruce M Carlson. 2014. Human Embryology & Developmental Biology [M]. 5th ed. Philadelphia: Elsevier Saunders.

Gary C Schoenwolf, Steven B Bleyl, Philip R Brauer et al. 2015. Larsen's Human Embryology [M]. 5th ed. Philadelphia: Elsevier Churchill Livingstone.

Keith L Moore, TVN Persaud, Mark G Torchia. 2016. The Developing Human: Clinically Oriented Embryology [M]. 10th ed. Philadelphia: Elsevier.

Keith L Moore, TVN Persaud, Mark G Torchia. 2016. Before We Are Born: Essentials of Embryology and Birth Defects [M]. 9th ed. Philadelphia: Elsevier Saunders.

Li Jicheng (李继承), Zeng Yuanshan (曾园山). 2018. Histology and Embryology [M]. 9th ed. Beijing: People's Medical Publishing House.

T W Sadler. 2015. Langman's Medical Embryology [M]. 13th ed. Philadelphia: Wolters Kluwer Health.

Victor P Eroschenko. 2017. Atlas of Histology: with Functional Correlations [M]. 13th ed. Baltimore: Wolters Kluwer.

William K Ovalle, Patrick C Nahirney. 2013. Netter's Essential Histology [M]. 2nd ed. Philadelphia: Elsevier Saunders.

Schedule Table

Chapter		Contents	Lecutre Hours	Practical Hours
	1	Introduction to Histology	0.5	4
	2	Epithelial Tissue	1.5	
	3	Connective Tissue Proper	2	4
	4	Cartilage and Bone	2	
Histology	5	Blood	2	4
	6	Muscle	2	
	7	Nerve Tissue	2	2+2*
	8	Nervous System	2	4
	9	Circulatory System	2	

Continued

Chapter		Contents	Lecutre Hours	Practical Hours
Histology	10	Digestive Tract	2	4
	11	Digestive Glands	2	
	12	Lymphoid System	2	4
	13	Skin	2	
	14	Respiratory System	2	4
	15	Endocrine System	2	
	16	Urinary System	2	
	17	Male Reproductive System	2	4
	18	Female Reproductive System	2	
	19	Sense Organs	2	4+2*
Embryology	1	General Embryology	4	
	2	Development of Face, Palate, Digestive System and Respiratory System	2	
	3	Development of Urogenital System	2	
	4	Development of Circulatory System	4	
		Total	48	42

Noting：* is experimental exam

Course Contents

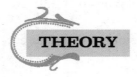

THEORY

I. Histology

Chapter 1　Introduction

1. The concepts of histology.
2. The four types of basic tissue.
3. The preparation of tissues for study.

fixation, embedding, sectioning and staining.

acidophilia, basophilia, neutrophilia, argyrophilia, metachromasia.

4. The methods used in histology.

light microscopy, electron microscopy, immunohistochemistry, enzyme histochemistry, cell and tissue culture.

Chapter 2　Epithelial Tissue

1. The characteristics of epithelium.

2. The classifications, typical locations and major functions of covering epithelia.

3. The specialized structures of epithelial cell surface (apical surface, lateral domain and basal domain).

4. The glandular epithelium and glands.

Chapter 3　Connective Tissue Proper

1. Types of connective tissue proper and their distributions.

2. Loose connective tissue.

cells, fibers and their structural features and functions.

intercellular substances, amorphous ground substance.

3. The basic structure and functions of the dense connective tissue, adipose tissue and reticular tissue.

Chapter 4　Cartilage and Bone

1. The definition and classifications of cartilage.

2. The structure and functions of hyaline cartilage, fibro cartilage and elastic cartilage.

3. Bone tissue.

(1) Bone cells.

osteoblast, osteocytes and osteoclasts.

(2) Bone matrix.

(3) Periosteum and endosteum.

(4) Structure of compact bone.

4. Osteogensis.

intramembranous ossification and endochondral ossification.

Chapter 5　Blood

1. The composition of plasma.

2. The structure and functions of blood cells.

erythrocytes, leucocytes and blood platelets.

3. The hemopoiesis.

origin and differentiate stages of blood cells.

major changes in developing hemopoietic cell.

types of bone marrow and the structure of red bone marrow.

Chapter 6　Muscle

1. The classifications of the muscle.

(1) Skeletal muscle.

cross striation, myofibrils, sarcomere, light band, dark band, H band, Z line, M line, thick and thin myofilament.

sarcoplasmic reticulum, transverse tubule system.

epimysium, perimysium and endomysium.

(2) Cardiac muscle.

the comparison of the structure between cardiac muscle and the skeletal muscle.

the structure and functions of the intercalated discs.

(3) Smooth muscle.

the basic structure and distribution of the smooth muscle.

Chapter 7　Nerve Tissue

1. The constituents of nerve tissue.

2. The structure and functions of neuron (cell body, dendrite, axon).

3. The classifications of neuron.

4. Nerve fiber.

(1) The classification of nerve fibers.

(2) The structure of myelinated nerve fiber, nodes of Ranvier.

(3) The organization within peripheral nerve.

epineurium, perineurium and endoneurium.

(4) The peripheral nerve endings.

5. Synapse.

(1) The definition and classifications of synapse.

(2) The components of chemical synapse.

presynaptic element, synaptic cleft, postsynaptic element.

6. Classifications and functions of neuroglia.

Chapter 8　Nervous System

1. Central nervous system.

(1) The general structure of the spinal cord, the cerebellum and the cerebrum.

(2) Meninges: dura mater, arachnoid and pia mater.

(3) Choroid plexus and cerebrospinal fluid.

(4) The structure and functions of blood brain barrier.

2. Peripheral nervous system.

the general structure of cerebrospinal ganglia and autonomic ganglia.

Chapter 9　Circulatory System

1. The components and functions of circulatory system.

2. Blood vessel.

(1) The basic structure of blood vessel wall.

(2) The structure and functions of large artery, medium-sized artery, small artery and arteriole.

(3) The general structure of the capillaries.

(4) The ultrastructure, function and distribution of three types of capillary (continuous, fenestrated, and sinusoidal capillaries).

(5) The differences in structure between veins and arteries.

(6) The components and functions of microcirculation.

3. Heart.

(1) The structure of the heart wall.

(2) The structure of cardiac skeleton and heart valves.

(3) The constituent, structure and functions of the impulse-generating and impulse-conducting system of the heart.

4. The classifications and structure of lymphatic vessels.

Chapter 10　Digestive Tract

1. The components and functions of digestive system.

2. The general structure of the digestive tract.

3. Oral cavity.

(1) Mucosa of oral cavity.

(2) The classifications of tongue papillae.

(3) The structure and functions of taste buds.

4. The structure and functions of the esophagus.

5. The structure and functions of stomach.

surface mucous cell, gastric glands, gastric mucosal barrier.

6. The structure and functions of the small intestine.

villi, intestinal epithelium, intestinal glands.

7. The structure and functions of the large intestine.

8. The structure and functions of the appendix.

9. The structure and functions of the gut-associated lymphoid tissue (GALT).

10. The principal endocrine cells of the gastrointestinal tract.

Chapter 11　Digestive Glands

1. The structure and functions of three pairs of major salivary glands (parotid, submandibular and sublingual glands).

2. The structure and functions of pancreas.

(1) Exocrine portion.

(2) Pancreatic islets (islets of Langerhans).

3. The structure and functions of liver.

(1) The structure and functions of heptatic lobule.

central vein, hepatocytes, space of Disse, hepatic sinusoids, bile canaliculi.

(2) The portal areas.

4. The structure and functions of the gall bladder.

Chapter 12　Lymphoid System

1. The components and functions of immune system.

2. The major cell types in immune system.

3. The structural features of diffuse lymphoid tissue and lymphoid nodule.

4. The classifications of lymphoid organs.

5. The structure and functions of thymus.

cortex and medulla, thymic (Hassall's) corpuscles, blood-thymus barrier.

6. The structure and functions of lymph nodes.

hilum, cortex, medulla.

7. The structure and functions of spleen.

white pulp, red pulp, marginal zone.

8. The structure and functions of tonsil.

Chapter 13   Skin

1. The general structure of skin.

2. The layers of epidermis.

3. The layers of dermis.

4. The distribution and functions of nonkeratinocytes.

5. The skin appendages.

(1) The structure of hairs.

(2) The glands of the skin.

Chapter 14   Respiratory System

1. The composition and functions of different parts of respiratory system.

2. The structure of trachea and primary bronchi.

3. Lung.

(1) Bronchial tree.

composition and transitional change in structures of conducting portion and respiratory portion;

(2) Alveoli.

structure and functions of type I alveolar cell, type II alveolar cell;

(3) The structure and function of blood-air barrier, pulmonary lobule, alveolar septum, alveolar pore and alveolar macrophage.

Chapter 15   Endocrine System

1. The composition of endocrine system.

2. The general structure of endocrine glands and endocrine cells.

3. The structure and functions of thyroid gland.

thyrocytes /follicular cells, parafollicular cell.

4. The structure and function of parathyroid gland.

chief cells, oxyphil cells.

5. The structure and functions of adrenal gland.

(1) Adrenal cortex.

zona glomerulosa, zona fasciculate and zona reticularis.

(2) Adrenal medulla.

6. The structure and functions of hypophysis.

adenohypophysis, neurohypophysis, hypophyseal portal system.

7. The structural and functional relationship between hypophysis and hypo-thalamus.

hypothalamus-neurohypophysis, hypothalamus-adenohypophysis.

8. The definition of the diffuse neuroendocrine system.

Chapter 16   Urinary System

1. The structure and functions of kidney.

(1) nephron.

Renal corpuscle and renal tubule.

(2) Filtration membrane/barrier;

(3) Collecting duct;

(4) Juxtaglomerular complex;

(5) Blood circulation of kidney.

2. The structure and functions of the ureter and urinary bladder.

Chapter 17   Male Reproductive System

1. The structure and functions of testis.

interstitial tissue, seminiferous tubules, spermatogenesis, spermiogenesis, Sertoli cell, Leydig cell,

2. The structure and functions of epididymis.

3. The structure and functions of ductus deferens.

4. The Structure and functions of prostate.

prostatic concretion.

Chapter 18   Female Reproductive System

1. The structure and functions of ovary.

(1) Ovarian follicles.

(2) Follicular growth.

(3) Follicular atresia.

(4) Ovulation.

(5) Corpus luteum.

2. The structure and functions of uterine tubes.

3. The structure and functions of uterus.

(1) Endometrium.

(2) Myometrium.

(3) Perimetrium.

(4) Menstrual cycle.

4. The structure and functions of uterine cervix and vagina.

5. The structure and functions of mammary gland.

Chapter 19   Sense Organs

1. The structure and functions of eyes.

fibrous layer, vascular layer, lens, vitreous body, retina, accessory structures of the eye.

2. The structure and functions of ears.

(1) External ear.

(2) Middle ear.

(3) Internal ear.

II. Embryology

Chapter 1　General Embryology

1. The definition of embryology.

2. The gametogenesis in the male and female.

3. The development of the first week.

(1) Normal site and phases of fertilization.

(2) Cleavage of zygote.

(3) Formation of blastocyst.

4. The development of the second week.

(1) Differentiation of embryoblast and trophoblast.

(2) Formation of bilaminar germ disc.

(3) Formation of cytotrophoblast, syncytiotrophoblast, amniotic membrane, amniotic cavity, yolk sac, extra embryonic mesoderm and extra embryonic coelom and connecting stalk.

(4) Appearance of prochordal plate.

(5) Implantation sites of blastocystes, decidua, and ectopic pregnancies.

5. The development of the third week.

(1) Appearance and fate of primitive streak and primitive node.

(2) Formation of germ layers.

(3) Neurulation.

formation of neural plate and neural tube, neural crest and its derivatives.

(4) Formation of notochordal process and notochord.

6. The development from the fourth to eighth week (Embryonic period).

(1) Folding of the embryo in the median plane.

(2) Folding of the embryo in the horizontal plane.

(3) Derivatives of ectoderm, mesoderm and endoderm.

7. The development from the third month to birth (Fetal period).

(1) Maturation of tissues and organs.

(2) Rapid growth of body.

(3) Expected date of delivery.

8. The placenta and fetal membrane.

(1) Placenta.

development of the placenta, placental circulation, the placental membrane, functions of the placenta.

(2) Umbilical cord.

(3) Amnion and amniotic fluid.

(4) Yolk sac (umbilical vesicle).

(5) Allantois.

(6) Chorion.

9. Multiple pregnancies.

(1) Formation of twins and types of twins.

(2) Types of placentas and fetal membranes in monozygotic and dizygotic twins.

(3) Conjoined twins.

(4) Other types of multiple births.

10. Teratology.

(1) Principles in teratogenesis.

(2) Classifications of birth defects.

(3) Genetic factors, environmental factors and multifactorial inheritance for congenital malformations.

Chapter 2   Development of Face, Palate, Digestive System and Respiratory System

1. The components and differentiation of pharyngeal apparatus.

2. The development of the face and palate.

(1) Five facial primordial.

(2) Development of primary palate and secondary palate.

(3) Congenital malformation.

cleft lip, cleft palate and oblique facial cleft.

3. The development of the digestive system.

(1) Formation and differentiation of primitive gut.

(2) Development of foregut, midgut and hindgut.

4. The congenital malformation of digestive tract, liver, gallbladder and pancreas.

5. Development and congenital malformation of respiratory system.

Chapter 3   Development of Urogenital System

1. The development of the pronephros, mesonephros and metonephros.

2. The development of the kidney, ureters, urinary bladder and urethra.

3. The development of gonads, genital ducts and external genitalia.

4. The relocation of the testis and ovary.

5. The congenital malformation of urogenital system.

Chapter 4   Development of Cardiovascular System

1. Early development of the heart and blood vessels.

(1) Establishment of the cardiogenic area and endothelial heart tubes.

(2) Vasculogenesis commences with the formation of blood island.

2. Later development of the heart.

(1) Circulation through the primordial heart.

(2) Partitioning of atrium, atrioventricular canal, ventricles.

(3) Partitioning of the truncus arteriorsus and conus cordis.

3. Fetal and neonatal circulation.

4. The congenital malformation of the heart and great vessels.

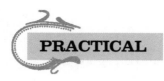

PRACTICAL

1. The structure, operation and care of a binocular light microscope.

2. The basic principle and process of paraffin section and HE staining.

3. Observing the following slides under light microscope.

(1) Epithelial tissue.

simple squamous epithelium, simple cuboidal epithelium, simple columnar epithelium, pseudostratified ciliated columnar epithelium and transitional epithelium.

(2) Connective tissue proper.

loose connective tissue, dense connective tissue, adipose tissue and reticular tissue.

(3) Cartilage and bone.

hyaline cartilage, fibrocartilage, elastic cartilage, bone tissue and cartilaginous ossification.

(4) Blood.

blood smear.

(5) Muscle.

skeletal muscle, cardiac muscle and smooth muscle.

(6) Nerve tissue.

Neuron and nerve fiber.

(7) Nerve system.

cerebrum, cerebellum and spinal cord.

(8) Circulatory system.

large artery, medium-sized artery and vein, small artery and vein, capillary and heart.

(9) Digestive tract.

esophagus, stomach, duodenum, jejunum, ileum, colon and appendix.

(10) Digestive glands.

salivary glands, liver, pancreas and gall bladder.

(11) Lymphoid system.

thymus, lymph node, spleen and tonsil.

(12) Skin.

skin of the human finger and scalp.

(13) Respiratory system.

olfactory mucosa, trachea and lung.

(14) Endocrine system.

thyroid, parathyroid gland, adrenal gland, pituitary gland and pineal body.

(15) Urinary system.

kidney, ureter and urinary bladder.

(16) Male reproductive system.

testis, epididymis, ductus deferens and prostate.

(17) Female reproductive system.

ovary, uterine tube, uterus, vagina and mammary gland.

(18) Sense organ.

eyelid, eyeball and inner ear.

4. Demonstrating electron micrographs as followings.

(1) Epithelial tissue.

microvillus and cilium (TEM) and microvillus and cilium (SEM).

(2) Connective tissue proper:

fibroblast (TEM), macrophage (TEM), mast cell (TEM), plasma cell (TEM) and collagen fiber (TEM).

(3) Cartilage and bone.

osteon and interstitial lamella (SEM) and osteoclast (TEM).

(4) Blood.

neutrophil (TEM), eosinophil (TEM), basophil (TEM) and blood platelet (TEM).

(5) Muscle.

sarcoplasmic reticulum (TEM), myofibril (TEM) and intercalated disc (TEM).

(6) Nerve tissue.

chemical synapse (TEM) and myelinated nerve fiber (TEM).

(7) Circulatory system.

continuous capillary (TEM) and fenestrated capillary (TEM).

(8) Digestive tract.

parietal cell (TEM) and chief cell (TEM).

(9) Digestive gland.

bile canaliculus and hepatocyte (TEM).

(10) Lymphoid system.

postcapillary venule (SEM) and splenic cord and splenic sinusoid (SEM).

(11) Respiratory system.

blood-air barrier (TEM) and type II alveolar cell (TEM).

(12) Urinary system.

filtration barrier (TEM).

5. Embryology.

(1) Models and video showing the main process of early stage of human embryo, fetal membrane, placenta and development of different organ and system.

(2) Observing slides of early stage of chick embryo and human placenta specimen.

BIOCHEMISTRY AND MOLECULAR BIOLOGY
生物化学与分子生物学

Chief Editors（主编）

Lü Lixia（吕立夏） Tongji University（同济大学）

Wang Xiuhong（王秀宏） Harbin Medical University（哈尔滨医科大学）

Li Ling（李凌） Southern Medical University（南方医科大学）

Yang Jie（杨洁） Tianjin Medical University（天津医科大学）

Deputy Chief Editors（副主编）

Zhang Wenli（张文利） Dalian Medical University（大连医科大学）

He Chunyan（何春燕） Wuhan University（武汉大学）

Li Dongmin（李冬民） Xi'an Jiaotong University（西安交通大学）

Li Jiao（李姣） Tongji University（同济大学）

Du Jian（都建） Anhui Medical University（安徽医科大学）

Li Gang（李刚） Tianjin Medical University（天津医科大学）

Editors（编委）（按姓氏拼音排序）

Dai Jianwei（戴建威） Guangzhou Medical University（广州医科大学）

Du Jian（都建） Anhui Medical University（安徽医科大学）

He Chunyan（何春燕） Wuhan University（武汉大学）

Kan Mujie（阚慕洁） Jilin University（吉林大学）

Li Dongmin（李冬民） Xi'an Jiaotong University（西安交通大学）

Li Gang（李刚） Tianjin Medical University（天津医科大学）

Li Jiao（李姣） Tongji University（同济大学）

Li Ling（李凌） Southern Medical University（南方医科大学）

Lü Lixia（吕立夏） Tongji University（同济大学）

Wang Xiuhong（王秀宏） Harbin Medical University（哈尔滨医科大学）

Yang Jie（杨洁） Tianjin Medical University（天津医科大学）

Zhang Jieping（张介平） Tongji University（同济大学）

Zhang Wenli（张文利） Dalian Medical University（大连医科大学）

Course Description

Biochemistry and Molecular Biology is defined as the science of the chemical and molecular basis of life. Its knowledge is essential to all life science. Normal biochemical processes are the basis of health. The major aim of it is the complete understanding of all the chemical processes associated with living cell at molecular level. It also helps medical students to understand the origin of life and to integrate biochemical and molecular knowledge into efforts to maintain health and to understand the biochemical and molecular mechanism underlying diseases and thus treat them effectively.

This rigorous course includes 4 main sections. All sections and chapters emphasize the medical relevance to biochemistry and molecular biology. Section I address the structures and functions of biological macromolecule, including protein, nucleic acid, enzyme and glycoconjugate. Section II describes many functions of metabolites in the cells and explains how various cellular reactions occur, linking to utilization and release of energy,synthesis and degradation pathways of carbohydrate, lipid, amino acid and nucleotide. Hemal and hepatic biochemistry are also included, focusing on carbohydrate metabolism of mature erythrocytes, biochemistry of porphyrins, bile pigments and biotransformation. Section III deals with genetic information transfer, covering DNA replication and repair, RNA biosynthesis, genome and gene expression regulation, protein synthesis. Section IV introduces the principle of common techniques of molecular biology, DNA recombination technology, gene diagnosis and gene therapy in addition to special topic on signaling transduction and growth factors, oncogene and suppressor gene.

The practical section of course will focus on basic techniques for biochemistry and molecular biology, including spectrometry, centrifugation, chromatography, electrophoresis, gene polymorphism detection which merges genomic DNA extraction, polymerase chain reaction, agarose gel electrophoresis and gene diagnosis. Km determination and the determination of blood lipid and glucose are also included.

Objectives

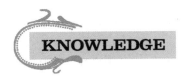

KNOWLEDGE

At the end of the course, the student should be able to:

1. Know the basic structure, chemical component, properties of common 20 amino acids present in proteins.

2. Describe the directionality and four levels of structures for proteins.

3. Identify the key concepts involved in protein structures, including peptide bond, motif, domain, subunit.

4. Explain the relationship between protein structure and functions.

5. Describe the physical-chemical properties of proteins.

6. Memorize the classification of nucleic acid, the chemical components of nucleic acid.

7. Describe the structures and functions of DNA and RNA, especially double helix model of DNA.

8. Describe the physical-chemical properties of nucleic acid and hybridization.

9. State the four principal mechanisms by which enzyme achieve catalysis.

10. Explain catalytic characteristics of enzymes, the significance of the activation of proenzeme (zymogen).

11. Describe the significance of Km and the factors affecting enzymatic activity: substrate concentration, enzyme concentration, temperature and pH.

12. Define the concept of isoenzyme and describe basic and clinical aspects of enzymology and regulation of enzymatic activity.

13. Explain the inhibition of enzyme activity, including irreversible and reversibleinhibition.

14. Describe the concept, structures and functions of glycoconjugate, glycoprotein and proteoglycan.

15. Explain the significance and key enzymes of glycolysis and gluconeogenesis, glycogenesis and glycogenolysis, aerobic oxidation, phosphate pentose pathway and tricarboxylic acid cycle and the regulation of key enzymes in those pathways.

16. State the significance of lactate cycle or Cori cycle as well as source and outlet of blood glucose. Be familiar with regulation of blood glucose by hormone.

17. Describe the synthesis and degradation of triglyceride as well as the process of β-oxidation of fatty acids.

18. Describe formation, utilization and significance of ketone bodies.

19. Memorize the classifications and functions of phospholipids.

20. Memorize key enzyme and materials in the synthesis of cholesterol and the fate of cholesterol.

21. Describe classifications, compositions and functions of plasma lipoprotein.

22. Define the concept of biological oxidation and respiratory chain organization, sequence and functions.

23. Recognize concept of oxidative phosphorylation as well as sites of ATP formation, ATP synthase, inhibitors and uncouplers of electron transfer chain.

24. Describe the degradation of amino acid: transamination, oxidative deamination and transdeamination, and union deamination.

25. Describe the process and significance of urea cycle as well as the sources and fates of ammonia, and transportation of ammonia in blood.

26. Memorize the carrier, kinds and function of one carbon unit.

27. Describe the special amino acid's metabolism.

28. Define the concept of de novo and salvage synthesis pathway, the origin atoms of purine ring and pyrimidine ring synthesized by the de novo synthesis pathway and the significance of de novo and salvage synthesis of purine and pyrimidine nucleotide.

29. Describe the degradation of purine and pyrimidine.

30. Explain the significance of glycolysis in mature erythrocyte and 2,3-BPG shunt.

31. Describe the synthesis of heme and its regulation.

32. Describe source, transportation, conversion of bile pigment in liver, excretion in intestine and bilinogen enterohepatic circulation.

33. Describe the source, classifications, transportation, conversion of bile acid in liver, excretion in intestine and bile acid enterohepatic circulation.

34. Describe the features and process of DNA replication, RNA transcription and

protein translation.

35. Describe the types of post-transcriptional processing of RNA.

36. State the types of post-translational modifications and positioning of protein.

37. Explain the molecular mechanisms of gene expression and regulation, the principles of genetic engineering.

38. Describe the concept, principle and strategy of gene diagnosis and gene therapy and its clinical application.

39. Define the concept, types and features of signal molecule and receptors.

40. State the classic signaling pathways, including membrane receptor mediated signaling pathway and intracellular receptor (nuclear receptor) mediated signaling pathway.

41. Define the concept, classification of oncogene and suppressor gene.

42. Explain molecular mechanism of oncogenes and suppressor genes.

43. Describe the concept and classification of growth factors and their receptors.

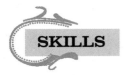

SKILLS

At the end of the course, the student should be able to:

1. Make use of conventional techniques/ instruments to perform biochemical analysis relevant to clinical screening and diagnosis.

2. Analyze and interpret investigative data.

3. Demonstrate the skills of solving clinical problems and decision making.

4. Interpret laboratory investigations for the diagnosis of gene polymorphism and to correlate the clinical manifestations/phenotype with the specific genotype.

Teaching and Learning Methods

Theory: Teaching biochemistry and molecular biology to undergraduate medical student is provided with the help of didactic lectures and tutorials that deal with the basic structure and components of macromolecule, metabolic pathway and regulation, genetic information transfer, special topics in biochemistry as well as introductory knowledge on molecular biology, including commonly used technique, principle of gene engineering, gene diagnosis and therapy.

Practical: Practical training make students know the basic principles, methods and techniques, strategies, and skills for biochemistry, basically covering spectrometry, centrifugation, chromatography and electrophoresis. Furthermore, gene polymorphism analysis strengthen students'better understanding of molecular biology. The student should pay more attention to biosafety in the laboratory, including dispose of lab waste.

Recommended Textbooks

Bhagavan NV, Ha Ch-Eun. 2015. Essentials of Medical BiochemistryWith Clinical

Cases [M]. 2nd ed. Philadelphia: Elsevier.

David L Nelson, Michael M Cox. 2013. Principles of Biochemistry [M]. 6th ed. New York: Lehninger.

Robert K Murray, Darryl K Granner, Peter A Mayes et al. 2012. Harper's Illustrated Biochemistry [M]. 29th ed. New York: McGraw-Hill Lange.

Schedule Table

Chapter	Contents	Hours
1	Introduction and protein's structure and function	6
2	Nucleic acid's structure and function	2
3	Enzyme and vitamin	6
4	Glycoconjugate	2
5	Metabolism of carbohydrates	8
6	Metabolism of lipids	6
7	Biological oxidation	4
8	Metabolism of amino acids	6
9	Metabolism of nucleotide	4
10	Hemal and liver biochemistry	3
11	DNA Biosynthesis	4
12	RNA Biosynthesis	4
13	Genome and Gene expression regulation	2
14	Protein Biosynthesis	6
15	Molecular biology techniques	4
16	Gene engineering	3
17	Gene diagnosis and therapy	2
18	Signaling transduction	4
19	Oncogene, suppressor and growth factor	2
Experiment 1	Use of the Spectrophotometer& Determination of Protein Concentration	3
Experiment 2	Determination of Km value of alkaline phosphatase	3
Experiment 3	Chromatography: (1) Using gel filtration column chromatography to separate hemoglobin and nucleoprotamine (demo); (2) Separating amino acids mixture by ion-exchange chromatography	3
Experiment 4	Centrifugation: The separation of monocytes by density gradient centrifugation	3
Experiment 5	SDS-Polyacrylamide Gel Electrophoresis of Proteins	3
Experiment 6	Effect of hormone on blood sugar and lipoprotein of rat	3
Experiment 7	Polymorphism analysis of ACE gene by extracting genomic DNA of buccal epithelial cells	6
Total		102

Course Contents

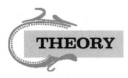

THEORY

Chapter 1   Introduction to Biochemistry

Definition of biochemistry, its central role in the life science, the relationship of biochemistry to health and disease to medicine.

Chapter 2   Protein Structure and Function

1. The amino acids are the building blocks of proteins. The 20 amino acids: structure and classification of amino acids,physicochemical properties of amino acids: ultraviolet absorption and chemical color reaction of amino acids.

2. Four levels of protein structure: the linkage of amino acids in protein and biologically active peptides,primary structure,secondary structure (the alpha helix, the beta sheet, beta turns, and random coil),motif, domain, tertiary structure,quaternary structure.

3. Structure-function relationship of proteins.

(1) Primary structure is the basis for spatial conformation of proteins, the similarity of primary structure of proteins often shares with the similarity of spatial structures and functions, the primary structure of proteins and molecular diseases, the primary structure of proteins providing importantly evolutionary information.

(2) The oxygen binding proteins: myoglobin and hemoglobin, the difference between their oxygen dissociation curve from their distinct protein conformation, the conformational variability of proteins and conformational diseases, eg, prion disease.

4. Classification of proteins: protein classification based on their shapes and solubility: globular proteins and fibrous proteins, protein classification based on their compositions and protein families.

5. Physical chemical properties of proteinand isolation.

(1) Physical-chemical properties of proteins: amphoteric dissociation of proteins; colloidal property of proteins; denaturation, precipitation and coagulation of proteins; the properties of special absorbance and color reactions.

(2) Principles of protein purification: changing protein solubility, purification methods based on molecular weight and size, purification methods based on charges of proteins.

Chapter 3   Nucleic acid structure and function

1. Structural units of nucleic acids-nucleotides: base, pentose and nucleosides, Nucleotides and nucleic acids have characteristic base and pentose; phosphodiester bonds

link nucleotides together to form nucleic acids.

2. Structures and functions of DNA: primary structure of DNA; secondary structure of DNA: DNA is a double helix that stores geneticinformation; polymorphisms of secondary structue of DNA; DNA can occur in different three-dimensional forms.

3. Structures and functions of RNA: mRNA, tRNA and rRNA; Messenger RNAs code for polypeptide chains; many RNAs have more complex three-dimensional structures.

4. Properties of nucleic acids: ultraviolet absorption, denaturation and renaturation of DNA,catalytic properties of RNA.

5. Nucleases.

Chapter 4　Enzyme

1. Structure and function of enzymes: composition of enzyme molecules, cofactors of enzyme, monomeric enzymes, oligomeric enzymes and multienzyme complex,active center of enzymes,isoenzymes.

2. Properties and catalytic mechanisms of enzymes.

(1) Properties of enzyme catalyzed reactions: highly catalytic efficiency of enzymes; specificity of enzymes, regulation of enzyme.

(2) Catalytic mechanisms of enzymes: formation of enzyme-substrate complex and induced-fit hypothesis; factors contributing to enzyme catalysis.

3. Enzyme Kinetics.

(1) Substrate concentration affects the rate of enzyme-catalyzed reactions: Michaelis-Menten equation, the significance of Km and Vmax.

(2) The effect of enzyme concentration, pH and temperature on the rate of enzyme-catalyzed reactions.

(3) The effect of inhibitors on the rate of enzyme-catalyzed reactions: irreversible enzyme inhibition, reversible enzyme inhibition (competitive inhibition, noncompetitive inhibition and uncompetitive inhibition).

(4) Activators of enzymes.

4. Regulatory enzymes: allosteric regulation, chemical modification, zymogens and their activations.

5. Nomenclature and classification of enzymes.

6. Clinical applications of enzymes: enzymes and pathogenesis, role of enzymes in diagnosis of diseases.

Chapter 5　Glycoconjugate

1. Molecular structures of glycans: linkage of monosaccharides in glycans.

2. Structures and functions of glycoproteins: classifications and structures of glycoproteins: N-linked, O-linked and GPI linked glycoproteins, effects of sugar chains on glycoproteins, abnormal glycoproteins and diseases.

3. Structures and functions of proteoglycans: GAGs,core proteins, linkage of GAGs and core proteins,functions of GAGs and proteoglycans.

Chapter 6　Carbohydrate Metabolism

1. Digestion and absorption of carbohydrates.

2. Anaerobic degradation of glucose: basic process of glycolysis, regulation of glycolysis, the significance of glycolysis.

3. Aerobic oxidation of glucose: oxidation of pyruvate to acetyl CoA, tricarboxylic acid cycle, the regulation of aerobic oxidation of glucose, the significance of aerobic oxidation of glucose.

4. Glycogenesis and glycogenolysis: basic process of glycogenesis, basic process of glycogenolysis, regulation of glycogenesis and glycogenolysis, glycogen storage diseases.

5. Gluconeogenesis: the basic process of gluconeogenesis, regulation of gluconeogenesis, the significance of gluconeogenesis, Cori cycle.

6. Pentose phosphate pathway (PPP): basic process and the significance of PPP.

7. Blood sugar and its regulation: blood sugar level and its regulation, abnormal blood sugar level.

Chapter 7　Lipid Metabolism

1. Fatty acids (FA) and derivatives of polyunsaturated fatty acids (PUFA): classification, nomenclature, and sources of FAs, eicosanoids: derivatives of PUFAs.

2. Digestion and absorption of dietary lipids.

3. Metabolism of fats: mobilization of fats, metabolism of glycerol, activation of FAs, transfer of activated fatty acyl into mitochondria, β-oxidation of fatty acids, ATP generated in fatty acid oxidation, formation, utilization of ketone bodies, significances of ketogenesis, biosynthesis of FAs, citrate pyruvate cycle, activation of acetyl CoA to malonyl CoA, palmitate synthetic process, elongation of palmitate to long-chain fatty acids; the synthesis of unsaturated fatty acids, synthesis of triacylglycerol, monoacylglycerol pathway, diacylglycerol pathway, regulation of fat metabolism.

4. Metabolism of phospholipids: metabolism of glycerophospholipids: synthesis of glycerophospholipids: diacylglycerol pathway, CDP-diacylglycerol pathway, degradation of glycerophospholipids, metabolism of sphingolipids: synthesis of sphingolipids, degradation of sphingolipids.

5. Metabolism of cholesterol: biosynthesis of cholesterol, regulation of cholesterol biosynthesis, conversion of cholesterol in vivo.

6. Metabolism of plasma lipoproteins: plasma lipids, classification, composition, and structure of lipoproteins, metabolism of lipoproteins, disorders of lipoprotein metabolism.

Chapter 8　Biological Oxidation

1. Electron transport chain (ETC): oxidation-reduction reactions, free energy changes in redox reactions, components of ETC, electron carriers function in order of increasing reduction.

2. Oxidative phosphorylation: chemiosmotic hypothesis, ATP synthesis, P/O ratio, inhibitors of oxidative phosphorylation, regulation of oxidative phosphorylation.

3. ATP and the other high energy compounds: ATP, creatine phosphate, acetyl CoA

and so on.

4. Selective transport across the inner mitochondrial membrane: transport of adenine nucleotides and phosphate, two shuttle systems for cytosolic NADH from glycolysis.

5. Other biological oxidations: reactive oxygen species (ROS); free radical scavenging enzymes;Cytochrome P450

Chapter 9   Protein Catabolism

1. Functions and Nutritional roles of proteins: functions of proteins,nitrogen balance; nutritional essential amino acids,physiological requirements and nutrition quality of dietary proteins.

2. Digestion, absorption and putrefaction of proteins: digestion of dietary proteins, absorption and transportation of amino acids, putrefaction of proteins.

3. Degradation of protein in cells: lysosomal pathway for proteins degradation, proteasome pathway for proteins degradation.

4. General catabolism of amino acids: deamination of amino acids: transamination, oxidative deamination of L-glutamate dehydrogenase,union deamination (coupled reaction of transaminases and L-glutamate dehydrogenase, purine nucleotide cycle), metabolism of α-keto acids, non-essential amino acids generated by amination, conversion into glucoses and lipids, supply energy.

5. Metabolism of ammonia: source of ammonia, transport of ammonia: alanine-glucose cycle,transport of ammonia by glutamine, formation of urea, regulation of urea biosynthesis and hyperammonemia.

6. Individual amino acid catabolism: decarboxylation of amino acids: gamma(γ)-Aminobutyric acid, Histamine, 5-Hydroxytryptamine,Polyamines, metabolism of one carbon units,metabolism of aromatic amino acids,metabolism of methionine, cysteine and cystine.

Chapter 10   Nucleotide Metabolism

1. Biomedical functions of nucleotides: building blocks of nucleic acids, storage and supplier of energy, mediator of physiological regulation, component of coenzyme, precursor for synthesis of some compounds, allosteric regulators and phosphate donors for covalent modification of enzymes, activated intermediates for metabolism, analogs of nucleosides and nucleotides as antimetabolites.

2. Degradation of nucleic acids.

3. Metabolism of purine nucleotides: biosynthesis of purine nucleotides: de novo synthesis of purine nucleotide: element sources of nucleotide, characteristics of de novo synthesis of purine nucleotides, synthesis of IMP, synthesis of AMP and GMP,regulation of de novo synthesis of purine nucleotides, salvage synthesis of purine nucleotides, degradation of purine nucleotides: uric acid, Gout.

4. Metabolism of pyrimidine nucleotides: biosynthesis of pyrimidine nucleotides: de novo synthesis of pyrimidine nucleotides: element sources of pyrimidine base, characteristics of de novo synthesis of pyrimidine nucleotides, synthetic pathway

of UMP; synthesis of CTP. Salvage synthesis of pyrimidine nucleotides: One-step synthesis,two-step synthesis,catabolism of pyrimidine nucleotides:NH_3, CO_2, β-aminoisobutyrate and β-alanine.

5. Deoxyribonucleotide biosynthesis: characteristics of ribonucleotide reductase, biosynthesis of deoxythymidine monophosphate(dTMP).

6. Biosynthesis of nucleoside diphosphate and nucleoside triphosphate.

7. Dysmetabolism of nucleotides and antimetabolites.

Chapter 11　Hemal and Liver Biochemistry

1. Metabolic characteristics of mature erythrocyte:Carbohydrates metabolism in mature erythrocyte. Heme biosynthesis: the process and regulation of heme biosynthesis.

2. Biotransformation: definition, reaction types and significance of biotransformation, influence factors of biotransformation.

3. Bile and bile acids:classification and physiological functions of bile acids, metabolism of bile acids, enterohepatic circulation of bile acids.

4. Metabolism of bile pigment and jaundice:production of bilirubin, transportation of bilirubin in the blood, transformation of bilirubin in the liver, conversion of conjugated bilirubin in the intestine, bilinogen enterohepatic circulation, hyperbilirubinemia and jaundice (hemolytic, hepatocellular and obstructive jaundice).

Chapter 12　DNA Replication

1. General features of DNA replication:Semi-conservative replication, bidirectional replication, semi-discontinuous replication,high fidelity of DNAreplication.

2. The enzymology of DNA replication:DNA polymerases, DnaA protein, DnaB protein (helicases), DnaC protein, single-stranded DNA-binding proteins, DNA topoisomerases, DnaG protein (primases), and DNA ligases.

3. DNA synthesis in prokaryotes: Initiation includes replication origin(oriC), replication fork and primosome formation. Elongation: leading strand synthesis,Lagging strand synthesis,Okazaki fragments. Termination: removal of RNA primer, filling in the gap by DNA polymerase I, sealing the nick by DNA ligase.

4. DNA synthesis in eukaryotes: initiation: many replication origins. Elongation: DNA polymeraseα and DNA polymerase δ , proliferating cell nuclear antigen(PCNA). Termination: telomeres.

5. Reverse transcription: complementary DNA (cDNA),Reverse transcriptase.

6. DNA damage and repair: types of mutation: point mutation, deletion, insertion and rearrangement, dynamic mutation. DNA Repair Systems: mismatch repair, photoreactivation repair, excision repair, SOS repair, recombination repair.

Chapter 13　RNA Synthesis（Genome and Gene expression regulation）

1. RNA polymerases and templates:DNA-dependent RNA polymerases in prokaryotes and eukaryotes, template strand and coding strand, asymmetric transcription.

2. RNA synthesis in prokaryotes: initiation: holoenzyme, promoter. Elongation: core enzyme, transcript bubble. Termination: ρ (rho)- dependent and ρ (rho)-independent termination.

3. RNA synthesis in eukaryotes:Pre-initiation complex: transcription factors, initiation: Phosphorylation of the CTD. Elongation: elongation factors. Termination:termination signals.

4. RNA processing: Modification of the 5′and 3′end: 5′cap and 3′poly A tail mRNA splicing: small nuclear RNAs (snRNAs); spliceosome. tRNA processing: Replacement of the 3′-terminal UU by CCA, modification of several bases, tRNA splicing. rRNA splicing.

5. Ribozyme.

6. Genome and gene expression regulation:The structure of chromosomes: chromatin of eukaryotic cells, nucleosome, bacterial chromosomes, principles of gene regulation: Housekeeping genes, constitutive gene expression, regulatory geneexpression. Operon, cis-acting elements, trans-acting factor, regulatory proteins, DNA-protein and protein-protein interaction, regulation of gene expression in prokaryotes: Universality of operon model; universality of repression mechanism, lactose(lac) operon in E. coli. Regulation of gene expression in eukaryotes: regulation of transcription for RNA pol I , RNA pol II and RNA pol III

Chapter 14　Protein Synthesis

1. The biosynthesis of protein synthesis: the genetic code, ribosome, amino acids, tRNA, enzymes: Protein factors.

2. Protein biosynthesis:Activation of amino acids. Initiation: Formation of the initiation complex in bacteria, initiation in eukaryotic cells. Elongation: ribosomal cycle. entrance(binding of coming Aminoacyl-tRNA), peptide bond formation, translocation. Termination:three termination codons, release factors (RF1, RF2, RF3). Polyribosome.

3. Posttranslational modifications: Folding of newly synthesized polypeptide chains: molecular chaperone, amino-terminal and carboxyl-terminal modifications, signal Sequences. Modification of individual amino acids: attachment of carbohydrate side chains, addition of prosthetic groups, proteolytic processing.

4. Protein sorting: sorting to the ER: signal sequences,signal recognition particle(SRP). Sorting to the mitochondria: amino-terminal signal sequence. Sorting to the nucleus: nuclear localization sequence(NLS).

5. Protein synthesis is inhibited by many antibiotics and toxins: puromycin, tetracyclines,cycloheximide, streptomycin,diphtheria toxin,ricin, interferon.

Chapter 15　Molecular Biology Techniques

1. Polymerase chain reaction (PCR): its concept, process, features, and its applications.

2. Molecular hybridization and blotting techniques: principle and application of Western blot, Northern blot, in situ hybridization and microarray.

3. The principle and application of restriction length fragment polymorphism analysis.

4. DNA sequencing using the Sanger dideoxynucleotide method.

5. Transgenic technology and gene targeting.

6. RNA interference(RNAi).

Chapter 16   Gene Engineering

1. Recombinant DNA technology: Action of restriction enzymes, DNA ligase, vectors, host cells.

2. Genetic engineering: Preparation of the target DNA, comparison of genomic and cDNA libraries, ligation of target DNA with a cloning vector, transformation of recombinant DNA into host cells, screening of the positive cloning cells that contain recombinant DNA, and expression of cloned genes in host cells.

Chapter 17   Gene Diagnosis and Gene Therapy

1. Gene diagnosis: Definition and its applications, including diagnosis of gene mutations,abnormal gene expressions, infectious agents, tumor mutations and forensic medicine.

2. Gene therapy: types of gene therapy (germline based and somatic cell based gene therapy), therapeutic strategies (gene replacement, gene correction, gene augmentation, gene inactivation) and basic process of gene therapy.

Chapter 18   Signaling transduction

1. Signal molecules: Extracellular signal molecules (neurotransmitter, endocrine hormones, local chemical mediators) and intracellular signal molecules.

2. Receptors: types of receptors (membrane receptors, ion channel receptors, G protein-coupled receptors, single transmembrane receptors, intracellular receptors) and characteristics of receptors.

3. Signal transduction pathways: G protein-coupled receptor mediated signal transduction pathway (G protein, Gs-cAMP-PKA pathway, Gq-IP$_3$/Ca^{2+} and DAG/ PKC signaling pathway), calcium signaling pathways, receptor tyrosine kinase mediatedsignal pathways, guanylate cyclases mediated signal pathways, TGF-β signal transduction pathways, intracellular receptor mediated signal pathways.

4. Signal transduction and medicine.

Chapter 19   Oncogene, suppressor and growth factor

1. Proto-oncogenes and oncogenes: definition, classification and mechanism.

2. Tumor suppressor genes: definition, classifications, and mechanism.

3. Growth factors:Definition, classification, function and their receptors.

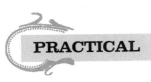

PRACTICAL

1. Spectrophotometry and measurement of protein concentration

(1) Principle of spectrophotometry.

(2) Principles of BAC assay, Bradford assay, Buriet'reaction for protein concentration determination.

(3) Correct operation of spectrophotometer and microplate reader.

(4) Biosafety and disposal of biomaterial.

2. Chromatography.

(1) Principle of chromatography.

(2) Correct operation of gel filtration column chromatography and ion-exchange chraomatography to do isolation from mixtures.

3. Electrophoresis.

(1) Principle of elctrotrophoresis.

(2) Principle of SDS-Polyacrylamide Gel Electrophoresis (PAGE).

(3) Correct running SDS-PAGE to separate proteins.

4. Centrifugation.

(1) Principle of Centrifugation.

(2) Correct operation of instrument of centrifugation.

(3) Preparative techniques, analytical measurements, care of centrifuges and rotors.

5. Kinetic Analysis of Enzyme.

Analysis of Km value of alkaline phosphatase.

6. Effect of insulin on blood sugar and lipoprotein in rat.

(1) Preparation of rat plasma.

(2) Measurement of blood sugar and lipoprotein.

7. Polymorphism analysis of angiotensin converting enzyme (ACE) gene by extracting genomic DNA of buccal epithelial cells.

(1) Buccal epithelial cells genomic DNA extraction.

(2) PCR amplification of ACE gene.

(3) Agarose Gel Electrophoresis analysis of PCR products.

PHYSIOLOGY

生 理 学

Chief Editors（主编）

Wang Liwei（王立伟） Jinan University（暨南大学）

Jiang Hong（姜宏） Qingdao University（青岛大学）

Liu Chuanyong（刘传勇） Shandong University（山东大学）

Deputy Chief Editors（副主编）

He Sichun（何斯纯） Jinan University（暨南大学）

Zhu Yi（朱毅） Tianjin Medical University（天津医科大学）

Editors（编委）（按姓氏拼音排序）

He Sichun（何斯纯） Jinan University（暨南大学）

Jiang Hong（姜宏） Qingdao University（青岛大学）

Liu Chuanyong（刘传勇） Shandong University（山东大学）

Wang Liwei（王立伟） Jinan University（暨南大学）

Wang Yuechun（王跃春） Jinan University（暨南大学）

Xu Geyang（许戈阳） Jinan University（暨南大学）

Zhou Zhuoyan（周卓妍） Jinan University（暨南大学）

Zhu Yi（朱毅） Tianjin Medical University（天津医科大学）

Course Description

Physiology is one of the important basic medical sciences and the foundation of medical practice. It is a study of the normal functions of cells, organs and systems of the living body, the mechanisms by which they are achieved and the regulation of functional activities. A firm grasp of its principles is essential not only for the study of successive courses, but also for students'future professional career after graduation.

Selection of the teaching material is in accordance with the necessity of medical education and emphasis is laid on basic theories and knowledge of physiology as well as on the training of basic techniques. During the course, it is encouraged to promote the ability of scientific critical thinking of the students. In order to improve the teachting efficiency, teaching is given in various ways including seminar, tutorial, self-study, as well as lecture. The problem-based learning, team-based learning and case-based learning are proposed to apply when necessary.

After complete the course, students should be able to: (1) describe the function of the major organs and systems of the human body; (2) explain the physiological control of these organ systems; (3) describe how these organ systems interact to maintain homeostasis.

Objectives

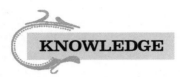

KNOWLEDGE

At the end of the course, student should be able to:

1. Describe the normal functions of all organ systems, regulatory mechanisms and interactions of the various organs for well co-ordinated total body function;

2. Understand the basic principles, mechanism and homeostatic control of all the functions of human body as a whole;

3. Explain the physiological aspects of normal growth and development;

4. Analyse the physiological responses and adaptation to different stresses during life processes;

5. Lay emphasis on the applied aspects of physiological function underlying disease.

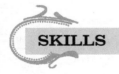

SKILLS

At the end of the course, the student should be able to:

1. Acquire the skills to do the experiments designed for study of physiological phenomena;

2. Interpret experimental/investigative data;

3. Distinguish between normal and abnormal experimental data and explain the data reasonably.

Teaching and Learning Methods

Physiology teaching includes theory teaching in classroom and practical teaching in laboratory. Theory teaching is given in various ways including seminar, tutorial, self-study, as well as lecture. Practical teaching will be given in laboratory, including basic experimental skill training and experiment designing and performing for study of physiological phenomena and the underlying mechanisms.

Recommended Textbooks

朱大年，王庭槐. 2014. 生理学［M］. 8 版. 北京：人民卫生出版社.

Arthur C Guyton, John E Hall. 1996. Human Physiology and Mechanisms of Disease [M]. 6th ed. London: Saunders.

Gillian Pocock, Christopher D Richards. 2006. Human Physiology: the Basic of Medicine [M]. 3th ed. Oxford: Oxford University Press.

John E Hall. 2015. Guyton and Hall Textbook of Medical Physiology [M]. 13th ed. Philadelphia: Elsevier.

Kim E Barrett, Susan M Barman, Scott Boitano et al. 2015. Ganong's Review of Medical Physiology [M]. 25th ed. Europe: McGraw-Hill Education.

Schedule Table (theory)

Chapter	Teaching Hours	Chapter	Teaching Hours
1. Introduction and Cellular Physiology	14	7. Formation and Excretion of Urine	8
2. Blood	6	8. Functions of the Nervous System	14
3. Circulation	16	9. Special Senses	6
4. Respiration	6	10. Endocrine	6
5. Gastrointestinal Function	6	11. Reproductive Function	4
6. Energy Metabolism and Body Temperature	4	Total	90

Course Contents

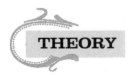

THEORY

Chapter 1　Introduction and Cellular Physiology

　　1. Definition of physiology.

　　2. Internal environment and homeostasis.

　　Body fluid compartments, definition of internal environment, homeostasis, regulation of body functions (neural regulation, humoral regulation, autoregulation, feedback, feed-forward).

　　3. Transports across cell membrane.

　　Diffusion (definition of diffusion, simple diffusion, facilitated diffusion, osmosis across selectively permeable membrane—net diffusion of water), active transport through the cell membrane (definition, primary active transport, secondary active transport), exocytosis (definition, processes), endocytosis (definition, types).

　　4. Signal transduction.

　　(1) Intercellular communication.

　　(2) Transmembrane signal transduction.

5. Membrane potentials.

Concept of membrane potentials, basic physics of membrane potentials, the resting membrane potential (characteristics, ionic basis), and local potential (characteristics). and the action potential (characteristics, ionic basis, conduction, "All-or-None" law).

6. Stimulus, response and excitation.

Stimulus, response, excitation, excitable cells, changes in excitability during action potential.

7. Muscle.

(1) Skeletal muscle.

Morphology of skeletal muscle (myofibrils, sarcotubules system), contractile responses (sliding mechanism of contraction, molecular basis of contraction, types of contraction, summation of contraction, relation between muscle length and tension, and velocity of contraction).

(2) Cardiac muscle.

(3) Smooth muscle.

8. Transmission between neuromuscular junctio.

Structures of neuromuscular junction (nerve terminal, synaptic cleft, motor end plate), transmission processes of the junction (quantal release of acetylcholine, end plate potential, destruction of the released acetylcholine).

Chapter 2　Blood

1. Constituents of blood.

2. Physical and chemical characteristics of blood.

3. Immune functions of blood.

4. Bone marrow and its haemopoietic function.

5. Physiology of red blood cells.

Characteristics (plastic deformation, suspension stability and osmotic fragility) and function of red blood cells, genesis of red blood cells (origin, materials and regulation), role of the spleen, hemoglobin (functions of hemoglobin, hemoglobin in the fetus, abnormalities of hemoglobin production, synthesis of hemoglobin, catabolism of hemoglobin).

6. Physiology of white blood cells.

Subtypes, characteristics, functions and genesis of white blood cells.

7. Physiology of platelets.

Characteristics, functions and genesis of platelets.

8. Blood clotting (hemostasis).

Response to injury, events in hemostasis, mechanism of blood coagulation, clot retr-action, and dissolution, anticlotting mechanisms, anticoagulants, abnormalities of hemostasis.

9. Blood types.

The ABO system, transfusion reactions, inheritance of A & B antigens, other agglutinogens, the Rh group, hemolytic disease of the newborn.

10. Lymph.

Composition, circulation and functions.

Chapter 3　Circulation

1. Origin of the heartbeat and the electrical activity of the heart.

(1) Origin and spread of cardiac excitation.

Anatomical structure, pacemakers, spread of cardiac excitation.

(2) Cardiac muscle cells.

Morphology (the intercalated discs), electrical activities (the resting potential, the action potential), physiological properties, contractile responses (excitation-contraction coupling, refractory period).

(3) The electrocardiogram (ECG).

Bipolar leads, unipolar (v) leads, formation and significance of normal ECG, ECG measurement.

(4) Cardiac arrhythmias.

Normal cardiac rate, abnormal pacemakers, implanted pacemakers, ectopic foci of excitation.

2. The heart as a pump.

(1) Mechanical events of the cardiac cycle.

Atrial systole, ventricular systole, pericardium, timing, length of systole and diastole, arterial pulse, atrial pressure changes and the jugular pulse, heart sounds, murmurs.

(2) Cardiac output Cardiac output in various conditions, factors controlling cardiac output, relation of tension to length in cardiac muscle, factors affecting end-diastolic volume, myocardial contractility, integrated control of cardiac output, oxygen consumption by the heart.

3. Dynamics of blood and lymph flow.

(1) and Function morphology Arteries and arterioles, capillaries, lymphatics, arteriovenous anastomoses, venules & veins, endothelium, vascular smooth muscle, angiogenesis.

(2) Biophysical considerations. Flow, pressure, resistance, applicability of physical principles to flow in blood vessels, laminar flow, shear stress average velocity, poiseuille-hagen formula, viscosity and resistance, critical closing pressure, law of laplace, resistance and capacitance vessels.

(3) Arterial & arteriolar circulation Velocity & flow of blood, arterial pressure, effect of gravity, methods of measuring blood pressure, auscultatory method, palpation method, normal arterial blood pressure.

(4) Capillary circulation.

Capillary pressure and flow, equilibration with interstitial fluid, active and inactive capillaries.

(5) Lymphatic circulation and interstitial fluid volume.

Lymphatic circulation, other functions of the lymphatic system, interstitial fluid volume.

(6) Venous circulation.

Venous pressure and flow, thoracic pump, effects of heartbeat, muscle pump, venous pressure in the head, air embolism, measuring venous pressure.

4. Cardiovascular regulatory mechanisms.

(1) Local regulation.

Autoregulation, vasodilator metabolites, localized vasoconstriction.

(2) Substances secreted by the endothelium.

Endothelial cells, prostacyclin and thromboxane A_2, endothelium-derived relaxing factor, other functions of NO, CO, endothelins, endothelin-1, regulation of secretion, cardiovascular functions, other functions of endothelins.

(3) Systemic regulation by hormones.

Kinins, adrenomedullin, natriuretic hormones, circulating vasoconstrictors.

(4) Systemic regulation by the nervous system.

Neural regulatory mechanisms, innervation of the blood vessels, cardiac innervation, vasomotor control, afferents to the vasomotor area, somatosympathetic reflex, baroreceptors, carotid sinus and aortic arch, buffer nerve activity, baroreceptor resetting, effect of carotid clamping and buffer nerve section, atrial stretch receptors, bainbridge reflex, left ventricular receptors, pulmonary receptors, clinical testing and stimulation, effects of chemoreceptor stimulation on the vasomotor area, direct effects on the vasomotor area, sympathetic vasodilator system, control of heart rate.

5. Circulation through special regions.

(1) Cerebral circulation.

Anatomic considerations, vessels, innervation, cerebrospinal fluid (formation and absorption, protective function), the blood-brain barrier, cerebral blood flow and its regulation, role of intracranial pressure, effect of intracranial pressure changes on systemic blood pressure, autoregulation, role of vasomotor & sensory nerves, blood flow in various parts of the brain, brain metabolism & oxygen requirements (uptake and release of substances by the brain, oxygen consumption, energy sources, glutamate and ammonia removal), stroke.

(2) Coronary circulation.

Anatomic considerations, pressure gradients and flow in the coronary vessels, variations in coronary flow, chemical factors, neural factors, coronary artery disease.

Chapter 4　Respiration

1. Pulmonary ventilation.

(1) Properties of gases.

(2) Anatomy of the lungs.

Air passages, bronchi and their innervation, pulmonary circulation.

(3) Mechanics of respiration Inspiration and expiration, respiratory muscles, artificial respiration, intrapleural pressure, bronchial tone, compliance of the lungs and chest wall, alveolar surface tension, surfactant, pulmonary volumes (tidal volume, inspiratory reserve volume, expiratory reserve volume, residual volume, pulmonary capacity (inspiratory capacity, functional residual volume, vital capacity, forced vital capacity, forced expiratory volume, total lung capacity), pulmonary ventilation, alveolar ventilation, dead space and uneven ventilation,

2. Gas exchange in the lungs and tissues.

Composition of alveolar air, diffusion coefficient, diffusion across the alveolocapillary membrane, factors affecting gas exchange, ventilation/perfusion ratio, pulmonary diffusion capacity.

3. Gas Transport Between the Lungs and the Tissues.

(1) Oxygen transport Oxygen delivery to the tissues, reaction of hemoglobin & oxygen, factors affecting the affinity of hemoglobin for oxygen, nitric oxide transport by hemoglobin, myoglobin.

(2) Carbon dioxide transport.

Buffers, fate of carbon dioxide in blood, chloride shift, summary of carbon dioxide transport.

4. Regulation of Respiration.

(1) Neural control of breathing.

Control systems, medullary systems, pontine and vagal influences.

(2) Chemical control of breathing.

Carotid and aortic bodies, chemoreceptors in the brain stem, ventilatory responses to changes in acid-base balance, ventilatory responses to CO_2, ventilatory response to oxygen lack, effects of hypoxia on the CO_2 response curve, effect of H^+ on the CO_2 response, breath holding, hormonal effects on respiration.

(3) Nonchemical influences on respiration.

Responses mediated by receptors in the airways and lungs (pulmonary stretch reflex, pulmonary inflation reflex, pulmonary deflation reflex, coughing and sneezing), responses in patients with heart-lung transplants, afferents from "higher centers", afferents from proprioceptors, respiratory components of visceral reflexes, respiratory effects of baroreceptor stimulation, effects of sleep.

5. Pulmonary circulation.

Pulmonary blood vessels, pressure, volume and flow, capillary pressure, effect of gravity, regulation of pulmonary blood flow.

6. Other functions of the respiratory system.

Lung defense mechanisms, pulmonary function in acid-base balance, metabolic and endocrine functions of the lungs.

chapter 5　Gastrointestinal Function

1. General considerations Organization, characteristics of smooth muscle, enteric nervous system, extrinsic innervation, peristalsis, basic electrical activity, regulation of motility, migrating motor complex.

2. Gastrointestinal hormones.

Enteroendocrine cells, gastrin, cholecystokinin-pancreozymin, secretin, gastric inhibitory peptide, other gastrointestinal hormones.

3. Mouth and esophagus.

Salivary glands, composition of saliva, control of salivary secretion, swallowing.

4. Stomach.

Anatomic considerations, gastric juice, mucosal barrier, pepsinogen secretion, hydrochloric acid secretion, ECL cells, gastric motility and emptying, hunger contractions, regulation of gastric secretion (cephalic phase, gastric phase, intestinal phase), regulation of gastric motility and emptying, peptic ulcer, other functions of the stomach.

5. Exocrine portion of the pancreas.

Anatomic considerations, composition and functions of pancreatic juice, regulation of the secretion of pancreatic juice.

6. Liver and biliary system.

Anatomic considerations, functions of the liver and gallbladder, compositionand functions of bile, regulation of biliary secretion.

7. Small intestine.

Intestinal mucus, intestinal secretion, intestinal motility, regulation of intestinal secretion and motility.

8. Colon.

Anatomic considerations, motility and secretion of the colon, transit time in the small intestine and colon, absorption in the colon, feces, intestinal bacteria, defecation, diarrhea.

9. Digestion and absorption Carbohydrates, proteins and nucleic acids, lipids, water and electrolytes, vitamins and minerals.

Chapter 6　Energy Metabolism and Body Temperature

1. Energy Metabolism.

Energy release, transform, transport, storage and utilization; energy metabolism rate, measurement of energy metabolism rate; the factors that influence energy metabolism; basal metabolism rate (BMR).

2. Body Temperature.

Core temperature and skin temperature, structure and function of skin, heat production, heat loss, regulation of heat production and loss, regulation of body temperature, changes during exposure to extreme heat and cold.

Chapter 7　Formation & Excretion of Urine

1. Functional anatomy.

Nephron, juxtaglomerular apparatus, blood vessels, lymphatics, capsule, innervation of the renal vessels.

2. Renal circulation.

Blood flow, pressure in renal vessels, regulation of the renal blood flow, functions of the renal nerves, autoregulation of renal blood flow, regional blood flow and oxygen consumption.

3. Glomerular filtration.

Concept of glomerular filtration rate (GFR), Measurement of GFR, substances used to measure GFR, glomerular filtration barrier, net filtration pressure, factors that affect GFR.

4. Tubular function.

General considerations, mechanisms of tubular reabsorption and secretion, Na^+, Cl^-, HCO_3^-, K^+ and Ca^{2+} reabsorption, glucose reabsorption, renal glucose threshold, glucose transport mechanism, additional examples of secondary active transport, substances secreted by the tubules, tubuloglomerular feedback and glomerulotubular balance.

5. Water excretion.

Proximal tubule, loop of Henle, Bartter's Syndrome, distal tubule, collecting ducts, vasopressin (antidiuretic hormone) aquaporins, the countercurrent mechanism, role of urea, water diuresis, water intoxication, osmotic diuresis, relation of urine concentration to GFR, "free water clearance".

6. Acidification of the urine and bicarbonate excretion.

H^+ secretion, fate of H^+ in the urine, reaction with buffers, ammonia secretion, pH changes along the nephrons, factors affecting acid secretion, bicarbonate excretion, implications of urinary pH changes.

7. Na^+ and Cl^- excretion.

Na^+ and Cl^- excretion, regulation of Na^+ excretion, effects of adrenocortical steroids, other humoral effects.

8. K^+ excretion.

H^+-Na^+ exchange, effects of aldosterone.

9. Diuretics.

10. Regulation of urine formation.

(1) Neural regulation.

(2) Humoral regulation.

Antidiuretic hormone, renin-angiotensin-aldosterone system, atrial natriuretic peptide.

11. Regulation of extracellular fluid composition and volume.

Defense of tonicity, defense of volume, defense of specific ionic composition, defense of H^+ concentration.

12. Clearance rate.

13. Filling and emptying of the bladder.

Anatomic considerations, micturition, reflex control, abnormalities of micturition, effects of deafferentation, effects of denervation, effects of spinal cord transection.

14. Effects of disordered renal function.

Proteinuria, loss of concentrating and diluting ability, acidosis, abnormal Na^+ metabolism uremia.

Chapter 8   Functions of the Nervous System

1. Functions of neuron and neuroglia.

(1) Neuron.

Dendrite (structures, functions), axon (structures, functions), nerve fibers (types, function, impulse conduction in nerve, axoplasmic transport), trophic action of nerve, neurotrophins.

(2) Neuroglia.

Subtypes, characteristics and functions.

2. Synaptic transmission.

(1) Definition of synapses, structures and types of synapses.

(2) Chemical synapse.

General processes of synaptic transmission, electrical events in postsynaptic neuron (excitatory postsynaptic potential, inhibitory postsynaptic potential, integrator), inhibition and facilitation at synapses (postsynaptic inhibition and facilitation, presynaptic inhibition and facilitation), synaptic plasticity.

3. Neurotransmitters and receptors.

Definition and general consideration, principal neurotransmitter and receptor systems.

4. Reflex.

Definition of reflex, reflex arc, general properties of reflexes, integration of reflex in central nervous system, mode of connection of central neurons, characteristics of central neurotransmission, central inhibition and facilitation.

5. Sensory function of the nervous system.

Sensory pathways; touch, proprioception temperature, pain; visceral pain and referred pain, sensory projection system; sensory area of cerebral cortex.

6. Roles of the nervous system in motor control.

(1) General principles and function of motor control system.

(2) Spinal cord.

Spinal motor neuron and motor unit, spinal shock, spinal integration, postural reflex (flexor reflex and crossed extensor reflex, stretch reflex, inverse stretch reflex, intersegmental reflex).

(3) Brainstem.

Inhibitory area and facilitatory area, decerebrate rigidity, attitudinal reflex (tonic labyrinthine reflex, tonic neck reflex), righting reflex.

(4) Cerebral cortex.

Motor area of cerebral cortex, pathways for motor control, flaccid paralysis, spastic paralysis.

(5) Basal ganglia.

General function, nigrostriatal system, Parkinson disease, Huntington disease.

(6) Cerebellum.

Functions of different parts of cerebellum.

7. The autonomic nervous system.

Anatomic organization of autonomic outflow, chemical transmission at autonomic junctions, responses of effector organs to autonomic nerve impulses, functional characteristics of the autonomic nervous system.

8. Roles of the nervous system in regulation of visceral activities.

Regulation of visceral activities by spinal cord, medulla oblongata, hypothalamus and cerebrum。

9. Neural basis of instinctual behavior and emotion.

Instinctual behavior, emotion, motivation, addiction.

10. Electrical activities of brain, sleep and wakefulness.

Spontaneous electrical activities of brain, evoked cortical potential, types of sleep, mechanisms underlying sleep and wakefulness.

11. Higher function of the nervous system.

Types and physiological basis of learning and memory, language and cognition.

Chapter 9   Special Senses

1. Vision.

(1) Functional anatomy of eye.

(2) Optics of eye.

Reduced eye, accommodation, near point, presbyopia, near reflex of the pupil, convergence reflex, pupillary light reflex, consensual light reflex, Argyll Robertson pupil, emmetropia, myopia, hyperopia, astigmatism, strabismus.

(3) Intraocular fluid.

Aqueous humor, intraocular pressure, glaucoma.

(4) Retina.

Anatomy and function of retina, types of photoreceptor, ionic basis of photoreceptor potentials, electroretinogram, photosensitive compounds, color vision, color blindness.

(5) Visual pathways and visual cortex.

Visual pathway and its lesion, visual cortex, depth perception.

(6) Other aspects of visual function.

Visual acuity, dark adaptation, light adaptation, visual field, monocular vision and binocular vision, diplopia, stereoscopic vision, fusion phenomenon, critical fusion frequency, after image.

2. Hearing and equilibrium.

(1) Hearing.

Functional anatomy of ear, physics of sound, roles of tympanic membrane, middle ear and cochlea in hearing, organ of Corti, auditory pathway and auditory cortex, tests for hearing and deafness.

(2) Equilibrium.

Structure and function of vestibular system, responses to rotational acceleration, responses to linear acceleration, spatial orientation, vestibular autonomic reaction, nystagmus, motion sickness.

3. Taste and smell.

Modalities, receptors, pathways, cortical and limbic areas associated with taste and smell, olfaction and memory and emotion.

Chapter 10   Endocrine

1. General aspects.

Endocrine and endocrine system, classification of hormones; general characteristics of hormone actions; mechanism of hormone action, control and regulation of hormone secretion.

2. Endocrine of hypothalamus and hypophysis.

Endocrine function of hypothalamus; hypothalamic regulatory peptides; hormones of adenohypophysis: growth hormone and prolactin; hormones of neurohypophysis: antidiuretic hormone and oxytocin.

3. Endocrine of pineal gland.

Melatonin.

4. Endocrine of thyroid.

Synthesis and metabolism of thyroid hormones; biologic actions of thyroid hormones; regulation of thyroid function.

5. Endocrine of adrenal gland:

Endocrine of adrenal cortex; hormones of adrenal cortex; biologic actions of corticosteroids; regulation of corticosteroid secretion; biologic actions and regulation of adrenal medullary hormones.

6. Endocrine functions of pancreas.

Physiological anatomy of pancreatic islet, hormones secreted by pancreatic islet, biologic actions of insulin and regulation of glucagon, of insulin and glucagon secretion.

7. Hormonal control of calcium metabolism and the physiology of bone.

Biologic actions of parathyrin and calcitonin, regulation of secretion of parathyrin and calcitonin, biologic actions and origin of vitamin D.

8. Endocrine functions of other tissues and organs.

Chapter 11　Reproductive System

1. Sex determination and differentiation and its disorders.

2. Puberty and gonadotrophins.

3. Male reproductive system.

Physiological anatomy, spermatogenesis and its regulation, composition of semen, endocrine function of testes, biologic actions and regulation of secretion of testicular hormones.

4. Female reproductive system.

Physiological anatomy of ovaries and its functions; biologic actions of ovarian hormones; ovarian cycle and menstrual cycle; ovulation and test for ovulation; menopause; fertilization and implantation; physiology of pregnancy; placenta, fetoplacental unit and hormones; physiology of labor; lactation.

5. Physiology of new born.

6. Sexual physiology and contraception.

Sexual mature, sexual reflexes, sexual act, sexual dysfunction, physiological basis of male and female contraception.

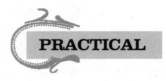

PRACTICAL

1. Basic techniques and requirements for physiological experiments in vitro and in vivo.

2. Basic techniques for testing or recording the functions of tissues, organs or systems (e.g. blood pressure, electrocardiogram, heart sounds, vision, hearing, etc.).

3. Stimulus, action potential and contraction of muscle (skeletal muscle and intestinal smooth muscle).

4. Pacemakers and heart beating.

5. Physiological regulation of respiration, blood pressure and urine formation.

6. Basic training in designing and performing physiological experiments.

MEDICAL MICROBIOLOGY
医学微生物学

Chief Editors（主编）
　Zhong Zhaohua（钟照华）　Harbin Medical University（哈尔滨医科大学）
　Tang Hua（汤华）　Tianjin Medical University（天津医科大学）
　Zhuang Min（庄敏）　Harbin Medical University（哈尔滨医科大学）

Deputy Chief Editor（副主编）
　Zhang Qingmeng（张庆猛）　Harbin Medical University（哈尔滨医科大学）

Editors（编委）（按姓氏拼音排序）
　Li Xiaoxia（李晓霞）　Tianjin Medical University（天津医科大学）
　Shang Qinglong（商庆龙）　Harbin Medical University（哈尔滨医科大学）
　Tang Hua（汤华）　Tianjin Medical University（天津医科大学）
　Teng Xu（腾旭）　Harbin Medical University（哈尔滨医科大学）
　Zhang Qingmeng（张庆猛）　Harbin Medical University（哈尔滨医科大学）
　Zhong Zhaohua（钟照华）　Harbin Medical University（哈尔滨医科大学）
　Zhuang Min（庄敏）　Harbin Medical University（哈尔滨医科大学）

Course Description

　　Microbiology is the study of microorganisms that exist as large and diverse groups of microscopic organisms, mainly including bacteria, viruses and fungi. Medical microbiology describes the microorganisms related to human infectious diseases involving biological characteristics, pathogenicity, immunity, laboratory diagnosis, prevention and treatment of these pathogens. Medical microbiology is one of fundamental courses for medical students who will be clinicians or associated medical professionals. Because of high-speed development in microbiological study and extensive relevance of human infectious diseases in recent years, this course mainly focuses on basic theory, basic knowledge and basic technical ability in order to foster students'abilities of problem solution in medical work.

Objectives

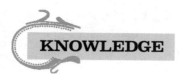

KNOWLEDGE

At the end of the course, the student shall be able to:

1. State the infective microorganisms of the human body and describe the pathogenesis of the related human diseases.

2. State the transmission modes of pathogens and opportunistic pathogens, including infection sources, transmission routes and susceptible population.

3. Describe the immunological mechanisms as host reaction to pathogen infection.

4. Practice in laboratory technologies for diagnosis of infectious diseases.

5. Master antimicrobial strategy in prevention and treatment of infectious disease, such as immunotherapy and vaccination program.

6. Apply methods of disinfection and sterilization to control hospital and community acquired infections.

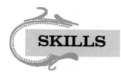

SKILLS

At the end of the course, the student shall be able to:

1. Design and implement laboratory methods for diagnosis of infectious diseases based on clinical manifestations and etiological knowledge.

2. Identify common infective microbes and choose proper antimicrobial medicines or vaccines in treatment or prevention of infectious diseases.

3. Use right way in collection, storage, transport and preparation of clinical specimens for laboratory diagnosis and microbiological identification.

Teaching and Learning Methods

Theory:

Lectures are presented with study guide as before-class preparation and slide show as on-class multi-media support. The relationship between pathogens and infectious diseases runs through the theory lesson, which is usually combined with knowledge of pathology, immunology and epidemiology.

Practice:

Based on the knowledge acquired in theory lesson, the laboratory technology for identification of pathogens and diagnosis of infectious diseases is introduced. Serial experiments including systemic and creative design are practiced according to the guide of teachers. Results are analyzed based on the background of the specimen provided.

Recommended Textbooks

Karen C Carroll, Janet S Butel, Stephen A Morse. 2016. Jawetz, Melnick, & Adelberg's
Medical Microbiology [M]. 27th ed. New York: McGraw-Hill Medical.

Patrick R Murray, Ken S Rosenthal, Michael A Pfaller. 2016. Medical Microbiology [M]. 8th
ed. Philadelphia: PA Elsevier.

Schedule Table

Chapter	Contents	Hours
	Introduction	1
1	Bacterial morphology and structure	3
2	Bacterial physiology	1
3	Phage	1
4	Bacterial Genetics	1
5	Drug resistance of bacteria	1
6	Bacterial infection and antibacterial immunity	3
7	Laboratory diagnosis, prevention and control of bacterial infection	2
8	Coccus	3
9	*Enterobacteriaceae*	3
10	*Vibrios*	0.5
11	*Helicobacter*	0.5
12	Anaerobic bacteria	2
13	Mycobacteria	2
14	*Haemophilus*	0.5
15	Zoonotic Bacteria	2
16	Coryneabacterium, Bordetella, Legionellae, Pseudomonads, Campylobacter, Stenotrophomonas, Acinetobacter, Moraxella, Aeromonas, listeria	1.5
17	Actinomycetes and Nocardia	Study by self
18	*Mycoplasma*	1
19	Rickettsia	1
20	*Chlamydiae*	1
21	Spirochete	1
22	General properties of viruses	3
23	Viral infection and antiviral immunity	2
24	Laboratory diagnosis, prevention and control of viral infections	2
25	Viruses associated with respiratory infections	2
26	Enterovirus	1
27	Acute gastroenteritis viruses	1

Continued

Chapter	Contents	Hours
28	Hepatitis viruses	2
29	Arbovirus	1.5
30	Viruses associated with hemorrhagic fever	1.5
31	Herpesviruses	2
32	Retroviruses	2
33	Rabies virus, Human papilloma virus, Parvoviruses, Poxvirus, Borna disease virus	1
34	Prion	1
35	Biology of fungi	1
36	Medical mycology	1
37	Exp.1 Basic methods of microbiological laboratory	4
38	Exp.2 Isolation and Identification of Pyogenic cocci	6
39	Exp.3 Laboratory diagnosis of pathogenic enterobacteria	6
40	Exp.4 Isolation and identification of influenza virus	4
41	Exp.5 Real-time PCR for Diagnosis of M. pneumonia	4
	Total	80

Course Contents

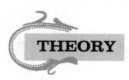

THEORY

Introduction.
1. Development history of microbiology.
2. Classification of microbes.
3. Unique differentiating features of eukaryotes and prokaryotes.
4. Relationship between microbes and human.

Chapter 1　Bacterial Structures

1. Basic structures and special structures of bacteria.
2. Structures and functions of cell wall; peptidoglycan; lipopolysacchride (LPS); outer membrane; teichoic acid.
3. Characteristics of cell wall of gram-positive bacteria and gram-negative bacteria.
4. Cell membrane: mesosome.
5. L forms of bacteria.
6. Capsule: glycocalyx and slime layer.
7. Flagellum.
8. Fimbriae (pilus): ordinary pilus and sex pilus.

9. Endospore, sporulation.

10. Size and shape of bacteria.

11. Mechanisms of gram stain.

12. Methods for bacterial morphology observation.

Chapter 2　Bacterial Physiology

1. Requirements for bacterial growth.

2. Bacterial growth curve; observation of bacteria growth.

3. Energy metabolism of bacteria; products of metabolism.

4. Techniques for bacterial cultures.

5. Classification of culture media.

6. Sterilization; disinfection; antisepsis; cleaning; asepsis.

7. Physical methods of sterilization and disinfection.

8. Pasteurization; fractional sterilization; sterilization by pressured steam; autoclave; filtration.

9. Disinfectants.

10. Bacterial taxonomy: genus; species.

Chapter 3　Bacteriophage

1. Phages; virulent phages; temperate phages; lysogenic phage.

2. Lysogenic bacterium; lysogeny; prophage; lysogenic conversion.

Chapter 4　Bacterial Genetics

1. Genetic variation; phenotypic variation.

2. Pathogenic island, PAI.

3. Plasmid; replicon; conjugative and non-conjugative plasmid; resistance plasmid; R factor; fertility plasmid F factor; virulence plasmid.

4. Transposition; transposable element; transposase; insertion sequence, IS; inverted repeat; transposon, Tn; integron, In.

5. Classification and definition of gene transfer and recombination: transformation; conjugation; high frequency recombinant, Hfr; transduction; general transduction; transducing phage; abortive transduction; restricted transduction; lysogenic conversion; protoplast fusion.

6. Resistance transfer factor, RTF.

7. Significance of bacterial heredity and variation in medicine: Bacillus Calmette-Guerin(BCG); gene engineering.

Chapter 5　Drug Resistance of Bacteria

1. Types of antibiotics base on chemical structure and characters.

2. Functional mechanisms of antibiotics; functional mechanisms of β-lactam antibiotics.

3. Genetics mechanisms of bacterial drug resistance.

4. Biochemical mechanisms of bacterial drug resistance.

Chapter 6   Bacterial Infection and Antimicrobial Immunity

1. Normal flora and its physiological functions.

2. Microecology; microeubiosis; microdysbiosis; dysbacteriosis.

3. Opportunistic pathogens.

4. Bacterial pathogenicity; virulence; median lethal dose, LD_{50}; median infective dose, ID_{50}.

5. Invasiveness related factors of bacteria; adhesin; bacterial biofilm, BF.

6. Toxigenicity; definition and characteristics of exotoxin and endotoxin; types and functions of exotoxin; pathophysiologic reaction and pathogenesis of endotoxin.

7. Innate immunity and adaptive immunity.

8. Extracellular bacteria; intracellular bacteria; anti-intracellular bacterial Immunity.

9. Exogenous infection and endogenous infection; bacterial transmission.

10. Types of bacterial infections; types of systemic bacterial infections: toxemia; endotoxemia; bacteremia; septicemia; pyemia.

11. Types of hospital infection; Nosocomial infection.

Chapter 7   Laboratory Diagnosis, Prevention, and Control of Bacterial Infection

1. Principles for specimen collection and handling.

2. Laboratory diagnosis strategy for bacterial infections; detection for antigens; nucleic acid detection; drug resistance test; serological test; animal test.

3. Artificial immunization: biological products for artificial passive immunization and artificial active immunization; vaccines: attenuated and killed vaccines; toxoid; antitoxin; BCG; subunit vaccine; comparison of attenuated and killed vaccines.

4. Programmed immunization.

Chapter 8   Coccus

1. Biological characteristics of *Staphylococcus aureus*.

2. Enterotoxins; toxic shock syndrome (TSST-1); exfoliative toxin; scalded skin syndrome; leucocidin.

3. *Staphylococcus* protein A (SPA); coagulase (+) or coagulase (–).

4. Biological characteristics of *Streptococcus pyogenes* and *Streptococcus pneumoniae*.

5. Scarlet fever; streptococcal toxic shock syndrome; rheumatic fever; acute glomerulonephritis; hemolysin.

6. Streptolysin O; hyaluronidase; streptokinase (SK); streptodornase (SD); Dick test.

7. Biological characteristics, pathogenesis and prevention of *N. gonorrhoeae* and *N. meningitides*.

8. Sexually transmitted disease, STD.

Chapter 9   *Enterobacteriaceae*

1. Biological characteristics of *Echerichia Coli*; ETEC; EAEC; EHEC; EPEC.

2. Biochemical reaction of *Enterobacteriaceae*.

3. Virulent factors of *Shigella*; diseases caused by *Shigella*.

4. Prevention of bacterium dysentery.

5. Biological characteristics of *Salmonella. typhi*, including classification, virulent factor, diseases and detection of pathogen.

6. Diagnosis and prevention of *Salmonella. typhi*.

Chapter 10 *Vibrio*

1. Biological characteristics of *Vibrio. cholerae*, including classification, virulent factor, diseases and detection of pathogen.

2. Detection of *Vibrio. cholerae*; pathogenicity, diagnosis and prevention of *Vibrio. parahaemolyticus*.

Chapter 11 *Helicobacter*

Relation between *Helicobacter pylori* and stomach cancer.

Chapter 12 Anaerobic Bacteria

1. Biological characteristics of *Clostridium. tetani*, including the form, staining, antigenic structure, culture, resistance, virulent factor, diseases and detection of pathogen.

2. Biological characteristics, virulent factor and disease of *Clostridium. perfringens*.

3. Virulent factor and disease of *Clostridium. botulinum*; prevention and control of tetanus.

4. Prevention of *C. botulinum*.

5. Virulent factor and disease of *Clostridium. difficile*.

Chapter 13 *Mycobacterium*

1. Biological characteristics of *mycobacterium*, including the form, staining, antigenic structure, culture, resistance, virulent factor, diseases and detection of pathogen.

2. Interpretation of tuberculin Test.

3. Staining and detection of *Mycobacterium leprae*.

Chapter 14 *Haemophilus*

Pathogenicity of *Haemophilus. influenza*.

Chapter 15 Zoonosis Bacteria

1. Biological characteristics of *Bacillus. anthracis*; virulent factor and disease; detection and prevention.

2. Biological characteristics, virulent factor and disease of *Yersinia. pestis*.

3. Biological characteristics of *Brucella*, including the form, staining, antigenic structure, culture, resistance, virulent factor and diseases; prevention of *Brucella*.

Chapter 16 Other Bacteria

1. Staining, antigenic structure, culture, virulent factor, diseases and detection of *C. diphtheria*.

2. Immunity and pathogenicity of *C. diphtheriae*; Schick test.

3. Pathogenicity of *Bordetella*, *Legionellae*, *Pseudomonads*, *Campylobacter*, *Stenotrophomonas*, *Acinetobacter*, *Moraxella*, *Aeromonas*, *Listeria*.

Chapter 17　*Actinomyces* and *Nocardia*

Diseases causing by *Actinomyces* and *Nocardia*.

Chapter 18　*Mycoplasma*

1. Definition of *Mycoplasma*; pathogenicity of *Mycoplasma*.
2. Immunity of *Mycoplasma*.

Chapter 19　Rickettsia

1. Definition of Rickettsia.
2. Infection source of query fever; pathogenicity of the other Rickettsia.

Chapter 20　*Chlamydiae*

1. Definition of *Chlamydiae*, life cycle of Chlamydia.
2. Detection and prevention of Chlamydia.

Chapter 21　Spirochete

1. Biological characteristics, pathogenicity and detection of *Leptospira* and *Treponema*.
2. Classification of Spirochaete; diagnosis and prevention of Spirochaete.

Chapter 22　General Properties of Viruses

1. Definition and biological features of virus.
2. Virion structure and component.
3. Viral replication circle, abortive infection, defective virus.
4. Effects of physical and chemical factors on viral replication.
5. Interference phenomenon and variation in viral infection.

Chapter 23　Viral Infection and Antiviral Immunity

1. Viral infection process and transmission routes.
Horizontal transmission and vertical transmission.
2. Types of viral infection.
Chronic viral infection, latent viral infection and slow virus infection.
3. Viral pathogenesis.
(1) Direct effects of virus on host cells.
(2) Immunopathologic injuries in virus infected host.
4. Interferon and its antiviral activity.
5. Specific and non-specific antiviral immune response.
6. Neutralizing antibody and its role in antiviral response.
7. Cell responses to viral infection.
8. Viral immune escape.

Chapter 24　Laboratory Diagnosis, Prevention and Control of Viral Diseases

1. Laboratory tests.
(1) Requirements of sample collection and transport.

(2) Isolation and culture of virus.

(3) Serological diagnosis of viral infection.

(4) Detection of viral antigens, nucleic acids and other virion components.

(5) Quantitation of virus and viral infectivity (PFU, $TCID_{50}$ and ID_{50}).

(6) Quick diagnosis of viral infection.

2. Prevention and treatment of viral infection.

(1) Artificial active immunization and the associated biological products.

(2) Artificial passive immunization and the associated biological products.

(3) Antiviral medicines and their bioactivities.

Chapter 25　Respiratory Vciruses

1. Respiratory viruses and related diseases.

2. Biology of influenza viruses like morphology, structure, typing and variation and immune features.

3. Pathogenicity and immune features of Measles virus.

4. Key points of prevention and treatment in Measles virus infection.

5. Pathogenicity of Mumps virus.

6. Biology of Coronavirus, the pathogenesis of SARS/MERS-Cov and the prevention and treatment for the related diseases.

7. Pathogenicity of Rubella virus, Respiratory Syncytial virus, Parainfluenza virus and Rhinovirus.

Chapter 26　Enterovirus

1. Species and common features of human Enterovirus.

2. Biology, typing, pathogenicity, immune features of poliovirus; Prevention and treatment of Poliovirus infection.

3. Pathogenicity of Coxsackievirus, ECHO virus and new Enterovirus (68, 70, 71).

4. Biology and pathogenicity of human Rotavirus and Norovirus.

5. Prevention and treatment of related acute gastroenteritis.

Chapter 27　Acute Gastroenteritis Viruses

1. Rotaviruses: biologic properties, pathogenesis, immunity and laboratory diagnosis.

2. Other gastroenteritis viruses (calicivirus, astrovirus, enteric adenovirus).

Chapter 28　Hepatitis Viruses

1. Classification and characteristics of hepatitis viruses.

2. HAV: biologic properties, pathogenesis, immunity, laboratory diagnosis, treatment and prevention.

3. HBV: structure, genome, replication cycle, antigen and antibodies, pathogenesis and immunity, laboratory diagnosis (acute infection; chronic infection; surface and core variants), treatment and prevention.

4. Main biological characteristics, transmission, detection and prevention of

hepatitis C, D and E.

5. Other hepatitis viruses (GBV-C, HGV, TTV).

Chapter 29　Arbovirus

1. Classification, common characteristics of arbovirus in China.

2. Main biological characteristics, related diseases, detection, prevention and treatment of Japanese Encephalitis Virus, JEV.

3. Main biological characteristics, epidemiology, pathogenicity, immunity and detection of dengue Virus, DENV.

4. Pathogenicity and epidemiology of forest encephalitis virus.

5. Other arbovirus (severe fever with thrombocytopenia syndrome virus, West Nile virus).

Chapter 30　Viruses Associated With Hemorrhagic Fever

1. Diseases caused by Hemorrhagic viruses; epidemiology, pathogenesis, immunity and laboratory diagnosis of hemorrhagic fever with renal syndrome (HFRS).

2. Hantavirus: structure, pathogenesis, immunity, serological assays.

3. Etiology, epidemiology, pathogenesis, immunity and laboratory diagnosis of Xingjiang Hemorrhagic Fever (XHF) and Ebola virus.

Chapter 31　Herpesviruses

1. Classification, related diseases, culture, common characteristics , detection and pathogenesis of herpes viruses.

2. HSV: Biologic properties, pathogenicity (pathology, primary infection and latent infection), disease (oropharyngeal disease, genital herpes, encephalitis, neonatal herpes, skin infection and infections in immunocompromised hosts), diagnostic laboratory tests, principles of treatments and prevention.

3. Pathogenicity of VZV; form and culture of CMV; antigen type, host cell and related disease of EBV.

Chapter 32　Retroviruses

1. Classification and common characteristics of retroviruses.

2. Structure, replication, variation, transmission, culture, pathogenicity, diagnosis and detections of HIV.

Chapter 33　Rabies Virus, Human Papilloma Virus, Parvoviruses, Poxvirus, Borna Disease Virus

1. Biological properties of Rabies virus; prevention and control of Rabies virus infection; Negri body.

2. Related disease of HPV; relationship with cervical cancer.

3. Pathogenicity of Parvoviruses, Poxviruse, Borna disease virus.

Chapter 34　Prion

Biologic properties, pathogenesis (Kuru, Creutzfeld-Jakob disease, Gerstmann-

Srraussler-Scheinker syndrome), diagnosis and prevention.

Chapter 35   Biology of Fungi

Morphology, pathogenicity, immunity, laboratory diagnosis, treatment and prevention of fungi.

Chapter 36   Medical mycology

1. Cutaneous mycoses: manifestation, etiologic agents, treatment, prevention.
2. Subcutaneous mycoses.
3. Systemic Mycose.
4. Opportunistic Mycoses: Candidiasis, Cryptococcosis, Others.

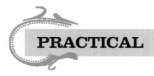

PRACTICAL

Exp. 1   Basic methods of microbiological laboratory.
1. Gram stain.
2. Bacterial culture and growth state observation.
3. Use of oil-immersion microscope.
Exp.2   Isolation and identification of pyogenic cocci.
1. Isolation and culture of bacteria.
2. Pure culture.
3. Antibiotic susceptibility test.
4. Coagulase test.
Exp.3   Laboratory diagnosis of pathogenic enterobacteria.
1. Streak pate method.
2. Gram stain.
3. Widal's reaction.
4. Serological identification of Salmonella.
Exp.4   Isolation and identification of influenza virus.
1. Hemagglutination test (HT).
2. Hemagglutination inhibition test (HIT).
Exp.5   Real-time PCR for diagnosis of *M. pneumonia*.
1. Procedure of PCR and real-time PCR experiments.
2. Applications of PCR and real-time PCR in pathogen diagnosis.

HUMAN PARASITOLOGY
人体寄生虫学

Chief Editors（主编）
Wang Fang（王放） Jilin University（吉林大学）
Liu Peimei（刘佩梅） Tianjin Medical University（天津医科大学）

Deputy Chief Editor（副主编）
He Ronghua（赫荣华） Jilin University（吉林大学）

Editors（编委）（按姓氏拼音排序）
He Ronghua（赫荣华） Jilin University（吉林大学）
Liu Peimei（刘佩梅） Tianjin Medical University（天津医科大学）
Wang Fang（王放） Jilin University（吉林大学）
Zheng Jingtong（郑敬彤） Jilin University（吉林大学）

Course Description

Parasitology is a subject which introduces students to understand the parasites that are relevant to human health. This course mainly includes helminthes, protozoans and arthropods. It emphasizes the morphology, life cycle, pathogenic factor and method for diagnosing parasites, as well as the way to prevent and treat diseases and parasites. In addition, the research development in parasite genomics, vaccines and antiparasitic agents are also need to understand. The most important task of parasitology is to grasp the basic concepts of parasitology, master the classification of parasites and hosts, understand the transmission routes of parasitic diseases and the way of parasites entering the human body (i.e. the way of infection), and familiar with the most important parasitic diseases worldwide and the harm effect to human health.

The purposes for parasitological learning are to master the basic theory of parasitology and to provide theoretical basis for clinical diagnosis. Therefore parasitology is an essential course in the clinical medical curriculum.

Objectives

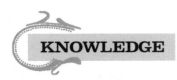

KNOWLEDGE

At the end of the course, the MBBS students shall be able to:

1. To understand the morphology of common parasites.
2. To state the relationship between parasite and host.
3. To describe the effects caused by parasitic diseases.
4. To identify parasite by laboratory diagnosis.
5. To state or indicate the methods of transmission of parasite and their sources, including insect vectors responsible for the transmission of the infection.
6. To describe the mechanisms of immunity to infection.
7. To describe suitable antiparasitic agents for treatment of parasitic infection.
8. To establish foundation for clinical medicine, preventive medicine and the control of parasitic diseases.

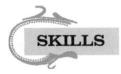

SKILLS

At the end of the course, the student should be able to practice the following experiments: the identification of helminthes, protozoans and arthropods; the identification of vectors responsible for transmission of parasitic infection.

Teaching and Learning Methods

Theory: Teaching parasitology to medical students is provided with the help of lectures and tutorials that deal with the basic information of parasitology. Moreover, tutorials and seminars are used on selected topics.

Practical: Practical training asks for medical students to do the experiments of identifying morphology of helminthes, protozoans and arthropods. Practical demonstrations and individual practical training are also used.

Recommended Textbooks

Burton J Bogitsh, Clint E Carter, Thomas N Oeltmann. 2013. Human Parasitology [M]. 4th ed. Boston: Academic Press.

Gao Xingzheng (高兴政). 2011. Medical Parasitology [M]. 2nd ed. Beijing: Peking University Medical Press.

Li Yonglong（李雍龙）, Zhu Xinping（诸欣平）, Su Chuan（苏川）. 2008. Human Parasitology [M]. Beijing: People's Medical Publishing House.

Wu Guanling（吴观陵）. 2005. Parasitology [M]. 3rd ed. Beijing: People's Medical Publishing House.

Schedule Table

Chapter	Contents	Hours	Chapter	Contents	Hours
1	Human parasitology introduction	2	12	Taenia solium &Taenia saginata	2
2	Protozoa Introduction	1	13	Hymenolepis nana & Echinococcus granulosus	2
3	Lobosea & Flagellata	3	14	Seminar-Zoonotic parasite	2
4	Sporozoa & Ciliatea	4	15	Nematoda-Introduction	1
5	Trematoda-Introduction	1	16	Ascaris lumbricoides	1
6	Fasciolopsis buski	1	17	Enterobius vermicularis & Hookworm	2
7	Clonorchis sinensis	2	18	Filaria & Trichuris trichiura	2
8	Paragonimus westermani	2	19	Medical Arthropoda-Introduction	2
9	Schistosome & Cercarial dermatitis	2	20	Arachnida	2
10	Cestoda-Introduction	1	21	Insecta	2
11	Spirometra mansoni & Diphyllobothrium latum	3		Total	40

Course Contents

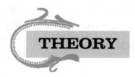

THEORY

Chapter 1　Human Parasitology Introduction

1. The conception of commensalisms, mutualism and parasitism.

2. The conception of parasite, host, intermediate host, final host, reservoir host, paratenic host, life cycle, infective stage and zoonosis.

3. The conception of endoparasite, ectoparasite, obligatory parasite, facultative parasite, permanent parasite, temporary parasite, opportunistic parasite and accidental parasite.

4. The importance of parasitic zoonoses.

5. The mutual adaptation between parasite and host: pathogenicity and immunity are phenomena of mutual adaptation of parasite and host.

6. The conception of sterilizing immunity, non-sterilizing immunity, premunition and concomitant immunity.

7. The general characteristics of parasite diseases.

8. Infectiousness: the key links of parasite diseases (source of infection, spreading channel and persons who are easy to be infected).

9. The factors influencing prevalence: living condition, poor nutrition, regional, ethnic customs and climate conditions.

10. The category of parasitology: medical protozoology, medical helminthology and medical arthropodology.

Chapter 2　Protozoa–Introduction

1. The general classfication of protozoa.
2. The morphology of protozoa: trophzoite and cyst.
3. The life cycle of protozoa.
4. The pathogenesis of medical protozoa.
5. The laboratory diagnosis of protozoa.

Chapter 3　Lobosea & Flagellata

1. The morphology of Amoebae.
2. The differences of *Entamoeba histolytica* and *Entamoeba coli*.
3. The basic process of life cycle, pathogenesis and laboratory diagnosis of Amoebae.
4. The epidemiological features, prevention and treatment of amoebiasis.
5. The morphology of *Leishmania donovani*, *Giardia Duodenalis* and *Trichomonas vaginalis*.
6. The basic process of life cycle, pathogenesis and laboratory diagnosis principle of *Leishmania donovani*, *Giardia Duodenalis* and *Trichomonas vaginalis*.

Chapter 4　Sporozoa & Ciliatea

1. The general characteristics of Class Sporozoa and Ciliatea.
2. The morphology of *plasmodium*: the exoerythrocytic stage and erythrocytic stage.
3. The life cycle of *plasmodium*: in human and in mosquito.
4. The pathogenesis and laboratory diagnosis of *plasmodium*.
5. The epidemiological features, prevention and treatment of malaria.
6. The morphology of *Toxoplasma gondii*.
7. The basic process of life cycle, pathogenesis and laboratory diagnosis of *Toxoplasma gondii*.
8. The epidemiological features, prevention and treatment of *Toxoplasma gondii*.
9. The morphology of *Balantidium coli*.
10. The basic process of life cycle, pathogenesis and laboratory diagnosis of *Balantidium coli*.

Chapter 5　Trematoda–Introduction

1. The position of trematoda in animal kingdom.
2. The characteristics of trematodes.
3. The morphology of trematodes.
4. The life cycle of trematodes.

5. The epidemiological features, prevention and treatment of trematodiasis.

Chapter 6　Fasciolopsis buski

1. The morphology of *Fasciolopsis buski*.
2. The form and structure of adult and egg of *Fasciolopsis buski*.
3. The life cycle, pathogenesis and laboratory diagnosis of *Fasciolopsis buski*.
4. The epidemiological features, prevention and treatment of fasciolopsiasis.

Chapter 7　Clonorchis sinensis

1. The morphology of *Clonorchis sinensis*: Trematode in liver.
2. The life cycle, pathogenesis and laboratory diagnosis of *Clonorchis sinensis*.
3. The epidemiological features, prevention and treatment of clonorchiasis.

Chapter 8　Paragonimus westermani

1. The morphology of *Paragonimus westermani*: Trematode in lung.
2. The life cycle, pathogenesis and laboratory diagnosis of *Paragonimus westermani*.
3. The epidemiological features, prevention and treatment of paragonimiasis.

Chapter 9　Schistosome & Cercarial dermatitis

1. The morphology of Schistosome: Trematode in blood vessel.
2. The form and structure of adult and egg of *Schistosoma japonicum*.
3. The life cycle, pathogenesis and laboratory diagnosis of *Schistosoma japonicum*.
4. The epidemiological features, prevention and treatment of schisosomiasis.
5. The pathogenesis of cercarial dermatitis.

Chapter 10　Cestoda–Introduction

1. The position of cestoda in animal kingdom.
2. The characteristics of cestodes.
3. The morphology of cestodes.
4. The life cycle of cestodes.
5. The epidemiological features, prevention and treatment of cestodiasis.

Chapter 11　Spirometra mansoni & Diphyllobothrium latum

1. The morphology *of Spirometra mansoni*.
2. The life cycle, pathogenesis and laboratory diagnosis of *Spirometra mansoni*.
3. The epidemiological features, prevention and treatment of sparganosis mansoni.
4. The morphology *of Diphyllobothrium latum*.

Chapter 12　Taenia solium &Taenia saginata

1. The morphology characteristics and main differences between *Taenia solium* and *Taeniasaginata* in scolex, neck, immature proglottid, mature proglottid, gravid proglottid and cysticercus cellulose.
2. The life cycle, pathogenesis and laboratory diagnosis of *Taenia solium* and *Taenia saginata*.

3. The epidemiological features, prevention and treatment of taencasis and cysticercosis.

Chapter 13   Hymenolepis nana & Echinococcus granulosus

1. The morphology of *Hymenolepis nana*.
2. The life cycle, pathogenesis and laboratory diagnosis of *Hymenolepis nana*.
3. The epidemiological features, prevention and treatment of hymenolepiasis nana.
4. The form of adult, larva and egg of *Echinococcus granulosus*.
5. The life cycle, pathogenesis and laboratory diagnosis of echinococcosis.

Chapter 14   Seminar–Zoonotic parasite

1. List the parasites that can cause zoonosis.
2. List the laboratory diagnosis of zoonotic parasites.

Chapter 15   Nematoda–Introduction

1. The position of nematoda in animal kingdom.
2. The general characteristics of nematodes.
3. The life cycle, pathogenesis and laboratory diagnosis of nematodes.
4. The epidemiological features, prevention and treatment of nematodosis.

Chapter 16   Ascaris lumbricoides

1. The morphology of *Ascaris lumbricoides*.
2. The life cycle, pathogenesis and laboratory diagnosis of *Ascaris lumbricoides*.
3. The epidemiological features, prevention and treatment of ascariasis.

Chapter 17   Enterobius vermicularis & Hookworm

1. The morphology of *Enterobius vermicularis*(pinworm), *Ancylostoma duodenale* and *Necator americanus* (hookworm).
2. The life cycle, pathogenesis and laboratory diagnosis of *Enterobius vermicularis*, *Ancylostoma duodenale* and *Necator americanus*;
3. The epidemiological features, prevention and treatment of enterobiasis and ancylostomiasis.

Chapter 18   Filaria & Trichuris trichiura

1. The morphology of *Wuchereria bancrofti* and *Brugia malayi* (Filaria).
2. The life cycle, pathogenesis and laboratory diagnosis of filaria.
3. The epidemiological features, prevention and treatment of filariasis.
4. The morphology of *Trichuris trichiura*(whipworm).
5. The life cycle, pathogenesis and laboratory diagnosis of *Trichuris trichiura*.
6. The epidemiological features, prevention and treatment of trichocephaliasis.

Chapter 19   Medical Arthropoda–Introduction

1. The position of arthropoda in animal kingdom.
2. The harmful effects of arthropods on human health.

Chapter 20　Arachnida

1. Arachnida: the morphology of *Hard tick*, *Soft tick* and *sarcoptes scabiei*.
2. The relationship of arthropods and human diseases.
3. The life cycle, pathogenesis and laboratory diagnosis of Class Arachnida.

Chapter 21　Insecta

1. Insecta: the morphology of mosquitoes, flies, lice and fleas.
2. The relationship of arthropads and human diseases.
3. The life cycle, pathogenesis and laboratory diagnosis of mosquitoes, flies, lice and fleas.

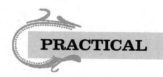

PRACTICAL

1. The identification of the adult and the egg morphology characteristics of medical protozoa.

Slide sample: *Entamoeba histolytica*, *Entamoeba coli*, *Trichomonas vaginalis*, *Malarial parasites*, *Toxoplasma gondii* and *Leishmania donovani*.

2. The identification of the adult and the egg morphology characteristics of medical trematodes.

Slide sample: *Clonorchis sinensis*, *Paragonimus westermani*, *Fasciolopsis buski* and *Schistosoma japonicum*.

3. The identification of the adult and the egg morphology characteristics of medical cestodes.

Slide sample: *Taenia solium*, *Taenia saginata* and *Hymenolepis nana*.

4. The identification of the adult and the egg morphology characteristics of medical nematodes.

Slide sample: *Ascaris lumbricoides*, *Enterobius vermicularis*(pinworm), *Ancylostoma duodenale*, *Necator americanus* (hookworm) and *Trichuris trithiura*(whipworm).

5. The identification of the adult and the egg or larva morphology characteristics of medical arthropods.

Slide sample: *Hard tick, Soft tick, Sarcoptes scabiei*, mosquitoes, flies, lice and fleas.

MEDICAL IMMUNOLOGY
医学免疫学

Chief Editors（主编）
Dai Yalei（戴亚蕾） Tongji University（同济大学）
Yao Zhi（姚智） Tianjin Medical University（天津医科大学）
Zhang Lining（张莉宁） Shandong University（山东大学）

Deputy Chief Editors（副主编）
Lu Linrong（鲁林荣） Zhejiang University（浙江大学）
Li Fang（李芳） Dalian Medical University（大连医科大学）

Editors（编委）（按姓氏拼音排序）
Dai Yalei（戴亚蕾） Tongji University（同济大学）
Li Fang（李芳） Dalian Medical University（大连医科大学）
Lu Linrong（鲁林荣） Zhejiang University（浙江大学）
Yao Zhi（姚智） Tianjin Medical University（天津医科大学）
Zhang Lining（张莉宁） Shandong University（山东大学）

Course Description

The immune response is the body's major defense against infectious factors. This section of the course, will present some of the fundamental characteristics of human immunology. During this course, students will learn about the ability of human body to mount innate and adaptive immune responses, the role of T and B lymphocytes, antibody structure, autoimmunity, and hypersensitivity. This course is very close with microbiology course, so students will also learn how to prevention of infectious disease with immunization.

This course will focus on mechanisms of host immune response and the scientific approaches that are used to investigate these processes. It includes basic immunology and clinical immunology sections. The first section will mainly teach on how immune system recognizes and responds to antigens, which covers the nature of antigens, components of immune system, principles of immune response, effector molecules and subgroups of immune cells derived from immune response, regulation of immune response, immunopathology, etc. The second section will teach on how an inappropriately developed immune response leads to diseases and the study of diseases caused by disorders of the immune system (failure, aberrant action, and malignant growth of the cellular elements of the system). It also involves diseases of other systems, where immune reactions play a part in the pathology and clinical features.

OBJECTIVES

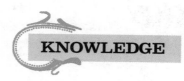

KNOWLEDGE

The aim of this course is to give an in-depth knowledge in immunology and training in the methods used in the field. At the end of the course, the students should obtain the knowledge of the fundamentals in immunology, including molecules of the immune system, cells and cell interactions in the immune response; effector functions, immunity and transplantation; tolerance and allergy, autoimmune disease.

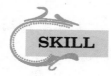

SKILL

At the end of the course, the student should have a specialized knowledge and understanding of aspects of the scientific basis of immune related disease, developed skills in the analysis of arguments and data from clinical aspects and in the use of problem-oriented approaches to contemporary scientific issues in medicine.

Teaching and Learning Methods

Theory: Teaching immunology to undergraduate medical student is provided with the help of lectures and short video that deal with student understanding the theoretical basis. Case study (PBL) will help student analysis the mechanisms of important immune-related diseases, including immunopathogenesis, laboratory diagnosis, treatment and clinical aspects immunity.

Practical: Practical training asks students to know the basic principles, methods and techniques, strategies, and skills for laboratory diagnosis of immune functional changes. The student is advised to pay attention to biosafety in the laboratory.

Recommended Textbooks

Abul K Abbas, Adrew H Lichtman, Shiv Pillai. 2015. Basic Immunology: Functions and Disorders of the Immune System [M]. 5th ed. Philadelphia pennsylvania: Saunders Elsevier.

Abul K Abbas, Adrew H Lichtman, Shiv Pillai. 2015. Cellular and Molecular Immunology [M]. 8th ed. Singapore: Elsevier Pte Ltd.

Thao Doan, Roger Melvold, Susan Viselli et al. 2012. Immunology [M]. 2nd ed. Philadelphia: Lippincott.

Schedule Table

Chapter	Contents	Hours	Chapter	Contents	Hours
1	Induction to the immune system	2	12	Immunological regulation	2
2	Antigen and antibody	4	13	Immunity at epithelial barriers and in immune privileged tissues	2
3	Soluble recognition and effector molecules	2	14	Immunity to microbes	1
4	Inflammatory response related molecules	2	15	Immunization and vaccines	1
5	Host barriers and innate immune cells	2	16	Hypersensitivity and allergy	2
6	Innate immunity	2	17	Autoimmunity and autoimmune diseases	4
7	Major histocompatibility complex and their genes	2	18	Immunodeficiency	2
8	Antigen capture and presentation to lymphocytes	2	19	Transplantation immunity	2
9	T lymphocyte development and cell-mediated immunity	4	20	Tumor immunity	2
10	B lymphocyte development and humoral immunity	4	21	Immunological techniques and measurement of immune functions (Laboratory practical)	14
11	Immunological tolerance	2		Total	60

Course Contents

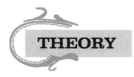

THEORY

Chapter 1   Induction to the immune system

1. Concept of immunity.

Innate immunity, adaptive immunity.

2. The immune system.

Immune organs, immune cells, immune tissues, lymphocyte homing and recirculation.

3. Overview of immune responses.

Innate immune responses, adaptive immune responses, properties of adaptive immune response.

4. Overview of immune responses to microbes.

Early innate immune response, adaptive immune response, decline of immune response, immunological memory.

5. Overview of history of immunology.

Chapter 2   Antigen and antibody

1. Concept of antigen and antibody.

2. Properties of antigen.

(1) Basic properties of antigen, basic structure of antigen, type of epitopes, type of antigen, whether T helper required for B cell activation.

(2) Affiliation between antigen and host,

(3) The source of antigen,

(4) Superantigen.

3. Type of receptors to capture antigen.

(1) Preformed receptors: PRR, MHC, others.

(2) Somatically generated receptors: TCR, BCR.

4. Properties of antibody.

(1) Basic structure, accessory molecule, hydrolytic fragment, diversity of antibody,

(2) Antibody functions: recognizing antigen, activating complement, binding to Fc receptor, neonatal immunity.

5. Human immunoglobulin isotypes.

IgM, IgD, IgG, IgA, IgE.

6. Antibody generation and their binding types.

(1) Antibody preparation.

(2) Antibody types: polyclonal antibody, monoclonal antibody, genetic engineering antibodies.

Chapter 3　Soluble recognition and effector molecules

1. Concept of complement.

Complement system, complement nomenclature, property of complement.

2. Complement activation.

The classical pathway, the alternative pathway, the mannose-binding lectin pathway, regulation of complement activation.

3. Complement functions and its clinic.

4. Other soluble effector molecules.

Pentraxins, collectins, ficolins: antibacterial peptide, lysozyme, β-lysin.

Chapter 4　Inflammatory response related molecules

1. Concept of inflammatory response.

2. Cytokines and their receptors.

Common property of cytokines, category of cytokine, category of cytokine receptors, cytokine functions, cytokine applications.

3. Human leukocyte differentiation antigen (HLDA).

Cluster of differentiation, HLDA functions.

4. Cell adhesion molecules.

(1) Immunoglobulin superfamily.

(2) Integrin family.

(3) Selectin family.

(4) Adhesion molecule functions.

(5) Adhesion molecule applications.

Chapter 5　Host barriers and innate immune cells

1. Barriers to infection.

Physical barriers, chemical and environmental barriers, biological barriers.

2. Cells of the innate immune system.

(1) Development of innate immune cells.

(2) Phagocytes: monocytes, macrophages, neutrophils.

(3) Dendritic cells.

(4) Natural killer cells.

(5) Innate-like lymphocytes: NKT, γδT, B-1 B cell.

(6) Others: basophils, mast cells, eosinophils.

Chapter 6　Innate immunity

1. Concept of innate immunity.

2. Components of innate immunity.

(1) Barriers, phagocytosis and killing, natural killer cell and its immune responses.

(2) Inflammation to exclude microbes.

(3) Systemic and pathologic consequences of inflammation.

(4) Microbial evasion of innate immunity.

(5) Role of innate immunity in stimulating adaptive immune response.

3. Innate immune response phages.

Immediate innate immunity, early induced innate immune response, initial adaptive immune response.

Chapter 7　Major histocompatibility complex and their genes

1. Concept of major histocompatibility complex.

2. Property of major histocompatibility complex.

MHC gene encoding locus and their structures, genetic features of MHC, peptide binding to MHC molecules.

3. MHC classes and their functions.

(1) MHC class I molecules, MHC class II molecules.

(2) MHC functions.

4. MHC with clinic.

Chapter 8　Antigen capture and presentation to lymphocytes

1. Capture of protein antigens by antigen-presenting cells (APC).

(1) Antigen-presenting cells and their category.

(2) Professional APC: Dendritic cell, macrophages, B cell.

2. Processing and presentation of protein antigen.

(1) Processing of internalized antigen for display by MHC class II molecules.

(2) Processing of cytosolic antigen for display by MHC class I molecules.

(3) Cross-presentation of internalized antigens to CD8+ T cells.

(4) Physiologic significance of MHC-associated antigen presentation.

Chapter 9   T lymphocyte development and cell–mediated immunity

1. T cell lineage.
(1) Thymus structure.
(2) αβ T cell development, γδ T cell development ,
(3) NKT cell origin.
2. Markers on the surface of T cell.
(1) TCR-CD3 complex, CD4/CD8,
(2) Co-stimulatory molecules: CD28, CTLA-4, ICOS, PD-1, CD2, CD40L,
(3) Other receptors: LFA-1/ICAM-1, cytokine receptors.
3. Subgroups of T cells.
(1) Categorized by activating stage: naïve T cell, effector T cell, memory T cell,
(2) Categorized by CD4 or CD8: $CD4^+$ T cell, $CD8^+$ T cell.
(3) Categorized by their functions: helper T cell (Th1, Th2, Th17, Tfh), cytotoxic T lymphocyte (CTL), regulatory T cell (Treg).
4. Phases of T cell responses.
(1) Recognition of MHC-associated peptides.
(2) Immunological synapse formation.
(3) Signal transduction and activation.
(4) Clonal expansion and differentiation.
(5) Decline of the immune response.
(6) Memory T cells formation.
5. Effector mechanisms of T cell-mediated immunity.
(1) $CD4^+$ T cell: Th1, Th2, Th17, Tfh.
(2) $CD8^+$ T cell: CTL.
(3) Regulatory T cell.
(4) Memory T cell.

Chapter 10   B lymphocyte development and humoral immunity

1. B cell lineage.
(1) Bone marrow.
(2) B cell development.
2. Markers on the surface of B cell.
(1) BCR-Igα/Igβ complex.
(2) Co-receptors: CD19/CD21/CD81
(3) Co-stimulatory molecules: CD40, CD80/CD86, LFA-1/ICM-1,
(4) Other molecules: CD20, CD22, CD32, cytokine receptors.
3. Subgroups of B cells and their functions.
B-1 B cell, B-2 B cell.
4. B cell responses to antigens.
(1) B cell activation with T-dependent antigen.
Recognition of antigen, signal transduction and activation, B cell proliferation and formation of antibody-secreting plasma cells, memory B cells generation, primary and secondary humoral immune response.

(2) B cell activation with T-independent antigen.

TI-1 antigen induced B cell response, TI-2 antigen induced B cell response, the difference of subsets of B cells response to T-independent antigen.

5. Effector mechanisms of humoral immunity.

Neutralization of microbes and microbial toxins, mediating opsonization and phagocytosis, activation of complement system, neonatal immunity, antibody feedback to regulation of humoral immune response by Fc receptor.

Chapter 11　Immunological tolerance

1. Concept of immunological tolerance.

2. Tolerance formation.

3. Immunological tolerance.

(1) T lymphocyte tolerance: central T cell tolerance, peripheral T cell tolerance.

(2) B lymphocyte tolerance: central B cell tolerance, peripheral B cell tolerance.

(3) Tolerance induced by foreign protein antigen.

4. Self-tolerance and autoimmune diseases.

Chapter 12　Immunological regulation

1. Concept of immunological regulation.

2. The formation of immunoregulation.

(1) Interaction with immune molecules.

Antigen-antibody, cytokine-cytokine receptor,

(2) Interaction receptors on the surface of immune cells.

Inhibitory receptor-active receptor, FcγRIIb-BCR,

(3) Interaction between immune cells.

Th1-Th2, Treg,

(4) Others regulations.

Activation-induced cell death (AICD), Fas/FasL, neuroendocrine immune regulation.

Chapter 13　Immunity at epithelial barriers and in immune privileged tissues

1. Concept of immunity at epithelial layer.

2. Immunity in the gastrointestinal system.

(1) Innate immunity and adaptive immunity in the gastrointestinal tract,

(2) Mechanisms of oral tolerance.

Property of the mucosal response, balance of commensal bacteria, local responses to commensals, mucosal DC regulate the induction of tolerance.

(3) Diseases related to immune responses in the gut.

3. Immunity in the cutaneous system.

(1) Innate immunity and adaptive immunity in the skin.

(2) Diseases related to immune responses in the skin.

4. Immune privileged tissues.

Eye, brain, testis, mammalian fetus.

Chapter 14　Immunity to Microbes

1. Concept of immune response to microbes.
2. Immunity to extracellular bacteria.
(1) Innate immunity and adaptive immunity to extracellular bacteria.
(2) Injurious effects during immune responses to extracellular bacteria.
(3) Immune evasion by extracellular bacteria.
3. Immunity to intracellular bacteria.
(1) Innate immunity and adaptive immunity to intracellular bacteria.
(2) Immune evasion by intracellular bacteria.
4. Immunity to viruses.
(1) Innate immunity and adaptive immunity to viruses.
(2) Immune evasion by viruses.
5. Immunity to Fungi.
Innate immunity and adaptive immunity to fungi.
6. Immunity to parasites.
(1) Innate immunity and adaptive immunity to parasites.
(2) Immune evasion by parasites.

Chapter 15　Immunization and vaccines

1. Concept of immunization.
2. Types of immunization.
(1) Natural immunity: natural active immunization, natural passive immunization.
(2) Artificial immunity: Artificial active immunization, artificial passive immunization.
(3) Adoptive immunity.
3. Passive immunization.
(1) The biological products for passive immunization.
(2) The side effect of artificial passive immunization.
4. Active immunization.
(1) Vaccination and herd immunity.
(2) Strategic considerations of vaccine.
(3) The influence factor for effective vaccination.
Property of vaccine, features of host, Mode of vaccine entrance, adjuvant,
(4) The side effect of artificial active immunization.
5. Types of vaccine.
Inactivated vaccine, lived-attenuated vaccine, toxoid, subunit vaccine, conjugate vaccine, synthetic peptide vaccine, genetic engineering vaccine, etc.
6. Application of vaccine.
Planned immunization in China, anti-infection, anti-tumors.

Chapter 16　Hypersensitivity

1. Concept of hypersensitivity and allergy.

2. Causes of hypersensitivity diseases.

Reactions against self-antigens, reactions against microbes, reactions against environmental antigens.

3. Mechanisms and classification of hypersensitivity reactions.

(1) Type I hypersensitivity.

Localized reactions, systemic reaction, clinical syndromes.

(2) Type II hypersensitivity.

Interaction of antibody with cells, interaction of antibody with the extracellular matrix, antibody-mediated disruption of cellular function, clinical syndromes.

(3) Type III hypersensitivity.

Localized reactions, systemic reaction, clinical syndromes.

(4) Type IV hypersensitivity.

Contact dermatitis, delayed hypersensitivity, T cell-mediated cytotoxicity, clinical syndromes.

4. Therapeutic approaches for hypersensitivity disorders and allergy.

Anti-inflammatory agents, depletion of cells and antibodies, anti-cytokines therapies, agents inhibit inflammatory cell migration, regulatory T cell therapies.

Chapter 17 Autoimmunity and autoimmune diseases

1. Concept of autoimmunity and autoimmune diseases.

2. Mechanisms of autoimmunity.

(1) Genetic basis of autoimmunity, immunologic abnormalities leading to autoimmunity, the role of infections in autoimmunity, other factors in autoimmunity.

(2) The reason for loss of self-tolerance: pathogenesis, genetic factors, role of infections and other environmental influences.

3. Selected autoimmune diseases.

(1) Humoral-associated autoimmune diseases.

Systemic lupus erythematosus (SLE), Rheumatoid arthritis (RA).

(2) Cell-mediated autoimmune diseases.

Multiple sclerosis, Type I diabetes mellitus.

Chapter 18 Immunodeficiency

1. Concept of immunodeficiency.

2. Primary immunodeficiency.

(1) Defects in stem cells,

(2) Defects in innate immunity.

Defects in phagocytes and natural killer cells, defects in the complement system.

(3) Defects in adaptive immunity.

Defects in T cells, defects in B cells.

(4) Lymphocyte abnormalities associated with other diseases.

Severe combined immunodeficiency, other forms of SCID: ADA deficiency, defects in nucleotide metabolism, X-linked SCID.

Defects in T cell activation and function, antibody deficiencies.

3. Acquired immunodeficiency.

(1) The reason for loss of immune response.

Physiologic sequelae, therapeutic treatment, infection, cancer.

(2) Selected disease associated with loss of immune response.

Human immunodeficiency virus and the Acquired immunodeficiency syndrome (AIDS).

4. Treatment of immunodeficiency.

Passive supplementation, bone marrow transplantation, genetic engineering.

Chapter 19　Transplantation immunity

1. Concept of transplantation immunity.

(1) General principles of transplantation immunology.

(2) Type of transplantation.

Human tissue and organs: the nature of alloantigen, MHC alloantigen,

Nonhuman tissues and organs: Xenogeneic graft.

(3) Type of immune response between host and graft.

Host-versus-graft reaction (HVGR), Graft -versus- host reaction (GVHR).

2. Adaptive immune response to allografts.

(1) Recognition of alloantigen by T cell: direct recognition, indirect recognition.

(2) The role of co-stimulation in T cell response to alloantigen.

(3) The role of specific antibodies for alloantigen.

(4) the mixed lymphocyte reaction.

3. Pattern and mechanisms of allograft rejection.

(1) Hyperacute rejection.

(2) Acute rejection: cellular rejection, antibody-mediated rejection.

(3) Chronic rejection and graft vasculopathy.

4. prevention and treatment of allograft rejection.

(1) Increasing matched tissue on graft donor and recipient.

(2) Agents producing general immunosuppression.

(3) Strategies for antigen-specific depression of allograft reactivity.

5. Selected clinical experience in grafting.

(1) Blood transfusion.

ABO blood group antigen, Lewis antigen, Rhesus (Rh) antigen.

(2) Kindy transplantation.

(3) Bone marrow grafting.

(4) Immune-privileged sits.

Chapter 20　Tumor immunity

1. Concept of tumor immunity.

2. Tumor antigens.

Mutated gene expressed protein, abnormal expressed but unmuted cellular protein, antigens of oncogenic viruses, oncofetal antigens, altered glycolipid and glycoprotein antigens.

3. Immune mechanisms against tumor.

(1) Innate immunity: NK cells, macrophages, γδ T cells, cytokines.

(2) Adaptive immunity: antibodies, CTLs,

4. Evasion of immune responses by tumors.

Loss antigen expression, treated tumor antigen as self-antigen, antigenic modulation, tumor-induced immune suppression, tumor-induced privileged site.

5. Immunotherapy for tumors.

(1) Enhancing host immune responses to tumors.

Vaccination with tumor antigens, blocking inhibitory pathways, cytokine therapy, non-specific stimulation of the immune system.

(2) Passive immunotherapy for tumors.

Adoptive cellular therapy, therapy with anti-tumor antibodies.

6. The role of innate and adaptive immunity in promoting tumor growth.

Chronic inflammation, some infection, etc.

Chapter 21　Immunological techniques and measurement of immune functions

1. Concept of Immunological techniques.

2. Epitope detection by antibodies.

(1) Particulate antigens,

Direct agglutination, indirect or passive agglutination.

(2) Soluble antigens.

Radial immunodiffusion, double-diffusion, immunoelectrophoresis (IEP).

3. Epitope quantitation by antibodies.

Radioimmunoassay (RIA), Enzyme-linked immunosorbent assay (ELISA), Fluorescent immunosorbent assay (FIA).

4. Epitope detection on and in immune cells.

Immunofluorescene (IF), monoclonal antibodies, flow cytometry.

5. Assessment of immune function.

Phagocyte function, cell proliferation, cytotoxic T-lymphocyte assay.

PRACTICAL AND DEMONSTRATIONS

1. Phagocytosis of innate immunity.

(1) Lysozyme lysis test.

(2) Neutrophil phagocytic function test.

(3) Macrophage phagocytic function test.

2. Antigen and antibody reactions.

(1) Agglutination.

Direct/indirect agglutination reaction, indirect agglutination inhibition test.

(2) Precipitation reactions.

Single/double agar diffusion, countercurrent/rocket immunoelectrophoresis, immunological colloidal gold signature.

(3) Complement.

Hemolytic reaction of complement, complement fixation test.

3. Detection of lymphocyte functions.

(1) T and B lymphocyte isolation and identification.

Separation of lymphocytes, identify B lymphocytes by immunohistochemistry technique, analysis of T lymphocyte subgroups by FACS.

(2) T and B cell functional assay.

T cell proliferation test, hemolytic plaque formation test.

4. ELISA for measuring soluble immune molecules.

(1) Detection of the level of cytokine (INF-γ) in medium.

(2) Detection of the level of antigen/antibody in serum.

PATHOLOGY
病　理　学

Chief Editors（主编）
Wu Qiang（吴强）　Anhui Medical University（安徽医科大学）
Zhou Ren（周韧）　Zhejiang University（浙江大学）
Gao Peng（高鹏）　Shandong University（山东大学）

Deputy Chief Editors（副主编）
Wu Zhengsheng（吴正升）　Anhui Medical University（安徽医科大学）
Wang Yalan（王娅兰）　Chongqing Medical University（重庆医科大学）
Chen Li（陈莉）　Nantong University（南通大学）
Song Bo（宋波）　Dalian Medical University（大连医科大学）
Xin Ying（辛颖）　Jilin University（吉林大学）
Mao Zhengrong（毛峥嵘）　Zhejiang University（浙江大学）

Editors（编委）（按姓氏拼音排序）
Chen Li（陈莉）　Nantong University（南通大学）
Gao Peng（高鹏）　Shandong University（山东大学）
Mao Zhengrong（毛峥嵘）　Zhejiang University（浙江大学）
Song Bo（宋波）　Dalian Medical University（大连医科大学）
Wang Yalan（王娅兰）　Chongqing Medical University（重庆医科大学）
Wu Qiang（吴强）　Anhui Medical University（安徽医科大学）
Wu Zhengsheng（吴正升）　Anhui Medical University（安徽医科大学）
Xin Ying（辛颖）　Jilin University（吉林大学）
Zhou Ren（周韧）　Zhejiang University（浙江大学）

Course Description

　　Pathology is the study of disease principles that mainly discusses etiology, pathogenesis, pathological changes and their relation to clinical features and outcome. It bridges preclinical medicine and clinical practice. Pathological changes cover metabolic, functional and morphological abnormalities, among which morphological changes are maily focused on. There are two parts of the course: general pathology and systematic pathology. General pathology mainly discusses lesions which are common changes in disease courses, while systematic pathology introduces characteristic changes of a certain disease. During the study of this discipline, students will be expected to comprehend diseases in a hierarchical way, i.e. at the level of cell, tissue, organ, and at the level of total human body. Above all, pathology is a compulsory course for medical students.

Objectives

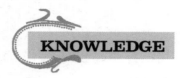

At the end of the course, the MBBS students shall be able to:

1. To master basic concepts and nomenclatures of lesions and their significances.

2. To master characteristic pathological changes of common diseases and their relations to clinical medicine.

3. To understand the etiology and pathogenesis of common diseases.

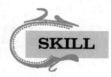

At the end of the course, students should be able to do the following experiments, the using of microscope and the method of observing the morphology at both gross and histologic levels.

Teaching and Learning Methods

Theory: Teaching work provides medical students with the help of lectures and tutorials that deal with the etiology, classifications, pathogenesis, and master the morphology, clinical characters, genetic features, prognosis, immunotype of major types of disorders of common diseases. The interaction between teachers and students is needed.

Practice: Practical training asks for medical students to know the principles, methods, techniques and strategies, and the skills for typical pathologic diagnosis. Students are advised to pay attention to master morphologic changes and their relations to clinical practice.

Recommended Textbooks

Chen Jie (陈杰). 2018. Textbook of Pathology [M]. Beijing: People's Medical Publis-hing House.

Kumar V, Abbas AK. 2015. Aster JC. Robbins Basic Pathology [M]. 9th ed. Philadelphia: WB Saunders.

Rubin R, Sttayer DS. 2013. Robbin's Pathology: Clinicopathologic Foundations of

Medicine [M]. 10th ed. Philadelphia:Lippincott Williams & Wilkins.

Zhai Qihui (翟启辉), Zhou Gengyin (周庚寅). 2009. Textbook of Pathology [M]. Beijing: Peking University Medical Press.

SCHEDULE TABLE

Chapter	Contents	Hours	Chapter	Contents	Hours
1	Introduction to pathology	1	10	Lymphatic and hematopoietic system	6
2	Cell and tissue adaptation and injury	6	11	Urinary system	9
3	Tissue repair	3	12	Immunopathology	4
4	Hemodynamic disorder	8	13	Genital system and breast	8
5	Inflammation	12	14	Endocrine system	4
6	Neoplasia	16	15	Nervous system	4
7	Cardiovascular system	10	16	Pathology of infectious disease and parasitosis	7
8	Respiratory system	10		Total	120
9	Digestive system	12			

Course Contents

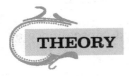

THEORY

Chapter 1   Introduction

1. The concept of pathology and its research objects and tasks.
2. The position and status of pathology in medicine.
3. The research methods and techniques of pathology.
4. The history of pathology.

Chapter 2   Cell and Tissue Adaptation and Injury

1. The concept, type and significance of adaptation including atrophy, hypertrophy, hyperplasia and metaplasia.

2. Major causes, mechanisms and patterns of cell and tissue injury. The concept, pathogenesis and morphologic changes of reversible cell injury (cellular swelling, fatty change, hyaline change, amyloid change, mucoid degeneration, pathological pigments deposition and pathological calcification).

3. The patterns of irreversible cell injury. The concept, types, morphologic changes (nuclear changes should be highlighted) and consequences of necrosis. The comparison between necrosis and apoptosis.

4. The concept and hypothesis of cell aging.

Chapter 3　Tissue Repair

1. The cell cycles.

2. Stem cells and its roles in the regeneration.

3. Tissue regeneration: concepts of regeneration and repair, regeneration processes and patterns of different tissues and their own characteristics, mechanisms of cellular regeneration.

4. Granulation tissue: the component, morphology, function and collagenization of granulation tissue.

5. Scar formation: the component and function of scar tissue.

6. The process of repair by connective tissue: angiogenesis, proliferation and migration of fibroblasts, extracellular matrix deposition and tissue remodeling.

7. Cutaneous wound healing: three main phases of cutaneous wound healing, healing by first and second intentions.

8. Fracture healing: hematoma, soft tissue callus, bony callus, bone remodeling.

9. Pathologic aspects of repair: age, nutritional status, infection and foreign matter, local blood circulation, innervation, ionizing radiation, and cautioned reduction and fixation of fracture.

Chapter 4　Hemodynamic Disorder

1. The concept, causes, pathological changes and consequence of hyperemia.

2. The concept of homeostasis and thrombosis.

3. The condition, types, morphology, process, mechanisms and consequence of thrombosis.

4. The concept and consequences of embolism.

5. The concept, cause, condition, types, morphology and consequences of the infarction.

Chapter 5　Inflammation

1. Overview of inflammation: definitions of inflammation, etiology, general changes in metabolism, function and morphology, focal and systemic clinical appearances.

2. Acute inflammation: vascular reactions, mediators of inflammation, types, courses and diagnosis.

3. Chronic inflammation: morphology and the clinical appearances. Definition and pathological features of granuloma.

Chapter 6　Neoplasia

1. Overview of neoplasm.

2. The definition, morphological features, differentiation and dysplasia of neoplasm.

3. The growth, invasion and spread of neoplasm.

4. The grading and staging of neoplasm.

5. The clinical effects of neoplasm on the host.

6. The comparison between benign and malignant tumors.

7. The nomenclature and classification of neoplasm.

8. Precancerous lesion, dysplasia and carcinoma in situ.

9. The molecular mechanism and pathogenesis of neoplasia.

10. Short introduction to common neoplasms.

Chapter 7   Diseases of Cardiovascular System

1. Atherosclerosis and ischemic heart disease (IHD): risk factor, pathogenesis, general lesions, characteristic morphology at different arteries and subsequent changes with clinical significances, coronary heart disease (angina pectoris, myocardial infarction (MI), sudden cardiac death (SCD), myocardial fibrosis).

2. Hypertension: risk factors, pathogenesis, vascular lesions and damages to involved organs.

3. Rheumatism and rheumatic heart disease: pathogenesis, morphology and effects.

4. Infective endocarditis: causes, pathogenesis and morphology.

·5. Vavular heart diseases, valvular stenosis and insufficiency.

6. Cardiomyopathy.

7. Myocarditis.

8. Pericarditis and other Pericardial Diseases.

9. Congenital heart disease: ASD, VSD, Fallot's bicuspid aortic valve, PDA.

10. Tumors of heart.

11. Diseases of blood vessels other than atherosclerosis.

Chapter 8   Diseases of Respiratory System

1. Introduction to chronic obstructive pulmonary disease: the definition, causes, morphology, clinical course of chronic bronchitis. The definition, types of emphysema, morphology, pathogenesis and clinical course of emphysema. The definition, pathogenesis, morphology and clinical course of bronchiectasis.

2. Introduction to cor pulmonale: the definition; disorders that predispose to cor pulmonale; morphology; clinical course of Cor pulmonale.

3. Introduction to pulmonary infections pneumonias: the pathogens, pathology (congestion, red hepatization, gray hepatization and resolution), clinical course and complications of lobar pneumonias. The pathogens, pathology, clinical course and complications of lobular pneumonia. The morphology, gross pathology clinical course and complications of bronchopneumonia.

4. Introduction to pneumoconiosis: basic changes of silicosis.

5. Introduction to respiratory tumors: the morphology, histologically of non-small cell lung carcinoma (NSCLC), squamous cell carcinoma, adenocarcinomas, large cell lung carcinomas and small cell lung carcinomas of lung cancer. The methods to diagnose lung cancer. The pathology characters about the histologic types of nasopharyngeal carcinoma.

6. Introduction to acute respiratory distress syndrome (ARDS).

Chapter 9　Diseases of Digestive System

1. Pathology of the gastro-intestinal tract:

(1) Carcinoma of the esophagus: etiology, pathological changes, metastasis and clinical-pathological correlation.

(2) Peptic ulcer: etiology, pathogenesis, pathological changes and complications.

(3) Gastritis: classification and pathological changes.

(4) Carcinoma of the stomach: etiology, pathological changes, metastasis and clinical-pathological correlation.

(5) Appendicitis: etiology, pathogenesis, pathological changes and classification.

(6) Colonic carcinoma: etiology, pathological changes, metastasis and clinical-pathological correlations.

(7) Ulcerative colitis: pathological changes and clinical-pathological correlation.

(8) Pancreatitis: etiology, pathogenesis, pathological changes and clinical-pathological correlation.

2. Pathology of the liver and biliary tract:

(1) Viral hepatitis: etiology, pathogensis, types, pathological changes and clinical-pathological correlation.

(2) Hepatocirrhosis: concept and classification, etiology, pathogenesis, pathological changes and its clinical features.

(3) Primary carcinoma of the liver: classification, etiology, pathological changes, metastasis and its clinical features.

Chapter 10　Diseases of Lymphatic and Hematopoietic System

1. Lymphoid neoplasms: concepts, types, biological behavior and its related clinical practice.

2. Hodgkin's lymphoma: etiology and pathogenesis, classification, the identified pathological changes and their relations to clinical practices.

3. Myeloid neoplasms: classification, pathogenesis, pathological changes and their relations to clinical features.

4. Histiocytic neoplasmes: classification, morphology, clinical features, prognosis.

Chapter 11　Disease of the Urinary System

1. Glomerular diseases: pathogenesis, pathological types , pathological changes and their relations to clinical syndromes.

2. Diseases affecting tubules and interstitial: etiology, pathogenesis, pathological changes and heir relations to clinical features.

3. Tumors: types and pathological changes of common tumors.

Chapter 12　Immunopathology

1. Autoimmune disease: pathogenesis, types, pathological changes and clinical practices.

2. The concepts of the rejection of transplant and the immune deficiency.

Chapter 13   Diseases of Genital System and Breast

1. Cervix: concepts, etiology, pathological features and the relation of pathological changes to clinical features of cancerous and precancerous lesions.

2. Corpus uteri: concepts, pathological features and the relation of pathological changes and the clinical features of the endometrial hyperplasia and endometrial carcinoma.

3. Hydatiform mole, invasive mole, choriocarcinoma: pathological features and their outcome.

4. Breast cancer: concepts, etiology, pathological features and their relations to clinical features.

Chapter 14   Diseases of Endocrine System

1. The major manifestation of anterior pituitary diseases, hyperpituitarism and hypopituitarism. The classification and main features of pituitary adenoma.

2. Thyroid diseases: thyroiditis, diffuse nontoxic goiter and Graves disease. The subtypes of thyroid carcinoma and their main features.

3. The major features of adrenocortical hyperfunction, adrenocortical insufficiency and neoplasm.

4. The types, pathogenesis and clinicopathologic correlation of diabetes mellitus. The features of insulinoma and gastrinoma.

Chapter 15   Diseases of Nervous System

1. The disorders of the nervous system: basic pathological changes , common complications, and clinical manifestations.

2. Infections of the nervous system: etiology, epidemiology, morphologic changes and clinical practices of epidemic cerebrospinal meningitis and epidemic encephalitis B.

3. Tumor: pathogenesis, classification and pathological changes.

4. Degenerative diseases and dementias.

5. Cerebrovascular diseases.

Chapter 16   Infectious Disease and Parasitosis

1. The etiology, pathogenesis, pathological changes, relationship between pathological characteristics and clinical manifestations of tuberculosis, typhoid fever, bacillary dysentery, leprosy, epidemic hemorrhagic fever, rabies, deep mycosis.

2. The etiology, pathogenesis, pathological changes, relationship between pathological characteristics and clinical manifestations of common parasitosis.

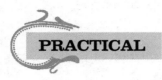

PRACTICAL

1. The way of using of microscopes.
2. Watch the autopsy demonstration.
3. The appearance of the lesions in common diseases.
4. Case discussion: the imitated clinicopathological conference.

PATHOPHYSIOLOGY
病理生理学

Chief Editors（主编）

Xu Zhelong（徐哲龙） Tianjin Medical University（天津医科大学）
Sun Liankun（孙连坤） Jilin University（吉林大学）
Wang Siying（汪思应） Anhui Medical University（安徽医科大学）

Deputy Chief Editors（副主编）

Xiao Xianzhong（肖献忠） Central South University（中南大学）
Li Cong（李骢） Dalian Medical University（大连医科大学）
Yao Xiaomei（姚小梅） Tianjin Medical University（天津医科大学）
Di Hongjun（邸红军） Tianjin Medical University（天津医科大学）

Editors（编委）（按姓氏拼音排序）

Di Hongjun（邸红军） Tianjin Medical University（天津医科大学）
Gong Yongsheng（龚永生） Wenzhou Medical University（温州医科大学）
Guo Lirong（郭丽荣） Jilin University（吉林大学）
He Xiaohua（何小华） Wuhan University（武汉大学）
Huang Qiaobing（黄巧冰） Southern Medical University（南方医科大学）
Li Cong（李骢） Dalian Medical University（大连医科大学）
Li Wenbin（李文斌） Hebei Medical University（河北医科大学）
Men Xiuli（门秀丽） North China University of Science and Technology
          （华北理工大学）
Sun Liankun（孙连坤） Jilin University（吉林大学）
Tian Fang（田芳） Zhengzhou University（郑州大学）
Tian Ye（田野） Harbin Medical University（哈尔滨医科大学）
Wang Siying（汪思应） Anhui Medical University（安徽医科大学）
Xiao Xianzhong（肖献忠） Central South University（中南大学）
Xu Zhelong（徐哲龙） Tianjin Medical University（天津医科大学）
Yao Xiaomei（姚小梅） Tianjin Medical University（天津医科大学）
Zhang Huali（张华莉） Central South University（中南大学）
Zhao Chenghai（赵成海） China Medical University（中国医科大学）

Course Description

Pathophysiology is a medical discipline that describes conditions typically observed during a disease state. Its main task is to study the general principles and mechanisms of disease development, alterations of metabolism and function in the body systems or individual organs, so as to explore the nature of disease, to provide theoretical basis for the prevention and treatment of disease. In medical education, pathophysiology is not only a medical foundation course, but also an important subject bridging basic and clinical medicine, playing an important role in the medical education system.

The origin of pathophysiology can be traced back to 18th century. Italian anatomist Morgagni (1682-1771) led the establishment of physiology research autonomous from medical research and created Organ Pathology. Modern pathophysiology began to develop as a distinct field of inquiry during the 19th Century by French physiologist Claude Bernard (1813-1878) that studied the causes, functional changes of clinical diseases. Combined with developments in the understanding of diseases, at present, pathophysiology is a required area of study for nearly all healthcare professional school programs (medical, dental, pharmacy, nursing, radiology, preventive medicine, public health and paramedic programs) in China, United States, Canada and other countries. Moreover, pathophysiology is an incredibly vital part of the medical field that will continue to grow in the upcoming future, due to the emergence of new diseases every year. Pathophysiology is also a comprehensive interdisciplinary subject correlated with many medical basic sciences.

Pathophysiology includes theoretical course and experimental course. For theoretical course, it includes two parts: basic pathological process and systemic pathophysiology. Pathophysiology mainly introduces the concept of disease and the general rules of occurrence and development of diseases. For basic pathological process, it focuses on alterations of function, metabolism and structure in the common set of features that may appear in a variety of diseases. For systemic pathophysiology, it focuses on the common pathological changes and mechanisms of each system in the development of diseases.

For experimental course, it mainly helps the students to establish a realistic scientific attitude, to observe and record the data from the experiments objectively, to analyze and summarize the data from the experiments systematically, to increase the chances of thinking and practice for students, to stimulate the independent thinking and innovation for students, to improve scientific idea and the exploring spirits for students.

The course utilizes lectures, experiments and case studies to interpret pathological processes, clinical information, diagnostic tests, signs and symptoms relating to mechanisms of disease, helping students achieve an understanding, both broad and specific, of how basic pathophysiologic concepts affect the organ systems above.

The purpose of this course is to make students understand the fundamental general and specific pathologic mechanisms involved in the onset and development of diseases, and master basic knowledge and basic skills. On this basis, students should be able, as a result, to describe how and why the signs or symptoms of various conditions appear so that the rational therapies of disease can be devised.

Objectives

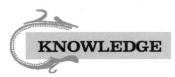

KNOWLEDGE

At the end of the course the students will be able to:

1. Understand the concept of disease and general rules of etiology and pathogenesis.

2. Master the alterations and mechanisms of function and metabolism of diseases.

3. Describe the clinical manifestations of a specific disease development, and explain the underlying mechanisms.

4. Culture students'skills of independent analysis, thinking and solving problems.

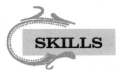

SKILLS

At the end of the course, the students will be able to:

1. Plan and interpret laboratory investigations for the diagnosis of common diseases and to correlate the clinical manifestations with the etiological agents.

2. Master the conventional surgical techniques.

3. Use the correct method of collection, storage and transport of clinical material for microbiological investigations.

4. Establish animal models for common diseases.

5. Analyze the occurrence and development of common diseases according to the data from the animal experiments.

Teaching and Learning Methods

Theory: Through lectures and tutorials, pathophysiology teachingseeks to help students learn the pathogenesis of diseases, and the underlying mechanisms of the alterations in body structure and function caused by diseases.

Practical: Lab teachings aim to help the students learnthe basic skills of animal operations, and to further understand the mechanisms for the initiation and development of diseases, and the alterations in body structure and function under pathophysiological conditions.

Recommended Textbooks

Stephen J. Mcphee. 2010. Pathophysiology of Disease [M]. 6th ed. New York: McGraw-

Hill Companies, Inc.

Sue E Huether. 2016. Understanding Pathophysiology [M]. 6th ed. Philadelphia: Elsevier Inc.

Sue E Huether. 2012. Understanding Pathophysiology [M]. 5th ed. New York: Mosby, Inc.

Schedule Table

Chapter	Contents	Hours	Chapter	Contents	Hours
1	Altered Cellular and Tissue Biology	1	12	Regulation of the Cardiovascular Function	2
2	Fluids and Electrolytes, Acids and Bases	6	13	Alterations of Cardiovascular Function	3
3	Stress and Disease	2	14	Function of the Pulmonary System	1
4	Biology of Cancer	2	15	Alterations of Pulmonary Function	2
5	Cancer Epidemiology	1	16	Function of the Renal and Urologic Systems	1
6	Pain, Temperature and Sleep	2	17	Alterations of Renal and Urinary Tract Function	2
7	Alterations in Cognitive Systems, Cerebral Hemodynamics, and Motor Function	2	18	Alterations of Female Reproductive System	0
8	Disorders of the Central and Peripheral Nervous Systems and Neuromuscular Junction	1	19	Alterations of Digestive Function	3
9	Alterations of Hormonal Regulation	2	20	Alterations of Musculoskeletal Function	0
10	Structure and Function of the Hematologic System	1		Total	36
11	Alterations of Hematologic Function	2			

Course Contents

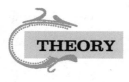

THEORY

Chapter 1　Altered Cellular and Tissue Biology

1. Cellular injury.
2. Cellular death.
3. Aging and altered cellular and tissue biology.
4. Somatic death.

Chapter 2　Fluids and Electrolytes, Acids and Bases

1. Distribution of body fluids and electrolytes.
2. Alterations of water movement.
3. Sodium, chloride and water balance.
4. Alterations in sodium, chloride and water balance.

5. Alterations in potassium and other electrolytes.

6. Acid-base balance.

7. Acid-base imbalances.

Chapter 3　Stress and Disease

1. Historical background and general concepts.

2. The stress response.

3. Stress, personality, coping, and illness.

Chapter 4　Biology of Cancer

1. Cancer terminology and characteristics.

2. The biology of cancer cells.

3. Clinical manifestations of cancers.

4. Diagnosis, characterization, and treatment of cancer.

Chapter 5　Cancer Epidemiology

1. Genetics, epigenetics, and tissue.

2. In utero and early life conditions.

3. Environmental-lifestyle factors.

Chapter 6　Pain, Temperature, and Sleep

1. Pain.

2. Temperature regulation.

3. Sleep.

Chapter 7　Alterations in Cognitive Systems, Cerebral Hemodynamics, and Motor Function

1. Alterations in cognitive systems.

2. Alterations in cerebral hemodynamics.

3. Alterations in neuromotor function.

Chapter 8　Disorders of the Central and Peripheral Nervous Systems and Neuromuscular Junction

1. Central nervous system disorders.

2. Peripheral nervous system and neuromuscular junction disorders.

Chapter 9　Alterations of Hormonal Regulation

1. Mechanisms of hormonal alterations.

2. Alterations of the hypothalamic-pituitary system.

3. Alterations of thyroid function.

4. Alterations of parathyroid function.

5. Dysfunction of the endocrine pancreas: diabetes mellitus.

6. Alterations of adrenal function.

Chapter 10　Structure and Function of the Hematologic System

1. Components of the hematologic system.
2. Mechanisms of hemostasis.
3. Anticoagulant system.

Chapter 11　Alterations of Hematologic Function

1. Alterations of erythrocyte function.
2. Alterations of leukocyte function.
3. Hemorrhagic disorders and alterations of platelets and coagulation.

Chapter 12　Regulation of Cardiovascular Function

1. The circulatory system.
2. The systemic circulation.

Chapter 13　Alterations of Cardiovascular Function

1. Diseases of the arteries.
2. Manifestations of heart disease.
3. Shock.

Chapter 14　Function of the Pulmonary System

Function of the pulmonary system.

Chapter 15　Alterations of the Pulmonary Function

1. Clinical manifestations of pulmonary alterations.
2. Pulmonary disorders.

Chapter 16　Function of the Renal and Urologic Systems

1. Regulation of renal blood flow.
2. Kidney function.
3. Test of renal function.

Chapter 17　Alterations of Renal and Urinary Tract Function

1. Urinary tract obstruction.
2. Urinary tract infection.
3. Glomerular disorders.
4. Acute kidney injury.
5. Chronic kidney disease.

Chapter 18　Alterations of Female Reproductive System (Self-Learning)

Chapter 19　Alterations of Digestive Function

1. Disorders of the gastrointestinal tract.
2. Disorders of the accessory organs of digestion.

3. Cancer of the digestive system.

Chapter 20   Alterations of Musculoskeletal Function (Self–Learning)

1. Musculoskeletal injuries.
2. Disorders of bones.
3. Disorders of joints.
4. Disorders of skeletal muscle.
5. Musculoskeletal tumors.

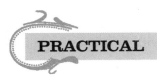

PRACTICAL

1. Hypoxia.
(1) Master the method of establishing the animal models of hypoxia caused by oxygen deficiency or carbon monoxide poisoning.
(2) Master with the mechanisms of hypoxic hypoxia and hemic hypoxia.
(3) Be familiar with the clinical manifestations during hypoxia.
2. Effects of hyperkalemia on the heart.
(1) Introduction to the ECG of hyperkalemia.
(2) Duplicate the animal model of hyperkalemia in rabbit.
(3) Observe the effects of hyperkalemia on the heart.
(4) Understand the characteristic of electrocardiogram (ECG) during hyperkalemia.
(5) Rescue the rabbit with hyperkalemia.
3. Experimental pulmonary edema.
(1) Introduction to the pathogenesis of edema.
(2) Duplicate an animal model of pulmonary edema in rabbit.
(3) Observe manifestations of pulmonary edema.
4. The duration of action of some barbiturates on mice.
Compare the sleeping time of different barbiturates and understand the characteristics of different barbiturates.
5. Analgesic effects of drugs on mice with twisting trunk method.
Observe and compare the analgesic action of the narcotic analgesics and antipyretic analgesics with twisting trunk method.
6. Hemorrhagic shock and treatment.
(1) Establish the animal model of hemorrhagic shock.
(2) Observe manifestations of hemorrhagic shock.
(3) Understand the pathogenesis and treatment of shock.
7. Experimental pneumothorax in rabbit.
(1) Duplicate pneumothorax model in rabbit.
(2) Observe the effects of pneumothorax on respiration, including its symptom, sign, mechanism and consequence.

(3) Master the changes of circulation in pneumothorax.

(4) Master the regulation of acid-base balance by blood gas analysis, and blood pressure detection.

8. Respiratory dysfunction in rabbit.

(1) Establish the animal model of obstructive hypoventilation and restrictive hypoventilation.

(2) Observe the manifestations of hypoventilation.

(3) Understand the blood gas in hypoventilation.

9. The effects of ammonia on the pathogenesis of rabbit hepatic encephalopathy.

(1) Master the methods to duplicate the animal model of acute hepatic encephalopathy through ligating subtotal liver lobes combined with infusion of solution compound NH_4Cl.

(2) Understand deeply the ammonia intoxication hypothesis on the pathogenesis of hepatic encephalopathy.

(3) Analyze and discuss why and how to reduce blood ammonia in hepatic encephalopathy and its significance.

PHARMACOLOGY
药　理　学

Chief Editors（主编）

Zhang Xiumei（张岫美）　Shandong University（山东大学）

Gao Jing（高静）　Jiangsu University（江苏大学）

Yao Jihong（姚继红）　Dalian Medical University（大连医科大学）

Zhang Xuemei（张雪梅）　Fudan University（复旦大学）

Deputy Chief Editors（副主编）

Lou Jianshi（娄建石）　Tianjin Medical University（天津医科大学）

Liu Huiqing（刘慧青）　Shandong University（山东大学）

Li hua（李华）　Dalian Medical University（大连医科大学）

Feng Yun（封云）　Jiangsu University（江苏大学）

Zhang Huiling（张慧灵）　Soochow University（苏州大学）

Editors（编委）（按姓氏拼音排序）

Feng Yun（封云）　Jiangsu University（江苏大学）

Gao Jing（高静）　Jiangsu University（江苏大学）

Li hua（李华）　Dalian Medical University（大连医科大学）

Liu Huiqing（刘慧青）　Shandong University（山东大学）

Lou Jianshi（娄建石）　Tianjin Medical University（天津医科大学）

Xü Xiao（许潇）　Jiangsu University（江苏大学）

Yao Jihong（姚继红）　Dalian Medical University（大连医科大学）

Zhang Huiling（张慧灵）　Soochow University（苏州大学）

Zhang Xiumei（张岫美）　Shandong University（山东大学）

Zhang Xuemei（张雪梅）　Fudan University（复旦大学）

Course Description

Pharmacology is a subject which studies the principles of interactions between drug and living organism which includes human body, cells and microorganisms and theil mechanisms. Pharmacology is one of the indispensable and professional basic courses for medical students. Pharmacology introduces the basic theories and principles of drug and then clinical relevance. The most important task of pharmacology is to explain the actions and its mechanisms of the drug, to provide the theoretical basis for clinic, enhancing the drug efficacy and reducing adverse drug reaction. The main parts of pharmacology include pharmacodynamics and pharmacokinetics. Pharmacodynamics explains the principal of the biochemical or physical actions of drugs on the body, including actions, mechanisms, indications, adverse reactions, contraindications of the drug. And pharmacokinetics reveals the principles of dynamic changes of drug in the body, mainly dealing with the change of drug concentration in human or animal body following administration, i.e., the changes of concentration in the dynamic system of absorption, distribution, metabolism and excretion (ADME). Pharmacology is based on physiology, biochemistry, pathology and pathogenic organisms. These studies lay a solid foundation for clinical courses.

The purposes for pharmacological learning are to master the basic theory of pharmacology and to provide theoretical basis for clinical rational drug use. Therefore pharmacology is an essential course in the clinical medical curriculum.

Objectives

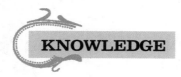

KNOWLEDGE

At the end of the course, the MBBS students shall be able to:

1. To master the basic principles of pharmacology.

2. To master the actions, action mechanisms, clinical uses, adverse reactions, and drug interactions of typical drugs.

3. To understand the process of drug in the body including absorption, distribution, metabolism and excretion, and the pharmacokinetic principles of typical drugs.

4. To master the actions, clinical uses and main adverse reaction of the common used drugs.

5. To master the important pharmacokinetic parameters of the common used drugs.

6. To be able to identify and monitor adverse drug reactions (ADRs) and appreciate the importance of ADR reporting.

7. To know the drugs used in systemic illnesses, infections and chemotherapy etc. with main mechanism(s) of action, pharmacokinetics, uses, side-effects and indications.

8. To understand the general principles of rational drug use.

9. To understand the methods in experimental pharmacology, principles of bioassay and be able to correlate drug effects with the actions of drugs at the receptors.

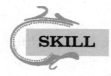

SKILL

At the end of the course, the student shall be able to practice the following experiments, the common used methods of pharmacological experiments, determination methods for pharmacological parameters (pA_2, pD_2 and $t_{1/2}$). the effects of some agent on blood pressure *in vivo*, the isolated heart, intestinal smooth muscle preparation and bronchial smooth muscle experiment and experimental design.

Teaching and Learning Methods

Theory: Teaching pharmacology to medical students is provided with the help of lectures and tutorials that deal with the principles of pharmacodynamics and pharmacokinetics of drugs.

Practicals: Practical training asks medical students to know the basic principles, methods and techniques, strategies, and skills by the typical pharmacological experiments and experimental design. The students are advised to pay attention to the regulation and biosafety of the pharmacological laboratory.

Recommended Textbooks

Bertram Katzung. 2016. Basic and Clinical Pharmacology [M]. 13th ed. New York: McGraw-Hill Medical.

Laurence Brunton, Bruce Chabner, Bjorn Knollman. 2016. Goodman and Gilman's the Pharmacological Basis of Therapeutics [M]. 13th ed. New York: McGraw-Hill Medical.

Lou Jianshi (娄建石). 2015. Pharmacology. Beijing: Qinghua University Press.

Richard A Harvey. 2013. Lippincott's Illustrated Pharmacology [M]. 5th ed. Philadelphia: Lippincott Williams & Wilkins.

Yang Baofeng (杨宝峰), Chen Jianguo (陈建国). 2018. Pharmacology [M]. 9th ed. Beijing: People's Health Publishing House.

Schedule Table

Chapter	Contents	Hours	Chapter	Contents	Hours
1	Introduction	2	13	Psychotropic drugs	3
2	Pharmacodynamics	4	14	Analgesics	2
3	Pharmacokinetics	4	15	Antipyretic-analgesic and anti-inflammatory drugs	3
4	Pharmacogenetics	2	16	Central nervous system stimulants	1
5	Introduction to autonomic pharmacology	2	17	Drugs used in the treatment of heart failure	3
6	Cholinoceptor activating and cholinesterase inhibiting agents	2	18	Antihypertensive drugs	3
7	Cholinoceptor antagonists	2	19	Antiarrhythmic drugs	2
8	Adrenoceptor agonists	2	20	Antianginal drugs	2
9	Adrenoceptor antagonists	2	21	Antiatherosclerotic drugs	2
10	Sedative and hypnotics	2	22	Diuretics and dehytrants	2
11	Antiepileptic drugs	2	23	Drugs acting on blood and hemopoietic system	3
12	Drugs used in the treatment of central nervous system degenerative diseases	2	24	Antitussives, expectorants and antiasthmatics	2

Continued

Chapter	Contents	Hours	Chapter	Contents	Hours
25	Drugs used in the treatment of gastrointestinal diseases	2	35	Broad-spectrum antibiotics	1
26	Drugs affecting uterine motility	1	36	Synthetic antimicrobial drugs	3
27	Histamine and antihistamine drugs	1	37	Antifungal drugs	1
28	Adrenocorticosteroids	3	38	Antiviral drugs	1
29	Drugs affecting the thyroid glands	2	39	Antituberculosis drugs	2
30	Antidiabetic drugs	2	40	Antimalarial drugs	2
31	Introduction to chemotherapeutic agents	2	41	Amebicides	1
32	β-Lactam antibiotics	3	42	Anthelmintic drugs	1
33	Aminoglycosides and polypeptides	2	43	Antineoplastic drugs	3
34	Macrolides, lincosamides and glycopeptides	2		Total	90

Course Contents

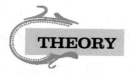

THEORY

Chapter 1　Introduction

1. The concepts of pharmacology, drug, pharmacodynamics and pharmacokinetics.
2. The nature and tasks of pharmacology.
3. History and development of pharmacology.
4. The role of pharmacology in clinical medicine and pharmacy.
5. Pharmacology in the research and development of new drugs.
6. The methods for pharmacology learning.

Chapter 2　Pharmacodynamics

1. The basic actions of drug.

The therapeutic effects and the adverse drug reactions.

Side reaction, toxic reaction (acute toxication, chronic toxication and special toxications such as carcinogenesis, teratogenesis and mutagenesis）, after effect, withdrawal reaction, allergic reaction, idiosyncrasy and drug dependence.

2. The dose-response relationship.

(1) Graded response: minimum effective concentration (C_{min}), threshold concentration, minimum effective dose, maximum efficacy (E_{max}), individual variability, and potency.

(2) Quantal response: Concentration for 50% of maximum effect (EC_{50}), toxic dose, minimum toxic dose, lethal dose, median lethal dose (LD_{50}) and therapeutic index(TI).

3. The mechanisms of drug action.

(1) Interaction of drug and receptors: Occupation theory, affinity index (pD$_2$) and antagonism parameter (pA$_2$).

(2) The types of receptors and the second messengers.

(3) G protein coupled receptors.

(4) Ligand-gated ion channel receptors.

(5) Recepter tyrosine Kinase.

(6) Intracellular receptors.

(7) Other enzyme receptors.

(8) cAMP, cGMP, IP$_3$, DAG, and Ca^{2+}.

4. The classifications of drugs according to the receptors: agonists and antagonists.

5. The regulation of receptors.

Chapter 3   Pharmacokinetics

1. The main modes and characteristics of drug permeation, and the effect of pH on drug permection.

2. The concepts of absorption and distribution, and its affecting factors: first-pass effect, bioavailability, blood plasma binding rate and apparent volume of distribution (Vd).

3. The concepts and main modes of drug metabolism, hepatomicrosomal enzymes, their inducers and inhibitors, and their effects on drug actions.

4. The concept of drug excretion and main routes, the passive tubular re-absorption and enterohepatic circulation.

5. The first-order elimination kinetics and zero-order elimination kinetics, typical time-concentration curve, compartment models and multiple dose kinetics.

6. The pharmacological importance of the elimination rate constant (K), half life ($t_{1/2}$), plasma clearance (Cl) and steady state concentration (C$_{ss}$).

Chapter 4   Pharmacogenetics

1. The effects of genetic factors on drug reactions.

(1) The effect of genetic factors on pharmacokinetics.

(2) The effect of genetic factors on pharmacodynamics.

2. The racial difference of drug reaction and metabolism.

Chapter 5   Introduction to Autonomic Pharmacology

1. The classifications of autonomic nervous system by their physiological function and transmitters.

2. The types of main transmitters.

3. Biosynthesis, storage, release and termination of noradrenaline and acetylcholine.

4. The types of main receptors.

5. The distribution and function of α- and β-adrenoceptor, M- and N-cholinergic receptor and other receptors.

6. The regulation of autonomic nerve system drugs on ANS: influence on receptors

directly or influence on the biosynthesis, transportation, storage and metabolism of the transmitters.

Chapter 6 Cholinoceptor Activating and Cholinesterase Inhibiting Agents

1. Concept and classifications of the cholinoceptor agonists.

2. Pharmacological effects of acetylcholine.

3. Pharmacological effects, clinical uses and adverse reactions of pilocarpine.

4. Reversible acetylcholinesterase inhibitors: pharmacological actions, *in vivo* process, characteristics and clinical applications.

5. Irreversible acetylcholinesterase inhibitors: mechanisms and symptoms of acute poisoning, principles of treatment and clinical applications of rescue alexipharmics (atropine and pralidoximes).

Chapter 7 Cholinoceptor Antagonists

1. The competitive blocking functions of atropine on M-cholinergic receptor, and its pharmacological characteristics, clinical applications, adverse effects, toxic symptoms and rescue principles.

2. The pharmacological characteristics, clinical applications of anisodamine and scopolamine, and the comparison with atropine.

3. The characteristics, uses, major adverse effects and contraindications of ganglion selective blockers.

4. The effects of skeletal muscle relaxants on N_m-receptor, the different modes of action between the non-depolarizing muscular relaxants and depolarizing muscular relaxants and their characteristics, applications and rescue principles.

Chapter 8 Adrenoceptor Agonists

1. The chemical structure and structure-effect relationship of adrenoceptor agonists.

2. The effects of MAO and COMT in the metabolism of CA and the main elimination ways.

3. Noradrenaline.

The major target receptors (α and β_1), the administration routes, effects on cardiovascular system, the clinical applications and the adverse reactions and their prevention and treatments.

4. Adrenaline.

The major target receptors (α and β), pharmacological functions, effects on cardiovascular system, clinical applications, side effects and contraindications.

5. Isoprenaline.

The major target receptors (β_1 and β_2), pharmacological functions, effects on cardiovascular system, adverse reactions and contraindications.

6. Dopamine.

The dose-effect relationship, pharmacological characteristics and applications.

7. The characteristics and applications of phenylephrine, dobutamine, amphetamine, cocaine and ephedrine.

Chapter 9　Adrenoceptor Antagonists

1. Phenoxybenzamine.

The major target receptors (α_1 and α_2), pharmacological characteristics, effects on cardiovascular system, clinical applications and adverse reactions.

2. Phetolamine.

The major target receptors (α_1 and α_2), pharmacological characteristics, effects on cardiovascular system, clinical uses and side effects.

3. The characteristics and applications of prazosin.

4. Nonselective β-adrenergic blocking agent—propranolol: pharmacokinetic characteristics, pharmacological effects, clinical uses, side effects and contraindications.

5. Selective β-adrenergic blocking agents—atenolol, etc.: pharmacological effects and clinical uses.

6. Antagonists with partial agonist activity—pindolol: pharmacological effects and clinical uses.

7. Antagonists of both α and β adrenoceptors—labetalol and carvedilol: pharmacological effects and clinical uses.

8. Reserpine: mechanisms.

Chapter 10　Sedative and Hypnotics

1. The effects, mechanism, clinical uses and adverse reactions of benzodiazepines.

2. The pharmacokinetics properties, uses and adverse reactions of diazepam and flurazepam.

3. The effects, mechanisms and clinical uses of barbiturates.

4. The properties of other sedative-hypnotic drugs.

Chapter 11　Antiepileptic Drugs

1. The classification of epilepsy and antiepilepsy drugs.

2. The actions, mechanisms, uses, adverse reactions and pharmacokinetics of phenytoin sodium.

3. The effects, mechanisms, uses, adverse reactions and pharmacokinetics of carbamazepine.

4. The effects and uses of ethosuximide, phenobarbital, primidone, sodium valproate and benzodiazepines.

5. The rational use of antiepileptics.

6. The pharmacological actions and clinical uses of magnesium sulfate.

Chapter 12　Drugs Used in the Treatment of Central Nervous System Degenerative Diseases

1. Parkinson's disease and Parkinson's syndrome.

Pathogenesis: dopamine theory and oxidative stress theory.

2. The pharmacological actions, mechanisms, clinical uses, adverse reactions, drug interactions and pharmacokinetics properties of levodopa.

3. The mechanisms and clinical uses of other dopaminomimetics.

(1) Decarboxylase inhibitors: carbidopa and benserazide.

(2) MAO-B inhibitor and antioxidants: selegiline.

(3) Dopamine receptor agonists: bromocriptine and pergolide.

(4) COMT inhibitors: tolcapone and enthacapone.

(5) The mechanisms and clinical uses of amantadine.

(6) The central anticholinergic drugs: mechanisms and clinical uses of trihexyhenidyl.

(7) The pathogenesis and strategy for senile dementia and Alzheimer's disease.

(8) The properties of acetylcholinesterase inhibitors: tacrine, donepezil, galanthamine, metrifonate and huperzine.

(9) The properties of M receptor agonists: xanomeline, milameline, sabcomedine.

(10) The properties of NMDA receptor antagonist: memantine.

Chapter 13　Psychotropic Drugs

1. Pathogenesis of psychotic disorders and classifications of antipsychiatric drugs.

Schizophrenia, mania, depression and anxiety.

2. The pharmacological actions, mechanisms, clinical uses and adverse reactions of chlorpromazine.

3. The action and uses of other antipsychiatric drugs.

Haloperidol, penfluridol, clozapine, risperidone and sulpiride.

4. The actions, mechanisms, uses and adverse reaction of lithium carbonate.

5. The classifications of antidepressants.

6. The effects, mechanisms, uses and adverse reactions of tricyclic antidepressants.

7. The properties of selective MAO-A inhibitors, noradrenaline reuptake inhibitors (NRIs), selective 5-HT reuptake inhibitors (SSRIs), serotonin and noradrealine reuptake inhibitors(SARIs) and noradrenergic and specific serotonergic antidepressants(NSSAs).

(1) Imipramine, amipramine, desipramine and nortripyline.

(2) Fluoxetine, fluovoxamine, paroxetine and sertraline.

(3) Wenlafaxin, duloxetine, and trazodone.

(4) Mirtazapine.

Chapter 14　Analgesics

1. The concept of pain and classifications of analgesics.

2. The opioid receptor and endogenous opioid peptides in pain regulation and analgesics.

3. The pharmacological actions, mechanisms, clinical uses and important adverse reactions of morphine.

4. The properties of codeine.

5. The characteristics of synthetic analgesics.

Pethidine, fentanyl, methadone and pentazocine.

6. The actions and uses of other narcotic analgesics: tramadol, dihydroetorphine, and rotundin.

7. The uses of opioid receptor antagonists: naloxone and naltrexone.

8. To understand steps analgesia therapy for cancer patients.

Chapter 15 Antipyretic–analgesic and Anti–inflammatory Drugs

1. To describe the relationships between the synthesis of PG and the action of analgesic-antipyretic and anti-inflammatory agents.

2. The shared pharmacological actions, uses and adverse reactions.

Inhibition of the synthesis of prostaglandin via inhibition of cyclooxygenase(COX).

3. The pharmacological effects, mechanisms of action, uses and adverse reactions of aspirin.

4. The properties of action and uses of acetaminophen.

5. The characteristics of other analgesic-antipyretic and anti-inflammatory agents.

Phenylbutazone, indomethacin, sulindoc, mefenomic acid, ibuprofen, naproxen, piroxicam and nimesulide.

6. The characteristics of selective COX-2 inhibitors: celecoxib.

Chapter 16 Central Nervous System Stimulants

1. The classifications of CNS stimulants.

2. The pharmacological effects and uses of caffeine.

3. The clinical uses of methylphenidate.

4. The properties of nikethamide and dimefline.

Chapter 17 Drugs Used in the Treatment of Heart Failure

1. The etiology and pathogenesiss of congestive heart failure.

2. The Pharmacological actions, mechanisms, clinical uses, adverse reactions of angiotensin-converting-enzyme inhibitor/angiotensin receptor blockers (ACEIs/ARBs).

3. The pharmacological actions, mechanisms, uses, adverse reactions of diuretics in the treatment of congestive heart failure.

4. The actions, mechanisms, uses, adverse reactions of β-blockers in the treatment of congestive heart failure.

5. The pharmacological actions, mechanisms, uses, adverse reactions and pharmacokinetics of digoxin.

6. The uses of aldosterone receptor antagonists.

7. The uses of vasodilators.

8. The uses of positive inotropes: dobutamine and phosphodiesterase inhibitors (inomrinone, milrinone).

9. The rational use and principles of agents in the treatment of heart failure.

Chapter 18 Antihypertensive Drugs

1. The etiology of hypertension.

2. The classifications of antihypertensive drugs.

3. The actions, mechanisms, uses, adverse reactions and pharmacokinetics of diuretics in the treatment of hypertension.

Thiazides, furosemide and indapamide.

4. The actions, mechanisms, uses, adverse reactions and pharmacokinetics of ACEIs and ARBs in the treatment of hypertension.

Captopril, enalapril, ramipril, losartan, and valsartan.

5. The actions, mechanisms, uses, adverse reactions and pharmacokinetics of calcium channel blockers in the treatment of hypertension.

Nifedipine, amlodipine and nitrendipine.

6. The actions, mechanisms, uses, adverse reactions and pharmacokinetics of β-blockers in the treatment of hypertension.

Propranolol, atenolol and carvedilol.

7. The actions, mechanisms, uses, adverse reactions of centrally acting α_2 agonists, peripherally acting α_1 blockers and direct vasodilators.

Clonidine, moxonidine, and sodium nitroprusside.

8. Hypertensive emergencies and treatment.

9. The new concept and principals in the treatment of hypertension.

(1) The rational treatment of hypertension and strategies for combination therapy in.

hypertension: monotherapy and multitherapy;individualization.

(2) Nonpharmacological management for hypertension.

Chapter 19　Antiarrhythmic Drugs

1. The physiological basis of antiarrhythmic treatment.

(1) Membrane potential of myocardial cell.

(2) Action potential phases and ions across membrane.

Physiological properties.

2. Pathogenesis mechanisms of arrhythmias and antiarrhythmic drugs.

3. The classifications of antiarrhythmic drugs.

4. The pharmacological actions, mechanisms, uses, adverse reactions and pharmacokinetics of class Ia, class II, class III and class IV antiarrhythmic drugs.

Quinidine, procanamide, propranolol, amiodarone, verapamil and diltiazem.

5. Properties of effects, mechanisms, uses, adverse reactions of class Ib, class Ic and miscellaneous drugs.

lidocanine, phenytoin, mexiletine, propofenone, sotolol, dofetilide and adenosine.

6. The rational use of antiarrhythmic drugs and the drug choice in the treatment of different types of arrhythmia.

Chapter 20　Antianginal Drugs

1. The etiology, pathophysiology and classifications of angina.

2. The pharmacological actions, mechanisms, uses, adverse reactions and pharmacokinetics of nitrates in the treatment of angina.

Nitroglycerin, isosorbidedinitrate, and isosorbide mononitrate.

3. The pharmacological actions, mechanisms, uses, adverse reactions and pharmacokinetics of β-blockers in the treatment of angina.

Propranolol, metoprolol, atenolol and carvedilol.

4. The pharmacological actions, mechanisms, uses, adverse reactions and pharmacokinetics of calcium channel blockers in the treatment of angina.

Nifedipine, verapamil and diltiazem.

5. The effects and uses of other drugs in the treatment of angina.

ACEIs/ARBs and nicorandil.

6. The rational use of antianginal drugs and treatment principles.

Chapter 21　Antiatherosclerotic Drugs

1. The etiology, lipoprotein transport, dyslipidaemia and pathophysiology of atherosclerosis.

2. The classifications of primary dyslipidaemia and therapeutic drugs.

3. The pharmacological actions, mechanisms, uses, adverse reactions and pharmacokinetics of statins in the treatment of atherosclerosis.

Lovastatin, simvastatin, pravastatin, atorvastatin and rosuvastatin.

4. The pharmacological actions, mechanisms, uses, adverse reactions and pharmacokinetics of fibric acids in the treatment of atherosclerosis.

Gemfibrazil, fenofibrate and benzafibrate.

5. The properties and uses of bile acid sequestrants, probucol, nicotinic acid and ezetimibe.

Chapter 22　Diuretics and Dehydrants

1. Kidney structure and function.

2. The physiological basis of diuretics.

3. The classifications of diuretics.

4. The pharmacological actions, mechanisms, uses, adverse reactions of loop diuretics.

Furosemide, ethacrynic acid and bumetanide.

5. The pharmacological actions, mechanisms, uses and adverse reactions of thiazide diuretics.

Hydrochlorothiazide, chlorothiazide and indapamide.

6. The pharmacological actions, mechanisms, uses, adverse reactions of potassium-sparing agents and aldosterone-receptor antagonists.

Triamtaerene, spironolactone and eplerenone.

7. The effects and uses of carbonic anhydrase inhibitors.

Acetazolamide.

8. The effects and uses of osmotic diuretics.

Mannitol.

Chapter 23　Drugs Acting on Blood and Hemopoietic System

1. The mechanisms of hemostasis and thrombosis.

2. Anticoagulants.

(1) The pharmacological effects, mechanisms, uses and adverse reactions of heparin.

Low molecular weight heparin: enoxaparin, tedelparin and logiparin.

(2) Thrombin inhibitors: argatroban, hirudin.

(3) Factor Xa inhibitors: rivaroxaban.

(4) The effects and uses of oral anticoagulants.

Coumarin, warfarin and dicumarol.

3. Fibrinolytics.

(1) The pharmacological effects, uses, adverse reactions of streptokinase, urokinase, and tissue-type plassminogen activator (tPA).

(2) Fibrinolytic inhibitors.

Effects and uses of aminomethylbenzoic acid.

4. Antiplatelet drugs.

(1) The classifications of antiplatelet drugs.

(2) The harmacological actions, mechanisms and uses of aspirin in the treatment of thrombosis.

(3) The pharmacological actions, mechanisms, uses of ridogrel, dipyridamol, epoprostenol, ticlopidine, clopidogrel, abciximab and lamifibanin the treatment of thrombosis.

5. Coagulants.

Effects and uses of vitamin K and thrombin.

6. Antianemic Agents.

(1) The classifications of anemia.

(2) The effects, mechanisms, uses, adverse reactions of iron supplements, vitamin B_{12}, folic acid, recombinant human erythropoietin, filgrastim and sargramostim.

7. Blood volume expander.

Effects and uses of dextran.

Chapter 24　Antitussives, Expectorants and Antiasthmatics

1. Background of bronchial asthma.

2. The classifications of antiasthmatics.

The pharmacological effects, mechanism of action and therapeutic applications of adrenergic agonists, glucocorticoids, leukotriene inhibitors, cromolyn sodium, theophylline and anticholinergic agents used in the treatment of asthma.

3. The pharmacological actions and clinical uses of antitussive drugs.

Chapter 25　Drugs Used in the Treatment of Gastrointestinal Diseases

1. The classifications of anti-peptic ulcer drugs.

2. The pharmacological effects and clinical uses of cimetidine and omeprazole.

3. The pharmacological effects and clinical uses of misoprostol, magnesium trisilicate and magnesium sulfate.

Chapter 26　Drugs Affecting Uterine Motility

1. The classifications of drugs affecting uterine motility.

2. The pharmacological effects, therapeutic applications and major adverse reactions of oxytocin.

3. The pharmacological effects, therapeutic applications and major adverse reactions of ergot alkaloid.

Chapter 27　Histamine and Antihistamine Drugs

1. The characteristics of the histamine receptor subtypes.

2. The comparison of characteristics of first and second generation of H_1-blockers: pharmacokinetics, pharmacodynamics, clinical uses and toxicity.

3. H_2-blockers.

The pharmacological effects, pharmacokinetics, clinical uses and adverse effects of cimetidine and ranitidine.

Chapter 28　Adrenocorticosteroids

1. The physiological effects of glucocorticoids.

Metabolism of sugar, protein, lipid, water and salt.

2. Action mechanisms of glucocorticoids.

3. The pharmacokinetics of glucocorticoids: various administration routes and principles, characteristics of transportation, activation and metabolism.

4. Pharmacological effects of glucocorticoids.

(1) Anti-inflammatory, anti-immune, anti-bacterial endotoxin, anti-shock actions and actions on cardiovascular system, central nervous system and other systems.

(2) Description of the favorable and unfavorable performance of these roles and performance of these possible reasons for the occurrence.

5. The clinical uses of glucocorticoids.

Severe acute infection(to relieve symptoms and gain more time), all kinds of inflammation, allergic reactions and autoimmune diseases, shock, certain blood diseases, replacement therapy and local treatment of skin diseases.

6. Adverse reactions.

Similar adrenocortical hyperthyroidism, long-term drug use lead to dysfunction, induced or exacerbated gastric ulcer, the extension of wound healing.

7. Mineralocorticoids Aldosterone: physiological and pharmacological effects, mechanism of action and clinical uses.

8. The characteristics of pharmacokinetics, clinical uses and toxicity of corticotrophin.

9. The characteristics of antagonists of adrenocortical agents.

Chapter 29　Drugs Affecting the Thyroid Glands

1. Biosynthesis, storage, secretion and regulation of thyroid hormones: thyroxine T_3 and T_4.

2. Mutual constraints among the hypothalamus, pituitary and adrenal glands.

3. The effects of thyroid hormones on promoting cellular growth and differentiation and energy metabolism, the clinical applications and adverse reactions.

4. Antithyroid drugs.

Thioamides: mechanisms of action, pharmacological effects and adverse reactions.

5. Iodine and iodides.

Endemic goiter and hyperthyroidism on the therapeutic effect, mechanisms of actions, clinical uses and toxicity.

6. Radioactive iodine in the diagnosis and treatment of hyperthyroidism.

7. Mechanisms and characteristics of adrenoceptor blocking agents.

Chapter 30   Antidiabetic Drugs

1. The classifications of diabetes mellitus.

Insulin dependent diabetes mellitus (IDDM) and insulin independent diabetes mellitus (NIDDM).

2. The chemistry, biosynthesis, secretion and degradation of insulin.

3. The development history of insulin, various preparations and dosing devices and accessories, pharmacokinetics; commonly used short-acting formulations points (such as ordinary insulin), medium effect (such as low protamine zinc insulin), long-lasting (such as protamine zinc insulin) and the principle of selection.

4. Mechanisms, physiological effects, pharmacological effects, clinical uses and adverse reactions of insulin.

5. Insulin secretagogues.

Sulfonylurea.

Pharmacokinetics, clinical uses, adverse reactions and drug interactions.

6. Biguanides.

Pharmacokinetics, clinical uses and adverse reactions.

7. Alpha-glucosides inhibitors.

Pharmacokinetics, clinical uses, adverse reactions.

8. Insulin sensitizing agents.

Thiazolidinediones: pharmacokinetics, clinical uses, adverse reactions.

Chapter 31   Introduction to Chemotherapeutic Agents

1. The basic concept about antimicrobial agents.

Antibacterial drugs, antibiotics, antimicrobial spectrum, antibiotic efficacy, minimal inhibitory concentration (MIC), minimum bacteriocidal concentration (MBC), chemotherapy index (CI), the post-antibiotic effect (PAE).

2. The classifications of antimicrobial agents.

3. The mechanisms of antimicrobial agents.

4. The mechanisms of antimicrobial agents' resistance and the principles of antimicrobial use.

Chapter 32   β–Lactam Antibiotics

1. The classifications of β-lactam antibiotics.

2. The pharmacological actionss, mechanisms of action, therapeutic applications, and major adverse reactions of penicillin.

Prevention and treatment of anaphylactic shock of penicillin.

3. The characteristics of antibacterial action and therapeutic applications of acid stable penicillins, penicillinase-resistant penicillins, broad spectrum penicillins and anti-pseudomonas aeruginosa broad spectrum penicillins.

4. The characteristics of antibacterial action and therapeutic applications of 1st, 2nd,

3rd and 4th-generation cephalosporins.

5. The therapeutic applications of β-lactam antibiotics and β-lactamase inhibitors.

Chapter 33   Aminoglycosides and Polypeptides

1. The antibacterial spectrum, mechanisms of antibacterial action and therapeutic applications of aminoglycosides.

2. The pharmacokinetics, bacterial resistance and the main adverse reactions of aminoglycosides.

3. The pharmacological effects and therapeutic applications of gentamicin and streptomycin.

4. The pharmacological effects, mechanisms of antibacterial action and therapeutic applications of polymyxin E.

Chapter 34   Macrolides, Lincosamides and Glycopeptides

1. The antibacterial spectrum, mechanisms of action, clinical uses, and the main adverse reactions of macrolides.

Erythromycin, azithromycin, roxithromycin and clarithromycin.

2. The antibacterial spectrum, mechanisms of antibacterial action, clinical applications and the main adverse reactions of lincomycins.

3. The pharmacological effect and therapeutic applications of vancomycin.

Chapter 35   Broad–spectrum Antibiotics

1. The concept of broad-spectrum antibiotics.

2. The antibacterial spectrum, mechanisms of antibacterial action, clinical applications and the main adverse reactions of tracyclines.

Tracycline, doxycycline, minocycline and tigecycline.

3. The antibacterial spectrum, mechanism of action, clinical applications and the main adverse reactions of chloramphenicols.

Chapter 36   Synthetic Antimicrobial Drugs

1. The classifications of quinolones and sulfonamides.

2. The antibacterial spectrum, mechanisms of antibacterial action, therapeutic applications, and the main adverse reactions of quinolones and sulfonamides.

3. The main sensitive bacteria and clinical applications to frequently used agents of quinolones (ciprofloxacin, norfloxacin, ofloxacin, pefloxacin, sparfloxacin, trovafloxacin and moxifloxacin) and sulfonamides.

4. The synergism mechanisms of sulfonamides and trimethoprim.

5. The antibacterial activities, therapeutic applications of metronidazole.

Chapter 37   Antifungal Drugs

1. Background knowledge of fungal infection.

2. The classifications of antifungal drugs.

3. The effects, mechanisms, clinical uses and adverse reactions of antifungal drugs.

Amphotericin B, triazole, imidazole and terbinafine and caspofungin.

4. Understanding the pharmacological characteristics and clinical uses of other antifungal drugs.

Chapter 38   Antiviral Drugs

1. Background knowledge of viral infection.

2. The classifications and mechanisms of antiviral drugs.

3. The effects, clinical uses and adverse reactions of antiviral drugs.

Amantadine, aciclovir, zidovudine, lamivudine, adefovir, dipivoxil, efavirenz and ribavirin.

4. Understanding the pharmacological characteristics and clinical uses of other antiviral drugs.

Chapter 39   Antituberculosis Drugs

1. Background knowledge of tuberculosis.

2. The classifications of antituberculosis drugs.

3. The effects, mechanisms, clinical uses and adverse reactions of the first-line antituberculosis agents.

Isoniazid, rifampicin, ethambutol, streptomycin and pyrazinamide.

4. The effects, clinical uses and adverse reactions of the second-line antituberculosis agents.

Sodium para-aminosalicylate, ethionamide, cycloserine, levofloxacin, rifapentine and rifandin.

5. The rational use of antituberculous drugs in the treatment of tuberculosis.

Chapter 40   Antimalarial Drugs

1. Background knowledge of plasmodium infection and malaria.

2. The classifications of antimalarial drugs.

3. The effects, mechanisms, clinical uses and adverse reactions of antimalarial drugs.
Chloroquine, artemisinin, quinine, primaquine and pyrimethamine.

Chapter 41   Amebicides

1. Background knowledge of amebiasis.

2. The classifications of amebicides.

3. The effects, mechanisms, clinical uses and adverse reactions of amebicides.
Diiodohydroxyquinoline, emetine, diloxanide and metronidazole.

Chapter 42   Anthelmintic Drugs

1. Background knowledge of worm infections.

2. The classifications of anthelmintic drugs.

3. The effects, mechanism, clinical uses and adverse reactions of anthelmintic drugs.

Diethylcarbamazine, piperazine, mebendazole, albendazole and pyruinium embonate.

Chapter 43   Antineoplastic Drugs

1. Background knowledge of neoplasm.

2. The classifications of antineoplastic drugs.

3. The classifications of drugs according to cancer cell kinetics (the concepts of cell cycle specific drug and cell cycle non-specific drugs).

4. The classification of drugs according to the structure and sources.

5. The classification of drugs according to the mechanisms of action.

6. Major common adverse effects of anti-neoplastic drugs.

7. The effects, mechanisms, clinical uses and adverse reactions of the cytotoxic antineoplastic drugs.

Alkylating agent, antimetabolites, plant alkaloids, antibiotics and other agents.

8. The pharmacological characteristics, clinical uses and adverse reactions of the non-cytotoxic antineoplastic drugs.

9. T he mechanisms of drugs resistance.

10. The rational use of antineoplastic drugs in the treatment of cancer.

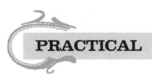

PRACTICAL

1. The common used methods of pharmacological experiments.

2. The determination methods for pharmacological parameters (pA_2, pD_2 and $t_{1/2}$).

3. The effects of some agents on blood pressure *in vivo*.

4. The experiment of analgesics.

5. The isolated heart preparation and experiment *in vitro*.

6. The effects of acetylcholine and atropine on intestinal smooth muscle *in vitro*.

7. The effects of histamine and antihistamine agents on bronchial smooth muscle *in vitro*.

8. The experimental design, preparation and accomplishment.

FORENSIC MEDICINE

法 医 学

Chief Editors（主编）

Chen Zhiming（陈志明） Jilin University（吉林大学）

Qi Baiyu（祁柏宇） Jilin University（吉林大学）

Deputy Chief Editors（副主编）

Chen Xiping（陈溪萍） Soochow University（苏州大学）

Lu Yingqiang（卢英强） Jilin University（吉林大学）

Zhang Mingyang（张明阳） Soochow University（苏州大学）

Editors（编委）（按姓氏拼音排序）

Chen Xiping（陈溪萍） Soochow University（苏州大学）

Chen Zhiming（陈志明） Jilin University（吉林大学）

Gao Tielei（高铁磊） Harbin Medical University（哈尔滨医科大学）

Liu Li（刘莉） Jilin University（吉林大学）

Lu Yingqiang（卢英强） Jilin University（吉林大学）

Peng Xue（彭雪） Harbin Medical University（哈尔滨医科大学）

Qi Baiyu（祁柏宇） Jilin University（吉林大学）

Xuan Zhaoyan（宣兆艳） Jilin University（吉林大学）

Yang Jin（杨津） Jilin University（吉林大学）

Zhang Mingyang（张明阳） Soochow University（苏州大学）

Course Description

Forensic medicine is a subject which studies and solves the medical problems in judicial practice. Forensic Medicine is one of the indispensable professional courses for medical students. Forensic Medicine introduces the basic theories and principles of death, postmorterm changes, injury, asphyxia, sudden death, poisoning , paternity testing, forensic mental illnesses and medical tangle. Forensic medicine belongs to applied medicine and needs to be based on the broad theoretical knowledge and technology of basic medicine and clinical medicine. At the same time, the development and achievements of forensic medicine will further enrich the medical knowledge, such as through the study of sudden death mechanism to explore the prevention of sudden death, through the analysis of medical tangle. to clarify the causes.

After graduation, medical students will become a doctor or engaged in medical-related work, they will often encounter some forensic related problem, a more systematic understanding and mastery of forensic knowledge and skills is necessary to improve the level of students'comprehensive knowledge and social adaptability.

Objectives

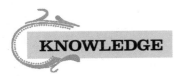

KNOWLEDGE

At the end of the course, the MBBS students shall be able to:

1. To master the basic theories and concepts of forensic medicine.
2. To understand the identification of a variety causes of violent death, including injury, asphyxia, poisoning, etc.
3. To understand the identification of sudden death.
4. To understand the mechanism of a variety of poisoning.
5. To understand the genetic polymorphism of various biological samples.

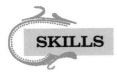

SKILLS

At the end of the course, the student shall be able to practice the following experiments:

1. Be able to record and assistant in forensic autopsy.
2. Be able to do the experiment of alcohol poisoning and organophosphorus pesticide poisoning.
3. Be able to do the experiment of blood grouping.

Teaching and Learning Methods

Theory: Teaching forensic medicine to medical students is provided with the help of lectures and turorials that deal with the basic concepts and mechanisms of death, injury and some diseases.

Practical: Practical training asks medical students to know the basic principles, methods and skills by the typical forensic experiments and experimental design and to pay attention to the regulation and biosafety of the forensic laboratory.

Recommended Textbooks

Jason Payne-James, Richard Jones, Steven B Karch, et al. 2011. Simpson's Forensic

Medicine [M]. 13th ed. London:Hodder Arnold.

Wang Baojie（王保捷）, Hou Yiping（侯一平）. 2013. Forensic Medicine [M]. 6th ed. Beijing: People's Health Publishing House.

Schedule Table

Chapter	Contents	Hours	Chapter	Contents	Hours
1	Introduction	2	8	Rape and infanticide	2
2	Death and postmortem changes	4	9	Forensic mental illness	1
3	Mechanical injury	6	10	Medical tangle	2
4	Mechanical asphyxia	4	11	Identification of the living and dead	4
5	Injury due to heat, cold and electricity	2	12	Outlook of forensic medicine	1
6	Sudden death	4		Total	36
7	Poisoning	4			

Course Content

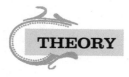

THEORY

Chapter 1　Introduction

1. The concept of forensic medicine, the relationship of forensic medicine and medicine, the responsibilities of forensic medicine, the relationship of doctor and forensic medicine.

2. Routine work of forensic scientist:crime scene investigation, the examination of the living, autopsy, the examination of the physical evidence, the examination of the documentary evidence.

3. Identification:the identification and experts, forensic identification report.

4. A brief history of forensic medicine: Chinese forensic history, foreign forensic history.

Chapter 2　Death and postmortem changes

1. The concept of death, cardiac death, breathing death, brain death and the criteria of brain death.

2. The death process, the concept and diagnosis of suspended animation , forensic death classification.

3. Postmortem changes.

4. Early postmortem changes:muscle flaccidity, rigor mortis, cadaveric spasm, livor

mortis, local desiccation, turbidity of cornea, autolysis.

5. Late postmortem changes:putrefaction, adipocere, mummification, cadaver tanned in peat bog, molded cadaver, maceration.

6. Postmortem injuries:carcasses destroyed by insects and animals, postmortem artifacts.

7. Postmortem interval.

Chapter 3　Mechanical injury

1. The concept and classification of mechanical injury.

2. The formation of mechanical injury:sharp instrument injury, blunt instrument injury and firearm injury.

3. Check and record mechanical injury.

4. The basic forms of mechanical injury:abrasion, bruise, wound, fracture, rupture of viscera, neurogenic shock, concussive injury.

5. Discrimination of antemorterm and postmortem injury.

6. Deduction of the cause of death, the age of mechanical injury, deduction of the inflicted weapon, the manner of death.

Chapter 4　Mechanical asphyxia

1. Concept and classification of asphyxia, postmortem findings in asphyxial deaths.

2. The concept, mechanism and body features of hanging, strangulation, and manual strangulation.

3. Concept, cause, process, body features of drowning death, diatom test, gettler test.

4. Asphyxia of oppression of the chest and abdomen.

5. Sex asphyxia, positional asphyxia, concept and characteristics.

Chaper 5　Injury due to heat, cold and electricity

1. Burn injury and burn death:the general features of burn dead body, the mechanism of burn death, the forensic identification of burn death, the differences of death from burn and cremated body.

2. Cold injury and cold death:the influencing factors of cold death, the process of cold death, the general features of cold dead body and the forensic identification of cold death.

3. Electrical injury:the influencing factors of electrical injury, the mechanism of electrocution, the morphological changes of electrical injury and electrocution, the concept and general features of electrical mark, the forensic identification of electrical death, the morphological changes of lightning death.

Chapter 6　Sudden death

1. The concept of sudden death, the clinical features of sudden death, the causes of sudden death , the incentives of sudden death , the forensic identification of sudden death,

2. The common diseases cause sudden death:diseases of cardiovascular system,

diseases of respiratory system, diseases of central nervous system, diseases of alimentary system, diseases of genitourinary system, diseases of endocrine system.

3. Miscellaneous sudden death:sudden infant death syndrome, sudden adult death syndrome.

Chapter 7　Poisoning

1. The concept of poisoning, the classification of poisons, the effects of poisons, the influencing factors of poisoning.

2. The mechanism and postmortem findings of antidepressant and sedative drugs poisoning, organophosphorus pesticide poisoning, carbon monoxide poisoning, alcohol poisoning, cyanide poisoning, opiates poisoning, rodenticide poisoning, some poisonous animal and plant poisoning, corrosive poisoning.

3. The forensic identification of poisoning:the sources of poison and the toxic and fatal dose, the samples required for toxicological analysis, the tolerance and idiosyncrasy, the doctor's duty in a case of suspected poisoning.

Chapter 8　Rape and infanticide

1. Rape: the concept of rape, the woman sexually mature judgment, virgin judgment, rape identification.

2. Infanticide: the cause of newborn death and their life time, the gestational age of the newborn, viability determination, identification of live births and stillbirths.

Chapter 9　Forensic mental illness

1. Normal and abnormal behavior, types of abnormal mental condition.

2. Mental health legislation and the criminal justice system.

3. Identification of statutory competence:criminal responsibility, competence to stand trial, competence of serving a sentence, ability to defend oneself against sexual abuse, competence of testimony, civil capacity, civil litigation capacity, labour capacity.

4. The effect of drink or drugs on responsibility.

5. Mental injury and mental disability.

Chapter 10　Medical tangle

1. The concept and classification of medical tangle.

2. The concept of medical malpractice and grading.

3. Identification of medical malpractice.

4. Malpractice prevention and treatment.

5. Medical malpractice administrative processing and supervision.

6. Medical malpractice damages and compensation.

7. The reasons and departments of common medical tangle.

Chaper 11　Identification of the living and the dead

1. Individuality of morphological characteristics and fingerprints.

2. Identitication from teeth.

3. Identification of the origin of tissue or samples.

4. The blood-stain patterns, priliminary test, conclusive test, species identification.

5. Identification by DNA profiling.

6. Tattoos and body piercing, identity of decomposed or skeletalized remains, facial reconstruction from skulls.

Chapter 12　Outlook of forensic medicine

1. The research of postmortem interval estimation.

2. The research of competition of causes of death.

3. The research of identification of the living and the dead.

4. The research of qualitative analysis of poisons.

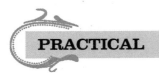

PRACTICAL

1. Preparation postmortem report in a case of death due to violence of any nature.

2. Preparation of a medico-legal report of an injured person due to mechanical violence.

3. Preparation postmortem report in a case of suspected poisoning and to preserve & dispatch viscera for chemical analysis.

4. Identification & drawing medico-legal inference from various specimen of injuries and some diseases.

5. Identification of a particular blood stain and its species origin.

6. Identification ABO & RH blood groups of a person.

MEDICAL GENETICS

医学遗传学

Chief Editors（主编）

Wen Dezhong（温得中） Jilin University（吉林大学）

Tang Hua（汤华） Tianjin Medical University（天津医科大学）

Deputy Chief Editors（副主编）

Yang Jianli（杨剑丽） Jilin University（吉林大学）

Cui Xueling（崔雪玲） Jilin University（吉林大学）

Wen Jianping（温剑平） Jilin University（吉林大学）

Editors（编委）（按姓氏拼音排序）

Cui Xueling（崔雪玲） Jilin University（吉林大学）

Peng Luying（彭鲁英） Tongji University（同济大学）

Song Chaoxia（宋朝霞） Jilin University（吉林大学）

Tang Hua（汤华） Tianjin Medical University（天津医科大学）

Wen Dezhong（温得中） Jilin University（吉林大学）

Wen Jianping（温剑平） Jilin University（吉林大学）

Yang Jianli（杨剑丽） Jilin University（吉林大学）

Zhao Jia（赵佳） Jilin University（吉林大学）

Course Description

Medical genetics is a rapidly advancing field of medicine. It is a course which is designed to provide an overview the phenotype, the pathology, and the genetic discipline of genetic diseases with the theory and the method of human genetics. To meet the need of medical genetics teaching for international medical students, we wrote the syllabus to guilde teaching and learning in Medical Genetics.

Schedule Table

Chapter	Contents	Hours	Chapter	Contents	Hours
1	Medical genetics introduction	2	7	Genetics of Cancer	4
2	Chromosomal basis heredity	2	8	Clinical cytogenetic	4
3	Patterns of single-gene inheritance	6	9	Genetic Variation in Individuals and Populations	4
4	Principle of clinical cytogenetic	4	10	The treatment of genetic disease	2
5	Multiple-factor inheritance	2	11	Genetic counseling and risk assessment	6
6	Epigenetic	4		Total	40
practical 1	preparation of chromosomes	8	practical 4	The sex determination test	4
practical 2	micronucleus test	4		Total	20
practical 3	sperm abnormal test	4			

Course Contents

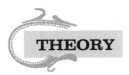

THEORY

Chapter 1   Introduction

Purpose and requirement:

In this chapter students should understand fundamental and terminology of medical genetics; know the harm of genetics diseases and its status, comprehend the researching category and characteristics.

Contents:

1. Medical genetics deals with the subset of human genetic variation that is of significance in the practice of medicine and in medical research.

2. Classification of genetic disorders:

(1) Single-gene disorders.

(2) Chromosome disorders.

(3) Multifactorial disorders.

3. Within human and medical genetics, there are many fields of interest: cytogenetic diseases involving chromosomal abnormalities; molecular and biochemical genetics involving the structure and function of individual genes; population genetics involving genetic variation in human populations and the factors that determine allele frequencies; clinical genetics involving the application of genetics to diagnosis and patient care; and Genetic counseling which combines the provosion of risk information while providing

psychological and educational support.

Chapter 2   chromosomal basis heredity

Purpose and requirement:

In this chapter students should understand fundamental and terminology of chromosomal and mast the mitosis and meiosis.

Contents:

1. Structure of human chromosomes: DNA double helix; Nucleosome; 30-nm-diameter fiber; loop of chromatin.

2. Mitosis: The process of mitosis is continuous, but five stages are distinguished: prophase, prometaphase, metaphase, anaphase, and telophase.

3. Meiosis: Meiosis is the type of cell division by which the diploid cell of the germ line gives rise to haploid gametes. Meiosis consists of one round of DNA synthesis followed by rounds of chromosome segregation and cell division. The two successive meiotic divisions are called meiosis I and meiosis II. Meiosis I is also known as the reduction division because it is the division in which the chromosome number is reduced from diploid to haploid by the pairing of homologs in prophase and by their segregation to different cells at anaphase of meiosis I. Meiosis II follows meiosis I without an intervening step of DNA replication. As in ordinary mitosis, the chromatids separate, and one chromatid of each chromosome passes to each daughter cell.

Chapter 3   Patterns of single-gene inheritance

Purpose and requirement:

In this chapter students should understand the typical patterns of transmission of single-gene disorders are discussed and mast heterogeneity, penetrance, expressivity, pleiotropy, and germline mosaicism.

Contents:

1. Allelic heterogeneity is an important cause of clinical variation. Many loci possess more than one mutant allele; in fact, at a given locus there may be several or many mutations. Sometimes, these different mutations result in clinically indistinguishable or closely similar disorders. But the inheritants of these mutants may be different. It is may be AD or AR. For example, sickle cell disease, the mutants of β-globin may be AD or AR.

2. For many phenotypes, pedigree analysis alone has been sufficient to demonstrate genetic heterogeneity. For example, congenital deafness, has long been known to occur in autosomal dominant, autosomal recessive, and X-linked forms. In recent years, pedigree analysis combined with gene mapping has demonstrated that there are at least two dozen loci responsible for 4 X-linked forms, 41 autosomal dominant forms, and 6 autosomal recessive forms.

3. The measurement of consanguinity is relevant in medical genetics because the risk of a child's being homozygous for a rare recessive allele is proportional to how related the parents are. The coefficient of inbreeding (F) is the probability that a homozygote has received both alleles at a locus from the same ancestral source; it is also the proportion of loci at which a person is homozygous or identical by descent.

4. Penetrance is the probability that a gene will have any phenotypic expression at all.

5. Expressivity is the severity of expression of the phenotype.

6. When a single abnormal gene or gene pair produces diverse phenotypic effects, such as which organ systems are involved and which particular signs and symptoms occur, its expression is said to be pleiotropic.

7. Mosaicism is defined as the presence in an individual or a tissue of at least two cell lines that differ genetically but are derived from a single zygote. A mutation occurring during cell proliferation, in either somatic cells or during gametogenesis, leads to aproportion of cells carrying the mutation. That is, to either somatic or germline mosaicism.

8. Maternal inheritance: a disease in a family that is only transmitted through the females. Those present in sperm are concentrated in the tail and do not contribute to the compliment of the fertilized zygote. Another unique feature of mtDNA diseases arises from the fact that a typical human cell including the egg cell contains only one nucleus, but hundreds of mitochondria. The upshot is that a single cell can contain both mutant mitochondria and normal mitochondria, and the balance between the two will determine the cell's health. The consequences of mitochondrial mutations, however, may be very different from those that occur in nuclear DNA.

Chapter 4　Principle of clinical cytogenetics

Purpose and requirement:

In this chapter students should understand the general principles of clinical cytogenetics and the various types of numerical and structral abnormalities observed in human karyotypes.

Contents:

1. Abnormalities of Chromosome Number: euploidy (Polyploidy) is the category of chromosome changes which involve the addition or loss of complete sets of chromosomes. Aneuploidy is the category of chromosome changes which do not involve whole sets. It is usually the consequence of a failure of a single chromosome (or bivalent) to complete division.

2. Structural aberrations: structural rearrangements are defined as balanced, if the chromosome set has the normal complement of chromosomal material, or unbalanced, if there is additional or missing material. Some rearrangements are stable, capable of passing through mitotic and meiotic cell dilisions unaltered, whereas others are unstable. To be stable, a rearranged chromosome must have normal structural elements, including a functional centromere and two telomeres.

3. Translocation: translocation involves the exchange of chromosome segments between two, usually nonhomologous, chromosomes. There are two main types: reciprocal and Robertsonian.

4. When the chromosomes of a carrier of a balanced reprocal translocation pair at meiosis, a quadrivalent (cross-shaped) figure is formed. At anaphase, the chromosomes usually segregate from this configuration in one of three ways, described as alternate, adjacent-1, and adjacent-2 segregation. Alternate segregation, the usual type of meiotic

segregation, produces gametes that have either a normal chromosome complement or the two reciprocal chromosomes; both types of gamete are balanced. In adjacent-1 segregation, homologous centromeres go to separate daughter cells, whereas in adjacent-2 segregation (which is rare), homologous centromeres pass to the same daughter cell. Both adjacent-l and adjacent-2 segregation yield unbalanced gametes.

Chapter 5　Chromosome disease

Purpose and requirement:

In this chapter, Students should be able to assay "karyotype" and describe the medical aspects of chromosome abnormalities, especially some specific syndromes, such as Down Syndrome, Fragile X Syndrome, Klinefelter Syndrome and Cri du Chat syndrome.

Contents:

1. Down syndrome (also named trisomy 21).

Karyotype: 46, XX(XY), +21

Clinical Feature: mental retardation, a flat face, sparse, an abnormal pattern of palm creases, straight hair, and short stature.

2. Cri du Chat syndrome.

also named $5P^-$ syndrome.

Clinical Feature: Low birth weight, abnormal larynx development, adults have small heads, round face, small chin; widely set eyes, poor muscle tone: difficulty walking and talking correctly, hyperactivity; aggression, tantrums and severe mental retardation.

3. Klinefelter Syndrome.

Karyotype:47, XXY.

Clinical Feature: reduced sexual maturity and secondary sexual characteristics, breast swelling, no sperm, slow to learn.

4. Fragile X Syndrome.

Clinical Feature: large ears, long face, and prominent jaw large testes and the learning difficulties.

Chapter 6　Multiple–factor inheritance

Purpose and requirements.

The chapter goals are to comprehend the multiple-factor hypothesis, give priority to the concepts about minor gene, additive effect, quantitative traits, quality traits, threshold, heritability, complex diseases and grasp the method of estimating heritability and recurrence risk of polygenetic diseases.

Contents:

1. Quantitative traits.

The characteristics of quantitative traits, the genetic basis of quantitative traits, the significance of polygenic inheritance.

2. The statistical analyses on quantitative traits.

Mean, variance, standard deviation, normal distribution.

3. Heritability.

Estimating the heritability from Twin studies.

4. Characteristics of inheritance of complex diseases.

Recurrence risk assessment of complex diseases.

Chapter 7　Epigenetics

Purpose and requirements.

The chapter goals are to comprehend epigenetic phenomena. The students are required to study epigenetic in hierarchies: In protein level, to comprehend histone modification and histone remodeler organization; In DNA level, to grasp DNA methylation; In RNA level, to study the main functions of non-coding RNAs in epigenetic field.

Contents:

1. Epigenetic phenomena.

Homozygous twins share a common genotype and are genetically identical but show significant phenotypic discordances.

Epigenetic: all heritable changes in gene expression and chromatin organization that are independent of the DNA sequence itself.

Significance: A supplementary of Genetics and admit acquired factors in individual development.

2. Histone modifications.

Mechanisms exist to "open up" or "condense" chromatin. The types of Histone modification. Give priority to Histones acetylating.

3. Histone remodeler.

Four families: SWI/SNF, ISWI, CHD, INO80; Rebuild or remove histones from DNA. ATP needed.

4. DNA methylation.

The function of DNMT1 (Methylate original site during DNA replication), DNMT2 (Unclear) and DNMT3 (Methylate new site).

CG Island: CpG cluster exists in upstream 5′of structural gene and methylation of CpG regulates gene expression.

5. Non-coding RNAs.

RNA which is not used for making proteins (non-coding RNA) can be cleaved and used to inhibit protein-coding RNA, such as miRNA, siRNA.

Chapter 8　Genetics of Cancer

Purpose and requirements.

The chapter goals are to comprehend the monoclonal origin hypothesis of tumor, multistep oncogenesis theory and two hit theory. The function of oncogene and tumor suppressor gene should be grasped well, and also the some basic concepts like proto-oncogene, cellular oncogene, virus oncogene.

Contents:

1. The evidences of monoclonal origin hypothesis, such as X chromosome evidence

and same mutation of genes which are involve in cancer.

2. Oncogenes.

Proto-oncogenes: to promote cell division, if mutate are activated improperly.

Oncogenes: proto-oncogenes mutate into oncogenes, which are activated improperly.

Virus oncogenes: discovery process of virus oncogenes and relationship between virus oncogenes and cell-oncogenes.

Cell-oncogenes: key genes are responsible for cell proliferation. Its expression and activity is controlled by cell accurately.

Cell-oncogenes in signal pathway: to introduce the cell proliferation signal pathway, in which cell-oncogenes take functions.

The pattern of proto-oncogenes mutate into cell-oncogenes, such as point mutations, amplification, viruses insertion, etc.

Tumor suppressive gene: Negative regulation during cell division. The functions and mutations of RB gene and P53 gene.

Introduce the Two hits theory and multistep oncogenesis theory.

Chapter 9   Genetic Variation in Individuals and Populations: Mutation and Polymorphism

Purpose and requirement.

Students must make sure the sorts of mutation which is the nature of genetically determined differences among individuals. And the Hardy -Weinberg equilibrium law also should be understood that the applications of the Law are in the estimation of gene frequency, genotype frequency, relative mating harmful effect and genetic hypothesis test.

Contents:

introduction: Understand the nature of genetically determined differences among individuals.

Mutation: is defined as any change in the nucleotide sequence or arrangement of DNA. Mutations can be classified into three categories.

1. Genome mutations: mutations that affect the number of chromosomes in the cell.

2. Chromosome mutations: mutations that alter the structure of individual chromosomes.

3. Gene mutations: mutations that alter individual genes.

Types of mutations and their consequences.

Nucleotide substitutions include missense mutations, chain termination mutation, RNA processing mutations, deletions and insertions, effects of recombination and dynamic mutations.

The Hardy-Weinberg Law.

If a population meets certain assumptions, however, there is a simple mathematical relationship known as the Hardy-Weinberg law for calculating genotype frequencies from allele frequencies.

know the assumptions of the Law.

Know the disturb Hardy-Weinberg Equilibrium.

Chapter 10   The treatment of genetic disease

Purpose and requirement:

In this chapter students should understand the purpose of the treatment of genetic disease is to eliminate or ameliorate the effects of the disorder, not only on the patient but also on his or her family.

Contents:

1. The current state of treatment of genetic disease.

1) Genetically complex diseases.

2) Single-Gene Diseases.

2. Special considerations in treating genetic disease, Long-term assessment of treatment is critical.

In genetic disease, perhaps more than in other areas of medicine, treatment initially judged as successful may eventually be shown to be imperfect.

3. Genetic heterogeneity and treatment.

The optimal treatment of single-gene defects requires an unusual degree of diagnostic precision; often one must determine not only the specific locus involved but also the particular class of allele at the locus.

4. Treatment strategies.

Genetic disease can be treated at many levels, at various steps away from the mutant gene.

(1) Therapy directed at the clinical phenotype.

(2) Treatment of metabolic abnormalities.

(3) Dietary restriction.

(4) Replacement.

(5) Diversion.

(6) Inhibition.

(7) Depletion.

5. The molecular treatment of disease.

(1) Treatment at the level of the protein.

(2) Enhancement of mutant protein function with small molecule therapy.

(3) Protein augmentation.

(4) Enzyme replacement therapy: extracellular augmentation of an intracellular enzyme.

(5) Enzyme replacement therapy: targeted augmentation of an intracellular enzyme.

(6) Increasing gene expression from the wild-type or mutant locus.

(7) Increasing gene expression from a locus not affected by the disease.

(8) Reducing the expression of a dominant mutant gene product: RNA interference.

(9) Modification of the somatic genome by transplantation.

(10) Stem cell transplantation.

(11) Nuclear transplantation.

Chapter 11　Genetic counseling and risk assessment

Purpose and requirement:

In this chapter students should understand genetic counseling is the process by which the patients or relatives at risk of an inherited disorder are advised of the consequences and nature of the disorder, the probability of developing or transmitting it, and the options open to them in management and family planning. This complex process can be separated into diagnostic (the actual estimation of risk) and supportive aspects.

Contents:

1. Genetic counselors.

A genetic counselor is an expert with a Master of Science degree in genetic counseling. In the United States, they are certified by the American Board of Genetic Counseling. In Canada, genetic counselors are certified by the Canadian Association of Genetic Counsellors. In China, genetic counseling is steered by the Chinese Board of Genetic Counseling (CBGC). Most enter the field from a variety of disciplines, including biology, genetics, nursing, psychology, public health and social work. Genetic counselors should be expert educators, skilled in translating the complex language of genomic medicine into terms that are easy to understand.

2. Patients.

Any person may seek out genetic counseling for a condition they may have inherited from their biological parents.

3. Families or individuals may choose to attend counseling or undergo prenatal testing for a number of reasons.

(1) Family history of a genetic condition or chromosome abnormality.

(2) Molecular test for single gene disorder.

(3) Increased maternal age (35 years and older).

(4) Increased paternal age (40 years and older).

(5) Abnormal maternal serum screening results or ultrasound findings.

(6) Increased nuchal translucency measurements on ultrasound.

(7) Strong family history of cancer.

(8) Predictive testing for adult-onset conditions.

4. Determining recurrence risks.

The estimation of recurrence risk is a central concern in genetic counseling.

(1) When a disorder is known to have single-gene inheritance, the recurrence risk for specific family members can usually be determined from basic Mendelian principles.

(2) Risk estimation by use of conditional probability when alternative genotypes are possible.

Course Description

Medical genetics, also known as human genetics, is the application of genetic knowledge in the medical field. Medical genetics through the study of the relationship between the occurrence and development of human diseases and genetic factors provide diagnosis, prevention and treatment for genetic disease contributing to the improvement of human health.

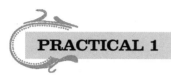

PRACTICAL 1

In vitro culture of human peripheral blood lymphocytes and preparation of chromosome samples.

Purpose and requirement:

1. Master in vitro culture of human peripheral blood lymphocytes and preparation of chromosome samples.

2. Master the methods of human chromosome observation.

Contents:

1. In vitro culture of human peripheral blood lymphocytes.

2. Preparation of chromosome samples.

3. Under a microscope , select finely disseminated , length of chromosome moderate Metaphase mitotic phase to observe; Count the number of chromosomes; According to the morphology of chromosomes and position of the kinetochore, differencing between male and female karyotype.

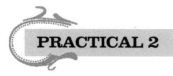

PRACTICAL 2

Polychromatic erythrocyte of mouse bone marrow micronucleus test.

Purpose and requirement:

1. Master the preparation method of polychromatic erythrocyte suspension.

2. Master the distinction mechanism of erythrocytes of eosinophils.

3. Master the method of micronucleus and eosinophils count calculation of micronucleus rate.

Contents:

1. The principle of polychromatic erythrocyte of mouse bone marrow micronucleus test.

2. The reagents and materials used in this experiment are introduced.

3. Introduce the process of filling and production of experimental operation steps.

4. Instruct students to complete the experiment operation.

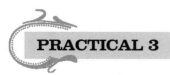

PRACTICAL 3

Sperm abnormalities in mice by chemical induction.

Purpose and requirement:

1. Master the preparation method of sperm abnormal test.

2. Master the morphology of normal sperm.

3. Master the morphology of abnormal sperm.

Contents:

1. The principle of Sperm abnormal test.

2. The reagents and materials used in this experiment are introduced.

3. Introduce the process of filling and production of experimental operation steps.

4. Guidance students to complete the experiment operation.

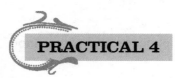

PRACTICAL 4

The sex determination test.

Purpose and requirement:

1. Master the principle of the sex determination test.

2. Master the preparation method of the sex determination test.

Contents:

1. The principle of the sex determination test.

2. The reagents and materials used in this experiment are introduced.

3. Introduce the process of filling and production of experimental operation steps.

4. Guidance students to complete the experiment operation.

CLINICAL PHARMACOLOGY
临床药理学

Chief Editor（主编）
Wei Wei（魏伟） Anhui Medical University（安徽医科大学）

Deputy Chief Editors（副主编）
Huang Min（黄民） Sun Yat-Sen University（中山大学）
Liu Zhaoqian（刘昭前） Central South University（中南大学）
Cui Yimin（崔一民） Peking University（北京大学）

Editors（编委）（按姓氏拼音排序）
Bi Huichang（毕惠嫦） Sun Yat-Sen University（中山大学）
Cui Yimin（崔一民） Peking University（北京大学）
Huang Min（黄民） Sun Yat-Sen University（中山大学）
Jiang Bo（江波） Zhejiang University（浙江大学）
Liu Zhaoqian（刘昭前） Central South University（中南大学）
Sun Wuyi（孙妩弋） Anhui Medical University（安徽医科大学）
Wei Wei（魏伟） Anhui Medical University（安徽医科大学）
Zhang Jing（张菁） Fudan University（复旦大学）
Zhang Lingling（张玲玲） Anhui Medical University（安徽医科大学）

Course Description

Clinical Pharmacology is the scientific discipline that involves all aspects of the relationship between drugs and humans. It is a multidisciplinary science that encompasses professionals with a wide variety of scientific skills including medicine, pharmacology, pharmacy, biomedical science and nursing. It is underpinned by the basic science of pharmacology, with added focus on the application of pharmacological principles and methods in the real world. It has a broad scope, from the discovery of new target molecules, to the effects of drug usage in whole populations.

Clinical pharmacology connects the gap between medical practice and laboratory science. The main objective is to promote the safety of prescription, maximise the drug effects and minimise the side effects. The course will focus on drug information, drug development, using PK-PD to determine optimal drug therapy, clinical drug effect assessment and other aspects of pharmacy practice related to clinical pharmacology.

Objectives

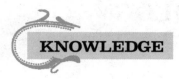

KNOWLEDGE

Upon completion of the course, students should be able to:

1. Use patient data and PK-PD principles to determine appropriate drug therapy and dosing.

2. Recognize and appropriately manage pharmacokinetic variability in patients with significant pharmacokinetic alterations in special populations.

3. Recognize and appropriately manage clinical pharmacogenetics, significant pharmacokinetic drug interactions and drug toxicology.

4. Perform therapeutic drug monitoring (TDM) in patients receiving drugs for which concentrations are measured in practice, and recognize physiological and laboratory markers of drug effect.

5. Recognize the preclinical development of new drugs and perform clinical trial of new drugs.

Teaching and Learning Methods

Theory: The lectures are conducted using a case-based format which promotes an active-learning environment. Other teaching styles such as didactic lectures, question-answer sessions and class discussions are used as appropriate.

Recommended Textbooks

魏伟. 2008. 临床药理学原理［M］. 2 版. 北京：科学出版社.

李俊. 2018. 临床药理学［M］. 6 版. 北京：人民卫生出版社.

Arthur J Atkinson Jr, Shiew-Mei Huang, Juan J L Lertora, et al. 2012. Principle of Clinical Pharmacology [M]. 3rd ed. New York: Academic Press.

Bertram G Katzung, Anthony J Trevor. 2014. Basic and Clinical Pharmacology [M]. 13th ed. New York: McGraw-Hill Education / Medical.

Peter N Bennett, Morris J Brown, Pankaj Sharma. 2012. Clinical Pharmacology [M]. 11th ed. New York: Churchill Livingstone.

Schedule Table

Chapter	Contents	Hours	Chapter	Contents	Hours
1	Introduction to Clinical Pharmacology	1	10	Clinical Treatment of Digestive Diseases	0.5
2	Drug Clinical Research	1	11	Drug Use in Pregnancy and Lactation Women	1
3	Drug Registration and Administration	1	12	Drugs Use in Neonates and Kids	1
4	Clinical Pharmacokinetics	1	13	Drugs Use in Elderly Patients	1
5	Therapeutic Drug Monitoring and Individualization of Drug Therapy	1	14	Clinical Analysis of Adverse Drug Reactions	2
6	Clinical Pharmacodynamics	1	15	Drug Abuse and Drug Dependence	1
7	Clinical Medication of Nervous System Diseases	1	16	Clinical Application of Antibacterial Drugs	1
8	Clinical Medication of Cardiovascular Diseases	1	17	Clinical Application of Antiviral Drugs	1
9	Clinical Medication of Endocrine and Metabolic Diseases	0.5	18	Clinical Application of Anti-malignant Tumor Drugs	1

Course Contents

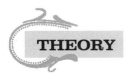

THEORY

Chapter 1　Introduction to Clinical Pharmacology

1. Concept of clinical pharmacology.
2. Important history events of modern pharmacology.
3. Development of clinical pharmacology.
4. The relationship between health, disease and drug.
5. General concept of clinical pharmacokinetics and clinical pharmacodynamics.
6. Hot spots in research of clinical pharmacology.

Chapter 2　Drug Clinical Research

1. Concept of new drugs.
2. Main contents of Good Clinical Practice (GCP).
3. Main contents and methods of phase I clinical trials.
4. Main contents and significance of phase II, III, IV clinical trials.
5. To determinate the minimum initial dose, the maximum tolerance dose of the tolerance test.
6. Bioequivalence tests and design of new drugs.

Chapter 3   Drug Registration and Administration

1. Concept of drugs, national essential drugs and over-the-counter medicines.
2. Registration classification, application and administration of drugs.
3. Selection principles of national essential drugs and over-the-counter medicines.
4. Management of drug classification.

Chapter 4   Clinical Pharmacokinetics

1. ADME factors.
2. Review of basic pharmacokinetic parameters.
3. Mathematical basis of clinical pharmacokinetics.
4. Dosing in liver disease and other disease states.
5. Applications of clinical pharmacokinetics.

Chapter 5   Therapeutic Drug Monitoring and Individualization of Drug Therapy

1. The history of therapeutic drug monitoring (TDM).
2. Concept of TDM.
3. The application of TDM.
4. TDM methods.
5. The methods of individualizing dosage therapy.
6. Population pharmacokinetics and PK/PD models.
7. Pharmacogenetics and individualized treatment.

Chapter 6   Clinical Pharmacodynamics

1. Drug selective effects, adverse reactions.
2. Dose-effect curve, time response curve and pharmacodynamic parameters.
3. Concept of receptor, agonist, antagonist, partial agonist, receptor regulations, synergistic and antagonistic effects.
4. Concept of biomarkers.
5. Influencing factors of drug actions.

Chapter 7   Clinical Medication of Nervous System Diseases

1. Clinical medication in cerebrovascular disease.
2. Clinical medication and pathogenesis of paralysis agitans.
3. General principles of treatment of epilepsy.
4. The mechanism of action of antiepileptic drug and clinical medication.
5. Clinical treatment of senile dementia.

Chapter 8   Clinical Medication of Cardiovascular Diseases

1. The clinical medication of hypertension.
2. The clinical medication of angina pectoris.
3. The clinical medication of arrhythmia.
4. The clinical medication of heart failure.
5. The clinical medication of atherosclerosis.

Chapter 9   Clinical Medication of Endocrine and Metabolic Diseases

1. Indications and adverse reactions of insulin.

2. The role, action mechanism and application characteristics of oral hypoglycemic agents.

3. The main pharmacological effects and clinical medication of thyroid hormones.

4. The action mechanism, application characteristics and major adverse reactions of anti-hyperthyroid drugs.

5. The causes of osteoporosis and the clinical medication.

Chapter 10   Clinical Treatment of Digestive Diseases

1. Classification, role, application and the main adverse reactions of therapeutic drugs for ulcer.

2. Gastrointestinal motility drugs, antidiarrheal drugs, laxative drugs.

3. Drugs for treating inflammatory bowel diseases.

4. Drugs for intestinal diseases.

5. Treatment principles of drug for liver disease.

6. Drugs for protecting liver.

7. Drugs for preventing and treating hepatic encephalopathy.

Chapter 11   Drug Use in Pregnancy and Lactation Women

1. The effect of drugs on pregnant women.

(1) Pharmacokinetics characteristics during pregnancy: absorption, distribution, metabolism and excretion.

(2) The principles of drugs use in pregnancy, and things to notice when using drugs.

2. The effect of drugs on fetal.

(1) Transport and metabolism of drugs in placenta.

(2) Pharmacokinetic characteristics in fetal: absorption, distribution, metabolism and excretion.

(3) Drugs damage to the fetus: teratogenic effects of drugs (A, B, C, D, X).

3. Drugs use in lactation women.

(1) Transport of drugs in breast milk and the influencing factors.

(2) The influence of drugs on lactation women and the influence of drugs on nursing infant.

Chapter 12   Drugs Use in Neonates and Kids

1. The characteristic of the pharmacokinetics and pharmacodynamics in neonates; the rational drug use in treating common diseases of neonates.

2. The principle and attention of rational drug use in neonates, infants and children.

Chapter 13   Drugs Use in Elderly Patients

1. The characteristic of the pharmacokinetics in elderly patients; the characteristic of the pharmacodynamics in elderly patients.

2. The principles of rational drugs selection and application in elderly patients.

Chapter 14　Clinical Analysis of Adverse Drug Reactions

1. Concept of adverse drug reaction (ADR).
2. Classification of ADR.
3. Concept of drug-drug interaction (DDI).
4. Mechanisms of DDI.
5. Prediction and clinical management of DDI.
6. ADR detection in clinical.

Chapter 15　Drug Abuse and Drug Dependence

1. Concept of drug abuse, drug dependence, drug tolerance and drug addiction.
2. Clinical manifestations of different types of drug dependence.
(1) Psychological dependence.
(2) Physical dependence.
(3) Cross-dependence.
3. Classification and characteristics of the dependent drug:
(1) Classification of the dependent drug.
(2) Characteristics of the dependent drug.
4. Harm, control and prevention of drug abuse.

Chapter 16　Clinical Application of Antibacterial Drugs

1. The status quo of clinical application for antimicrobial drugs.
2. The relationship between pharmacodynamics, pharmacokinetics and the curative effect, adverse reactions.
3. The basic principles of antibacterial drugs in clinical application.
4. Therapeutic drug monitoring of antimicrobial drugs.
5. The allergic reactions of antibacterial drugs.
6. The clinical application of antibacterial drugs.

Chapter 17　Clinical Application of Antiviral Drugs

1. The classification and clinical significance of antiviral drugs.
2. The clinical application of antiviral drugs.
3. Rational clinical application for the treatment of viral hepatitis.
4. Classification and clinical application of anti-HIV drugs.

Chapter 18　Clinical Application of Anti-malignant Tumor Drugs

1. Relationship between cell proliferation kinetics and tumor chemotherapy.
2. The classification and characteristics of anti-malignant tumor drugs.
3. The clinical application of anti-malignant tumor drugs.
4. The role, development and prospect of biological therapy in the treatment of malignant tumor.
5. The principle of combination therapy.

INSTRUCTION OF MEDICINE
医 学 导 论

Chief Editors（主编）
 Tang Hua（汤华） Tianjin Medical University（天津医科大学）
 Yuan Zhenghong（袁正宏） Fudan University（复旦大学）
 Chen Liyu（陈利玉） Central South University（中南大学）

Deputy Chief Editors（副主编）
 Wang Yun（王韵） Peking University（北京大学）
 Li Mingyuan（李明远） Sichuan University（四川大学）
 Li Guoxia（李国霞） Tianjin Medical University（天津医科大学）
 Zhang Guangling（章广玲） North China University of Science and Technology
  （华北理工大学）
 Zhong Zhaohua（钟照华） Harbin Medical University（哈尔滨医科大学）

Editors（编委）（按姓氏拼音排序）
 Bao Fukai（宝福凯） Kunming Medical University（昆明医科大学）
 Chen Liyu（陈利玉） Central South University（中南大学）
 Fu Li（傅力） Tianjin Medical University（天津医科大学）
 Guo Xiaokui（郭晓奎） Shanghai Jiaotong University（上海交通大学）
 Li Guoxia（李国霞） Tianjin Medical University（天津医科大学）
 Li Mingyuan（李明远） Sichuan University（四川大学）
 Peng Yihong（彭宜红） Peking University（北京大学）
 Tang Hua（汤华） Tianjin Medical University（天津医科大学）
 Wang Yun（王韵） Peking University（北京大学）
 Yuan Zhenghong（袁正宏） Fudan University（复旦大学）
 Zhang Guangling（章广玲） North China University of Science and Technology
  （华北理工大学）
 Zhong Zhaohua（钟照华） Harbin Medical University（哈尔滨医科大学）
 Zhu Fan（朱帆） Wuhan University（武汉大学）

Course Description

 Introduction of Medicine is a comprehensive medical subject which briefly describes
the origin and the development of medicine from the B. C. dates to the present, and it is

an interdisciplinary program which breaks the boundary of basic courses and clinical course, and it has its own development, content and research methods. *Introduction of Medicine* is organized chronologically, according to the dates that are associated with a discovery or breakthrough. The most important task of *Introduction of Medicine* is to provides a wide audience with a brief guide to important medical milestones, ideas, and thinkers, and explores the general rule of medical science development by insight into the relationship among natural science, society, culture, politics, economy and philosophy. *Introduction of Medicine* includes four parts: the origin and development of medicine, medical education and medical study, doctors and patients and health service system. The origin and development of medicine mainly introduces the basic concept of medicine, the history of Chinese and Western medicine development. Medical education and medical study mainly introduces medical education, health work policy, mission and medical personnel training. Doctors and patients mainly introduces the clinical work of the staff, object, medical interpersonal relationship and communication, clinical diagnosis and treatment concepts. Health service system explains the prevention and care, and legal issues in health care.

The purposes for *Introduction of Medicine* learning are to let students contact the clinic, the hospital, patient, clinical practice early, improve the students'interest in clinical medicine and the perceptual knowledge of medicine, and to let students establish a thinking of patient oriented, patient centered, whole heartedly serving the patient. It will help students project a positive professional attitude and promote the role of conversion from a medical student to a real doctor.

Objectives

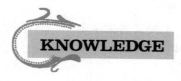

KNOWLEDGE

At the end of the course, the MBBS students shall be able to:

1. To master the basic concept and current situation and the connotation of medicine, and the students know how to study medicine.

2. To master the role of the doctor and the patient, and students know how to be a good doctor.

3. To understand the general hospital, students establish perceptions of hospital and clinic.

4. To master the symptoms, diagnosis and treatment, rehabilitation and prevention knowledge of human illness.

5. To master the communication skills with the patients.

6. To master the definition and ingredients of the health service system. To understand the models and development of the health system in some countries.

Teaching and Learning Methods

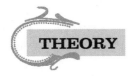

THEORY

1. Classroom lectures.

(1) Teachers apply various teaching methods such as heuristics teaching, contrasting teaching to facilitate students to learn *The Intruduction Of Medicine*.

(2) Students'self-directed learning is needed in the individual chapters. Teachers will first provide the emphasis of the chapters and key questions. Students could focus on them and give their answers. The answers should be handed in and evaluated.

(3) Multi-media teaching methods.

2. Seminars will be held. Students with small groups search for the related information regarding the topic, write review articles or book reports, and give their presentation in the seminar.

3. Students are encouraged to take part in the research group of teachers to have their early experience in medical research.

4. Students will investigate or visit the health care services system.

Recommended Textbooks

Charles Green Cumston. 1988. An Introduction to the History of Medicine: From the Time of the Pharaohs To the End of the XVIIIth Century [M]. New York: Dorset Press.

Clifford A Pickover.2013. The Medical Book: from Which Doctors to Robot Surgeons:250 Milestones in the History of Medicine [M]. New York: Sterling Milestones.

Roy Porter. 1997. The Greatest Benefit to Mankind: A Medical History to Humanity [M]. New York/London: W W Norton.

William Bynum. 2008. The History of Medicine: A Very Short Introduction [M]. New York: Oxford University Press.

Schedule Table

Chapter	Contents	Hours	Chapter	Contents	Hours
1	Introduction	2	5	Seminar: Prepare a presentation about the development of Medicine	4
2	The origin and development of medicine-Ancient Medicine	2	6	The intersection and conflict between Chinese and Western Medicine	2
3	Medicine in medieval times and renaissance period	2	7	Development of Modern Medicine	4
4	17th, 18th and 19th Century Medicine	4	8	Modern Medicine - Holistic Integrative Medicine	2

Continued

Chapter	Contents	Hours	Chapter	Contents	Hours
9	Modern Medicine - Personalized Medicine and Precision Medicine	2	12	Health service system	2
10	Modern medical education and medical study	4	13	Seminar: Prepare presentations about the relationship of Doctors and patients or health service system in different country	4
11	Doctors and patients	2		Total	36

Course Content

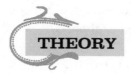

THEORY

Chapter 1　Introduction

1. Medicine.

(1) The definition and characteristics of medicine: Medicine is of art, sciences-based medicine and humanistic medicine.

(2) The major research fields, contents, classification and scope of medicine.

2. History and development of medicine: purpose and chronology.

3. Introduction of medicine includes four parts: the origin and development of medicine; medical education and medical study; doctors and patients; health service system.

Chapter 2　The origin and development of medicine –Ancient medicine

1. The origin of medicine: archaeological evidences, historical records.

2. Ancient oriental medicine.

(1) Ancient Egyptian medicine: Characteristics, papyrus, mummification and the medical significance, medical education in the ancient Egypt.

(2) Ancient Babylon and Assyrian medicine: Astrology.

(3) Ancient Indian medicine.

(4) Ancient Chinese medicine.

3. Ancient western medicine.

(1) Ancient Greece medicine:

1) Famous philosophers and their medical thinking: Empedocles, Hippocrates, Aristotle, Socrates, Plato, etc.

2) The main contents of "Hippocratic Collection" and significance.

(2) Medicine in the Alexandrian period (Hellenistic Medicine): Greek medicine flourishes in Alexandria with Herophilus and Erasistratus.

(3) Ancient Roman medicine:

1) Characteristics: Succeeding and developing the achievements of ancient Greece

medicine; Roman sanitation; the military settlements where had hospitals, establishment and development of hospital system.

2) Famous medical scientist: Claudius Galen and his medical achievements.

4. The characteristics of ancient medicine.

Chapter 3　Medicine in medieval times and renaissance period

1. Medieval medicine: were the period in between the Roman Empire (often said to have ended in AD476) and the Renaissance (often dated form 1453).

(1) The different ages: the Dark ages (476-l066), the High Middle Ages (1066-1453).

(2) The main factors which contribute to the slow development in medicine and science in the middle ages (Dark ages): the decline and fall of the Roman Empire, the influence of religion and scholasticism, pandemic of the infectious diseases, occupation of medicine by Greece and Roman aristocrat.

(3) Characteristics of Byzantine medicine.

(4) Arabian medicine: stages of development, the achievements at the zenith of Arabian medicine, famous physicians (Rhazes, Avicenna).

(5) The origin and development of medical schools as well as the medical education.

1) Rise of the earliest collegiate school: Collegiate school of Salernum and its significance.

2) Two universities which have a special interest at this period in connection with the development of medical studies and their characteristics of medical education: Bologna in Italy, and Montpellier in Southern France.

(6) Foundation of hospitals and pandemic of infectious diseases: origins of hospitals, leprosy and pesthouse, plague (Black Death Disease) and seaport quarantine.

2. Medicine in renaissance : often dated form 1453.

(1) Social and cultural background: the development of industrial and commercial capitalism, formation of handcraft workshop, spread of four great inventions of ancient China (gunpowder, paper, compass, and printing) in Europe, collapse of eastern Roman Empire, migration of Greek culture heritage to the west, abundance of knowledge about geography, emergence of humanism, advancement of astronomy.

(2) Revolution of medicine: emphasis of scientific practice.

(3) Establishment of human anatomy: Mondino de Luzzi, Leonardo da Vinci, Vesaliu A.

(4) Reforms of surgery: the achievements of Pare A.

(5) Advancements in medicine and new opinions about infectious diseases.

3. Characteristics of medical development in middle ages and the Renaissance.

Chapter 4　17th, 18th and 19th century medicine

1. The 17th century medicine.

(1) The natural science background of medical development and the representative figures: Bruno G., Dilderp V., Galileo Galilei, Kepler, Pietro da Cortona, et al.

(2) The main medical achievement in 17th century:

1) Acupuncture compendium.

2) William Harvey's discovery of circulatory system.

3) The discovery of the pancreatic duct by Wirsung.

4) The comprehensive description of the human lymphatic system by Thomas Bartholin and Olaus Rudbeck.

5) The discovery of sperm.

6) The invention and application of microscopes and the earliest discoveries of microbiome zoo within us.

7) The discovery of brunner's glands.

8) The discovery of *Sarcoptes Scabiei* initated a new era in medicine.

9) Three views of medical theory (iatrophysics; iatrochemistry; vitalism), clinical medicine-the first successful separation of twins joined at the abdomen.

(3) Other characteristics of 17th century medicine: the establishment of Institute of Medicine (IOM); the publication of medical journals; the beginning of medical international communication; the introduction of medicinal plants to Europe.

2. The 18th century medicine.

(1) The social background of medical development: the fast development of scientific techniques; the formation of the view of mechanical materialism.

(2) The main medical achievement in 18th century.

1) The invention of Pulse Watch: Sir John Floyer.

2) The progress of physiology: Galvsnism; the discoveries of Haller A Von, Bell C, Stephen H, et al.

3) The establishment of pathological anatomy: Albinus's tables of the human body, the idea of Morgagni G B about the sites (autopsy) and causes of disease.

4) A treatie on scurvy: James Lind. Cerebrospinal fluid: Cotugno. Exploring the Labyrinth (inner ear), Hunter's Gravid Uterus, Lavoisier's Respiration, the use of digitalis, phrenology, etc.

5) Hospitals : Johann Peter Frank. The bed side teaching: Boerharve H. Ambulance. Alternative Medicine.

6) The invention of percussion: Auenbrugger L.

7) The independence of obstetrics: the invention and application of obstetric forceps.

8) The application of statistics.

9) The improvement of the public health condition.

10) The vaccination invention: Edward Jenner.

3. The 19th century medicine.

(1) The first half of 19th century.

1) The social background: the advances of natural science and philosophy.

2) The main medical achievements:

Cytology and cellular pathology (Schleiden MJ, Schwann TH and Virchow R).

Comparative anatomy and embryology (Cuvier G, Baer K, et al.).

Pharmacology (the extraction of effective ingredient and production of chemical synthesized medicine).

The establishment of experimental pharmacology; physiology and experimental physiology.

Diagnostics (the invention of auscultation apparatus and mediate percussion).

3) The backward clinical medicine.

(2) The second half of 19th century.

1) The social background: the gradual rise of Japanese medicine and United States medicine.

2) The main medical achievements:

Bacteriology (the important contribution of Louis Pakoff's revealing phagocytosis, Widal's reaction).

The invention and application of anesthetization and sterilization; preventive medicine (sanitary survey, the foundation of reseasteur and Robert Koch to medicine and significance).

Immunology (Behring and Kitasato's discovery of diphtheria antitoxin, Metchnirch institutes of public health).

The emergence of forensic medicine ad nursing, the liberalization of psychotic patients, the foundation of International Red Cross (IRC).

4. The characteristics and development patterns of the 17th~19th century medicine.

Chapter 5　Seminar: Prepare a presentation about the development of Medicine

Noting: Choosing some main medical achievements in the 19th century medicine that is not mentioned in this book to talk about.

Chapter 6　The intersection and conflict between Chinese and Western Medicine

1. The social backgrounds in science, technology and ideology.

2. The main medical achievements of Chinese medicine:

(1) Medical writings and pharmacotraditional Chinese medical formulae.

(2) The new progress and innovation in the field of medicine, epidemiology and anatomical physiology.

(3) The achievements in the maturity and the heyday of Chinese medicine: the medical literature, medical journals and academic groups, clinical departments, pharmacology, medical systems, preventive health.

(4) The main achievement of contemporary Chinese medicine in the field of the prevention and cure of diseases, preclinical medicine, preventative medicine, medicine, combination between Chinese and Western medicine, etc.

(5) The achievements on medical books and prescription books.

3. The spread and development of Western medicine in China.

4. The impact of Chinese medicine abroad and its international prospects.

5. The combination between Chinese and Western medicine and the development trends of Chinese medicine in the future.

Chapter 7　Development of modern medicine

1. The social and cultural background: science and technology development.

(1) Specialization of medical science, pharmaceutical sciences, diagnostics and therapeutics, etc.

(2) The internationalization of medical development.

(3) Modernization of medical techniques.

(4) Intersection of the various medical subjects creates new borderline subjects.

(5) The network of modern medicine.

(6) Human genome project (HGP) and the post-genome era.

(7) Proteome project.

(8) The cancer genome project.

2. The branches of the modern medicine and their main research contents.

(1) Basic medicine: Biology, Anatomy, Physiology, Pathophysiology, Biochemistry, Microbiology, Parasitology, Immunology, Histology and Embryology, Pathology, Medical Psychology, Forensic Medicine, Pharmacology, Epidemiology, Protective Medicine, etc.

(2) Clinical disciplines: Internal Medicine, Surgery, Obstetrics & Gynaecology, Paediatrics, Diagnostics, Clinical Ecsomatics, Medical Imageology, Neurology, Psychiatry, Traditional Chinese Medicine, Integrated Traditional and Western Medicine, etc.

3. The advance and development trend in various subjects of modern medicine: Molecule Biology, Immunology, Genetics, Transplantation, Gene Therapy, Geratology, New Emerging Infection Diseases.

4. The evolution of the medical models.

(1) Definition of medical model.

(2) The characteristics and transitions of medical models: Spirtualism medical model, Nature philosophical medical model, Mechanistic medical model, Biomedical model, Bio-psycho-social medical model.

(3) The characteristics of modern medicine and the disadvantages of biomedical model.

(4) The significance of the transition in medical models.

5. The characteristics of modern medicine development.

6. The enlightenment from the development of modern medicine.

Chapter 8　Modern medicine - Holistic Integrative Medicine

1. Holistic Integration Medicine(HIM): a new form of medicine.

(1) Definition of Holistic Integration Medicine.

(2) The characteristics of Holistic Integration Medicine.

(3) The advantages of Holistic Integration Medicine compared to tranditional modern medicine.

(4) The significance of Holistic Integration Medicine.

2. The social and cultural background:

(1) The whole person: body, mind, soul and spirit.

(2) Science and technology development.

(3) The relationship of medicine and science.

(4) Physical and mental health.

3. The main research contents: patients, disease, clinical, doctors, both, both Chinese and Western medicine, prevention and treatment.

4. The methods to speed up the development of HIM.

Chapter 9　Modern medicine - Personalized Medicine and Precision Medicine

1. Personalized Medicine:

(1) The concept of Personalized Medicine.

(2) Social and cultural background.

(3) Human genome project (HGP) and the post-genome era.

(4) Gene Sequencing techniques.

(5) The Clinical reference of Personalized Medicine: Tumor molecule targeting individualized therapy.

(6) The prospects of Personalized Medicine.

2. Precision Medicine :

(1) The concept of Precision Medicine.

(2) Genetic testing technology.

(3) The pioneer of Precision Medicine: Nader Javadi.

(4) The difference of Precision Medicine and Personalized Medicine.

(5) The Clinical reference of Precision Medicine: Tumor molecule targeting individualized therapy.

(6) Short-term goal of Precision Medicine: cancer treatment.

(7) The prospects of Precision Medicine.

Chapter 10　Modern medical education and medical study

1. International medical education standards ("**Standards**" as the short form thereinafter) and their general requirements.

(1) History background of constituting the **Standards.**

(2) Purpose of constituting the **Standards.**

(3) Concept of the **Standards.**

(4) Basic contents of two **Standards** in the world (international standards in medical education by the World Federation for Medical Education [WFME] and Global Minimum Essential Requirements by the Institute for International Medical Education [IIME]).

2. Reform and development of medical education.

(1) The structures of medical education system, the categories of medical education process, its missions and characteristics.

(2) Challenges confronted by medical education, the reform contents of medical education and teaching.

(3) Medical education system and education reform in China.

3. The characteristics of medical study.

(1) The characteristics of study in college and the influencing factors.

(2) The characteristics of medical study.

(3) The principles of medical study.

4. The strategies and methods of medical study: the memory methods of medical knowledge, the training methods of medical thinking, the study methods of medical courses, the study methods in the medical internship, the training methods in research

ability, and training methods of complex makings.

Chapter 11　Doctors and patients

1. The role (character) of doctors.

(1) The features of doctor's role.

(2) The rights and obligations of a doctor, the duties of doctors.

(3) Occupational quality of doctors.

2. Role of patients: the need and expectation of patients, the rights and obligations of patients.

3. Medical interpersonal relationship and communication.

(1) Concept of communication, general skills of communication.

(2) How to communicate with patients better for doctors.

(3) Concept, model and influence factors of doctor-patient relationship, how to establish harmonious doctor-patient relationship, correctly dealing with interpersonal relationship in medical practice.

4. Problems related with law in clinical practice.

(1) Concept of hygiene law and regulation, legal liability (obligation) in hygiene laws.

(2) Concept and grade of medical malpractice (Medical Accidents), identity and procedure of expert evaluation (technology identification) on medical malpractice.

(3) Several conditions that don't belong to medical malpractice.

Chapter 12　Health service system

1. The health services system: the definition, ingredients and functions.

2. The health service system.

(1) The hospital and the medical care system.

1) The basic functions, the staff and classified methods of hospital.

2) The developing process of hospital.

3) The factors influencing the hospital development, including medical science, medical technology, nursing, medical education, medical insurance, the function of government, the ownership of hospitals, etc.

(2) The typical models of the international health system and the process of their reform.

3. The status of medical care in China.

(1) The policies of health service.

1) The forming and development of the policies after the establishment of P. R. China.

2) The forming and significance of the policies in the new stage.

(2) The health resource, including the health organization, the hospital beds, the personnel, health financing, etc.

(3) The main achievement of health service after the establishment of P. R. China.

(4) The health reform: the background, principles and tasks.

Chapter 13　Seminar: Prepare presentations about the relationship of Doctors and patients or health service system in different country